Advances in Medicine for Farm Animals

Advances in Medicine for Farm Animals

Editor: Mel Roth

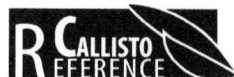

R CALLISTO REFERENCE

www.callistoreference.com

Callisto Reference,
118-35 Queens Blvd., Suite 400,
Forest Hills, NY 11375, USA

Visit us on the World Wide Web at:
www.callistoreference.com

ISBN: 978-1-64116-151-0 (Hardback)

Cataloging-in-Publication Data

Advances in medicine for farm animals / edited by Mel Roth.
    p. cm.
Includes bibliographical references and index.
ISBN 978-1-64116-151-0
1. Veterinary medicine. 2. Domestic animals. 3. Livestock. I. Roth, Mel.
SF745 .V48 2019
636.089--dc23

Table of Contents

Preface

This book aims to highlight the current researches and provides a platform to further the scope of innovations in this area. This book is a product of the combined efforts of many researchers and scientists, after going through thorough studies and analysis from different parts of the world. The objective of this book is to provide the readers with the latest information of the field.

The treatment, control and diagnosis of all health conditions in animals is under the domain of veterinary science. Studies in this field extend to both farm and wild animals. Farm animals are raised for the provision of meat, eggs, milk, leather, fur and wool. Good husbandry, appropriate feeding and hygiene contribute to the maintenance of animal health and welfare in the farm. Animals are susceptible to many different diseases and prone to various internal and external parasites. Certain examples of common animal diseases are classical swine fever, foot-and-mouth disease, etc. Some of these diseases can be prevented through vaccines. In other cases, antibiotics are used. This book strives to provide a fair idea about the discipline of veterinary medicine with respect to farm animals and to help develop a better understanding of the latest advances within this field. It includes some of the vital pieces of work being conducted across the world, on various topics related to this area of study. Scientists and students actively engaged in this field will find this book full of crucial and unexplored concepts.

I would like to express my sincere thanks to the authors for their dedicated efforts in the completion of this book. I acknowledge the efforts of the publisher for providing constant support. Lastly, I would like to thank my family for their support in all academic endeavors.

Editor

Assessment of reproductive and growth performances of pig breeds in the peri-urban area of Douala (Equatorial Zone)

J. Kouamo[1,*], W.F. Tassemo Tankou[1], A.P. Zoli[1], G.S. Bah[2] and A.C. Ngo Ongla[3]

[1]School of Veterinary Medicine and Sciences, University of Ngaoundere, P.O. BOX 454, Ngaoundere, Cameroon
[2]Regional Center of the Institute of Agricultural Research for Development (IRAD) Wakwa. P.O. BOX 65, Ngaoundere, Cameroon
[3]DDPIA, MINEPIA (Ministry of Livestock, Fisheries and Animal Husbandry), Yaounde-Cameroon

Abstract

The aim of this study was to evaluate the reproductive and growth performances of pig breeds in Douala, Cameroon. The reproductive performance of gilts and multiparous sows (38 per group) from 8 selected farms were monitored and controlled. Thereafter, piglets were controlled from birth to weaning age. The age at first service (AFS), fertility index (FI), fecundity, age at first farrowing (AFF), weight at first farrowing (WtFF) and litter size (LS) of gilts were 179.97 ± 25.40 days; 1.76 ± 0.77; 100 ± 0.00; 350.47 ± 40.58 days; 107.26 ± 31.85 kg and 7.18 ± 1.93 piglets, respectively. In sows, the FI, fecundity, LS and farrowing interval (FarI) were 1.13 ± 0.34; 100 ± 0.00; 9.03 ± 2.14 piglets and 179.63 ± 25.14 days, respectively. FI and LS were better in sows compared to gilts (P = 0.000). The sex ratio was 0.63. Local breed animals reared in semi-modern farms and fed mixed feed showed the lowest WtFF. In piglets, the average birth weight (kg), the average weaning weight (kg), age at weaning (days) and survival rate (%) until weaning were 1.32 ± 0.20, 10.60 ± 1.41, 56.86 ± 8.24 and 48.43, respectively. These results indicated that reproductive performance is strongly influenced by breed, feed and farm type.
Keywords: Douala, Feed, Fertility, Growth, Pig breed.

Introduction

Cameroon has about 19,400,000 inhabitants and pork is consumed by nearly 70% of the population (INS, 2011). The pig population is estimated at 1.7 million and the industry provides about 30,000 tons of pork per year. Pork production was estimated at about 48,960 tons in 2010 and is expected to peak 86,190 tons in 2015 (MINEPIA, 2011). The current production estimated (2.02 kg/person/ year) is low when compared to the demand of 5 kg pork/ person/year (MINEPIA, 2011). The low productivity is attributed mainly to the production system and the poor exploitation of production potential. To reduce importation of pork, the government of Cameroon has funded projects to promote the improvement of livestock productivity such as the Pig Industry Development Program (PSDB), Projects to improve Agricultural Competitiveness (PACA), and many others. Despite these efforts, pig production in Cameroon is still insufficient and is characterized by a traditional farming systems consisting of small pig production units. The farming conditions are often poor and farmers usually choose farming options with minimum investment and professional interventions while hoping to maximize profitability (Nyabusore, 1982). Under these conditions, little is known of the pig's performance and how they vary from one farm to another.

These small farms play an important role in the socio-economic lives of the local people. Pigs are a valuable source of capital, are used to meet the daily family needs, and are an important source of animal protein (Thorne, 1992). Despite the interest in increasing pork production there is lack of literature on pig productivity in Cameroon (Mopate-Logtene and Kabore-Zoungrana, 2010).

This study was conducted to assess the reproductive and growth performance of pig breeds in the peri-urban area of Douala (Equatorial Zone). Specifically we determined the reproductive performance of gilts/sows, the growth performance of their piglets, and evaluated the effect of rearing factors on these performances.

Materials and Methods

Area of the study

The study was conducted in peri-urban area of Douala; the Littoral region of Cameroon situated between 4° 3' 1" North and 9° 42' 0" East. The farms were located in Wouri Department, near several markets of Douala. According to the agro-ecological classification of Cameroon, Douala is characterized with a constant temperature of about 26°C and the rainy season starts from March and ends in October. Very heavy rains resulting in flooding usually occurs between June and October.

Design of study

A total of 76 pigs were randomly selected from eight farms from within the framework of PACA (Table 1).

*Corresponding Author: Dr. Justin Kouamo. School of Veterinary Medicine and Sciences, University of Ngaoundere, P.O. BOX 454, Ngaoundere, Cameroon. E-mail: justinkouamo@yahoo.fr

Table 1. Structure of the research population.

Breed	Gilts	Sows	Total
Large-white	19	20	39
Duroc	4	8	12
Landrace	13	8	21
Local	2	2	4
Total	38	38	76

All of these farms were sponsored by the World Bank in partnership with the Ministries of Agriculture and Rural Development (MINADER) and Livestock, Fisheries and Animal Husbandry (MINEPIA). PACA projects were funded by the World Bank and launched in the North West Region of Cameroon in 2010. These projects had the main objective to "increase the competitiveness of beneficiary producer organizations that are working in the maize, rice, plantains, pigs and poultry sectors". These projects were given a budget of 62 million Euros to spend over a period of five years, with aims to increase livestock production by 20% (MINEPIA, 2011).

Data collection on farm characteristics

Questionnaires were used to collect information on farm structure and management, as well as socio-economic characteristics of breeders. Three farming systems were identified: traditional (n=1; 12.5%), semi-modern (n=5; 62.5%) and modern (n=2; 25%). The traditional pig's farm (type 1) was located at about 300 m from homes and in most cases the walls and floors were constructed with planks. The farm was not protected from visitors and the hygiene practices were not standard. The farming conditions were often poor. Most of the work was performed by family members using inappropriate equipment as there were minimal investments and professional interventions. The semi-modern farms (type 2) were based on solid concrete floors but the walls (1.2 m high) were made up of temporary materials (bricks or wood) and located about 500 m from homes with limited access to visitors. The semi-modern pig sties were used for raising sows, lactating dams, the fatteners and boars. The heath care provided to the pigs was both prophylactic (vaccination against swine erysipelas) and curative. Labourers may be recruited but their labor time was not factored in, though wearing boots was a common practice on most farms. The modern farms (type 3) in the context of this study were well constructed buildings located more than 500 m from homes for biosecurity reasons. The floors were concreted and sloped gently to facilitate cleaning by washing with water. The buildings were partitioned to enable grouping of pigs per age whenever necessary. There were footbaths at each entrance and exit of the main building. Health care consisted of prophylactic and curative therapies against common pathologies such as swine erysipelas, salmonellosis, African swine fever, transmissible gastro-enteritis, vesicular stomatitis, and metabolic diseases associated with calcium, iron and vitamin deficiencies. Veterinarians were contracted to provide health services. Staffs were dressed with blue blouse and wore boots, gloves and masks.

Feeding

The animals were fed twice a day according to a predetermined schedule or standardized farming code provided by the supervisory ministry, MINEPIA (2011) and water was available *ad libitum*. Some of the farmer composed their own feed while others bought feed supplied by the Feed Mills Corporation of Cameroon (SPC). The nutritive value of the farmer composed feed was: 45 to 60% energy, 25 to 35% protein, 2 to 4% Calcium/Phosphorus and 1.5 to 2% mineral and vitamins complex (MVC). The feed of SPC consisted of 65 to 75% energy, 12 to 25% protein, 2-3% Calcium/Phosphorus and 1.5 to 2% MVC. The pigs received the same amount of feed and feed content depending of their age and weight. The raw materials were composed of maize, maize bran, waste from grinding mills, soya bean cake, cotton seed cake and groundnut cake, fish meal and bone meal.

Evaluation of the reproductive performance of gilts and sows

The pigs were bred by natural mating and the heats were detected with using breeding boars. The fertility index (FI: total number of mating for a conception), fecundity (% live piglets born per bred gilt or sow within 6 hours), age at first service (AFS), farrowing interval (FarI), litter size (LS), weight at first farrowing (WtFF), age at first farrowing (AFF) and the sex ratio (male/live piglets) were determined. Weight of adult pigs was estimated using a barometric tape (Zoometer) on the thoracic circumference while piglets were weighed on a weighing balance typeTTZ-200.

Piglet growth performance assessment

The piglets were weighed at birth (BWt) and at weaning (WWt). The age at weaning (AW) was recorded and the survival rate determined. Clinical signs of some diseases were recorded until weaning.

Statistical analysis

Data were analyzed using the Statistical Package for the Social Sciences software (SPSS-20). Analysis of Variance and Turkey HSD tests were used to compare different groups. Differences were significant at $P < 0.05$.

Results

Reproductive performance

Of the 76 gilts and sows monitored, a total of 607 live piglets were farrowed with a sex ratio of 0.63. Table 2 shows the overall of reproductive performance in gilts and sows. The FI and LS in sows were better than those of gilts ($P = 0.000$).

Effects of breed, the type of farm and feed on reproductive performance in gilts and sows

Since the number of farms involved in the project was low; in particular the fact that the "traditional system" was represented by a single farm (with only 3 sows/gilts), results and discussion have been limited the comparison to two types of farms (modern vs. semi-modern)

Tables 3 and 4 show the respective effects of some husbandry factors on reproductive performance of gilts and sows. The WtFF was heavily influenced by breed, farm type and the feeding. Local pig breeds reared in semi-modern farms and fed mixed feed had the lowest weight at WtFF. Gilts in modern or type 3 farms and fed on complete diet exhibited better LS while the Landrace sows have the best LS.

Growth performance and health profile of the piglets

Of all farrowed piglets, the average BWt (kg), the average WWt (kg), AW (days) and survival rate until weaning were 1.32 ± 0.20, 10.60 ± 1.41, 56.86 ± 8.24 and 48.43, respectively. These performances were influenced by breed, farm type and source of feed (Table 5). Of the 51.57% of piglets that died, 11.14% were from sudden death, and 88.86% were suffering from various diseases including: neonatal diarrhea (95%), Salmonella (15%), constipation (57%), infections respiratory (5%), gastrointestinal parasites (100%), sarcoptic mange (20.56%) and abscesses (12.12%).

Discussion

The AFS was in the range (137 to 281 days) described by Rozeboom *et al.* (1996), but less than that reported by Ayssiwede (2005) in Benin and Mopate-Logtene *et al.* (2009) in Central African Republic and the CDDR/SAILD (1996). This variation may be due to the heterogeneous type of farm and feeding systems considered in this study. The AFS of animals raised in modern farms was younger compared to those raised on semi-modern farms. Since animals raised on type 3 farms were fed on complete diet, it is most probably that complete and well balanced diets were responsible for gilts reaching puberty earlier than those fed the mixed feed and raised on type 2 farms (Ayssiwede, 2005). However, other environmental factors of semi-modern farms such as inadequate ventilation and facilities to control high ambient temperatures could result in drop in reproductive and growth performances (Quiniou *et al.*, 2000). Precocity could also be due to the grouping effects from the random combination with fattening animals as was observed more in the modern than semi-modern farms (Dovonou, 2002).

Table 2. Overall reproductive performance of gilts and sows (means±SEM).

Parameters	Gilts	Sows	P-value
AFS (days)	179.97±25.40		
FI	1.76±0.77[a]	1.13±0.34[b]	0.000
Fecundity (%)	100.00±0.00	100.00±0.00	
AFF (days)	350.47±40.58		
WtFF (kg)	107.26±31.85		
LS (piglets)	7.18±1.93[a]	9.03±2.14[b]	0.000
FarI (days)		179.63±25.14	

[a,b]Means within the same row with different indices are significantly different at *P*<0.05.

Table 3. Effect of breed, type of farm and feed on reproductive performance in gilts.

Parameters	AFS (days)	FI	Fecundity (%)	AFF (days)	WtFF (Kg)	LS (piglets)
Breed						
Large-white (n=19)	183.68±5.13[a]	1.67±0.29[a]	100.00±0.00	342.05±8.94[a]	96.47±6.23[a]	7.28±0.41[a]
Duroc (n=4)	184.50±13.13[a]	3.00±0.00[a]	100.00±0.00	365.75±7.75[a]	108.25±7.56[a]	6.50±1.26[a]
Landrace (n=13)	177.75±8.54[a]	1.70±0.17[a]	100.00±0.00	354.54±13.60[a]	128.46±8.75[b]	7.46±0.58[a]
Local (n=2)	149.00±10.00[a]	2.00±0.00[a]	100.00±0.00	373.50±15.50[a]	70.00±20.00[a]	6.00±1.00[a]
P- value	0.32	0.43		0.56	0.01	0.69
Type of farms						
Semi-modern (n=18)	189.76±6.24[a]	1.44±0.24[a]	100.00±0.00	342.83±8.73[a]	91.33±3.42[a]	6.33±0.36[a]
Modern (n=19)	169.16±4.61[b]	1.91±0.21[a]	100.00±0.00	355.68±10.05[a]	121.16±8.58[b]	7.89±0.46[b]
P- value	0.01	0.10		0.41	0.01	0.03
Feed						
Mixed (n=19)	191.39±6.10[a]	1.60±0.27[a]	100.00±0.00	345.26±8.61[a]	93.37±3.82[a]	6.47±0.37[a]
Complete (n=19)	169.16±4.61[b]	1.91±0.21[a]	100.00±0.00	355.68±10.05[a]	121.16±8.58[b]	7.89±0.46[b]
P - value	0.01	0.37		0.44	0.00	0.02

[a,b]Means within the same column with different indices are significantly different at *P*<0.05. n=number.

Table 4. Effect of breed, type of farm and feed on reproductive performance in sows.

Parameters	FI	Fecundity (%)	LS	FarI (days)
Breed				
Large-white (n=20)	1.15±0.08[a]	100.00±0.00	9.55±0.31[a]	184.63±4.85[a]
Duroc (n=8)	1.12±0.12[a]	100.00±0.00	6.86±0.96[b]	166.37±8.81[a]
Landrace (n=8)	1.12±0.12[a]	100.00±0.00	10.13±0.67[a]	172.37±10.23[a]
Local (n=2)	1.00±0.00[a]	100.00±0.00	7.00±2.00[c]	202.67±14.38[a]
P-value	0.95		0.00	0.10
Type of farms				
Semi-modern (n=21)	1.14±0.08[a]	100.00±0.00	9.00±0.53[a]	171.75±4.11[a]
Modern (n=15)	1.13±0.09[a]	100.00±0.00	8.93±0.51[a]	186.47±7.80[a]
P-value	0.86		0.81	0.19
Feed				
Mixed (n=23)	1.13±0.07[a]	100.00±0.00	9.09±0.49[a]	173.18±4.01[a]
Complete (n=15)	1.13±0.09[a]	100.00±0.00	8.93±0.51[a]	186.47±7.80[a]
P-value	0.98		0.83	0.11

[a,b,c]Means within the same column with different indices are significantly different at $P<0.05$. n=number.

Table 5. Effect of breed, type of farm and feed on growth performance in piglets.

Parameters	BWt (kg)	WWt (kg)	AW (days)	Mortality rate (%)
Breed				
Large-white (n=145)	1.35±0.02[a]	10.76±0.92[a]	57.34±0.69[a]	46.96[a]
Duroc (n=46)	1.37±0.03[a]	11.01±0.21[b]	58.30±0.97[a]	18.53[b]
Landrace (n=91)	1.26±0.01[b]	10.43±0.17[a]	56.12±0.91[a,b]	30.03[c]
Local (n=12)	1.18±0.03[b]	8.52±0.18[c]	51.25±2.23[b]	4.47[d]
P-value	0.000	0.000	0.041	0.000
Type of farms				
Semi-modern (n=162)	1.27±0.01[a]	10.22±0.10[a]	55.47±0.77[a]	51.76[a]
Modern (n=118)	1.38±0.02[b]	11.15±0.14[b]	60.07±0.21[b]	37.70[b]
P-value	0.000	0.000	0.000	0.000
Feed				
Mixed (n=175)	1.27±0.01[a]	10.24±0.09[a]	54.80±0.75[a]	60.70[a]
Complete (n=119)	1.38±0.02[b]	11.15±0.14[b]	60.07±0.21[b]	39.30[b]
P-value	0.000	0.000	0.000	0.000

[a,b,c,d]Means within the same column with different indices are significantly different at $P<0.05$. n=number.

Of the 38 gilts in this study, only 42.9% were successfully bred during their first heats. FI was better in sows compared to gilts. Multi-parity being an important fertility factor, FI tended to 1 with older sows (Labroue et al., 2000). It is recommended that gilts should be serviced during their 2nd and 3rd heat to avoid the risk of dystocia and increase birth weight of piglets and hence their viability (FAO, 2009).

The average AFF of gilts was within the range (348 to 487 days) reported by Aloeyi (1997) and Missohou et al. (2001) in Togo and Senegal, respectively; was slightly less than that described by Aumaitre et al. (1966) and Legault et al. (1996) in France but higher than that of local pigs in Benin (Ayssiwede, 2005) and in Central African Republic (Mopate-Logtene et al., 2009). This variation might have been due to breed and breeding environment. Reproductive performance is influenced by weight gain regardless of the farming system in place. The performance of the local pigs in Cameroon was low compared to some hybrids and exotic breeds (Keambou et al., 2010).

The average WtFF is comparable to that reported by Rozeboom et al. (1996), but much higher than the 62.3 kg and well below 158.1 kg obtained from local and improved breeds respectively (CDDR/ SAILD, 1996). In this study, the Local breeds have the lowest WtFF. This corroborates with the results of Rozeboom et al. (1996) who reported higher WtFF in exotic breeds than local breeds. Animals raised on modern farms and fed complete feed had the best WtFF due to the positive effect of feeding on the breeding conditions of animals. Messi (1982) stated that though the final weight of the animal depends on several factors such as breed, birth weight, management system and fattening period. Diet therefore plays an important role in the reproductive performance and growth of animals irrespective of breed, and thus the profitability of farm operations (Ayssiwede, 2005).

The LS of gilts is similar to that reported in Benin (Ayssiwede, 2005) and in Pala, Garoua and Bangui (Mopate-Logtene et al., 2009), but lower than the values found in Nigeria (Smith, 1982), Senegal (Lokossou, 1982; Missohou et al., 2001) and Europe (Eastwood et al., 2011). LS increased with age and parity as average LS was significantly higher in sows than gilts. The development of the female reproductive organs usually attains full potential after several parities. Landrace pigs were very prolific (CDDR/ SAILD, 1996) in Cameroon. According to Labroue et al. (2000), LS initially increases with parity and then decreases until 7th and 8th farrowing (Youssao et al., 2009). The age factor is followed by breed and farm type. Exotic breeds and hybrids are more prolific than local breeds (Keambou et al., 2010). Similarly, poor breeding conditions cause a decrease in the numerical and weight productivity in pigs (Youssao et al., 2008). However, other authors suggest that body conditions of gilt did not influence the LS during the first three parities (Rozeboom et al., 1996).

The FarI observed in this study is comparable to the 176 days reported in Togo (Aloeyi, 1997); higher than the 160 days in Franfce (Eastwood et al., 2011) but lower than the 188 and 246 days reported in Benin (Ayssiwede, 2005) and Madagascar (Razafimanantsoa, 1988), respectively. That the Cameroonian pigs were farrowing twice a year is a good indicator of the breeding potential that can be exploited in planning improvement program to increase pig population in Cameroon.

There were more male than female piglets per litter as has been previously reported (Solignac et al., 1989). However, Lougnon and Picard (1982) were of the opinion that this sex ratio is influenced by LS. In this study LS greater than 7 were dominated by males. Local breeds littered more male piglets, but whatever the breed, the number of male piglets littered was above 50% of the new born (Solignac et al., 1989). Though breeding system and livestock production

techniques may influence the proportion of male births (Ayssiwede, 2005).

The average BWt of the pigs were similar to those reported by Canope and Raynaud (1980) in Guadeloupe; lower than those of several authors (Razafimanantsoa, 1988; Missohou et al., 2001; Ayssiwede, 2005) but greater than the weight reported by Smith (1982) and Abdallah (1997) in Nigeria and the Central African Republic, respectively. These variations may be due to several factors including breed and the management systems of the various farms studied.

In a similar way, the WWt and AW were different from those reported in other studies in tropical countries (Bastianelli, 2002; Ayssiwede, 2005). The exotic breeds, despite the tropical rearing conditions, had better WWt than Local breeds. This study demonstrated that there is a positive correlation between growth and breeding conditions.

The mortality rate observed was higher than 15.9% reported by Solignac et al. (1989) in France but lower than the 67.5% obtained by Ayssiwede (2005) in Benin farms. Higher mortality rates amongst the exotic breeds could be linked to their poor adaptability to tropical conditions and inappropriate handling of dams during farrowing due to inexperience of farmers. In addition, overcrowding in the type 2 and 3 farms might have helped in the spread of certain diseases, resulting in high mortalities and fewer weaned piglets. Also diets that are not tailored to the breed's need may be a source of increase morbidity and mortality (Sambou, 2010).

Conclusion

The reproductive and growth performances of pigs in the peri-urban area of Douala were strongly influenced by breed, type of farm and source of feed. Simple changes in the management and breeding technique could possibly improve on these performances.

Reference

Abdallah, E. 1997. Elevage porcin en région périurbaine de Bangui (Centrafrique). Thèse: Méd. Vét., Dakar, pp: 32.

Aloeyi, K. 1997. Performances de reproduction du porc Large-white à la ferme BENA-Développement au Togo. Thèse de Doctorat, pp: 85.

Aumaitre, A., Legault, C. and Salmon-Legagneur, E. 1966. Aspects biométriques de la croissance pondérale du porcelet: influence du sexe, de l'année de naissance, du numéro et de la taille de la portée. Centre national de Recherches zootechniques, 78 - Jouy-en-Josas, pp: 15.

Ayssiwede, S. 2005. L'insémination artificielle porcine: une perspective pour l'amélioration de la productivité des porcs au Bénin. Mémoire de fin d'étude en DES-GRAVMT, pp: 85.

Bastianelli, D. 2002. L'élevage porcin traditionnel. Mémento de l'agronome, ministère des Affaires étrangères (MAE), Centre international en recherche agronomique pour le développement (CIRAD) et le groupe de recherche et d'échanges technologiques (GRET), pp: 1521-1527.

Canope, L. and Raynaud, Y. 1980. Etude comparative des performances de reproduction des truies des races créole et Large-White en Guadeloupe. Ann. Géné. Sel. Anim. 12, 267-280.

CDDR/SAILD. 1996. Elevage de porcs. Synthèse technique, pp: 14.

Dovonou, M.N. 2002. Performances zootechniques des races porcines au Sud Bénin et perspectives d'amélioration par croisement avec le Piétrain stress négatif. Mémoire de fin d'études, DES interuniversitaire. ULg: FMV/FUSAGx.

Eastwood, L., Beaulieu, D. and Leterme, P. 2011. Les performances des truies sont influencées par le rapport Oméga-3/Oméga-6 des acides gras de l'aliment. Journées Rech. Porcine, pp: 43.

FAO. 2009. Farmer's hand book on pig production (for small holders at village level), pp: 86 (33-43).

INS. 2011. Annuaire statistique du Cameroun. Recueil des séries d'informations statistiques sur les activités économiques, sociales, politiques et culturelles du pays jusqu'en 2010-2012, pp: 456.

Keambou, T.C., Manjeli, Y., Hako, B.A., Meutchieye, F. and Awono, J.C. 2010. Compared effects of a concentrate and a traditional diet on growth and economic performances of young local-breed pigs in North Cameroon. Rev. Elev. Méd. Vét. Pays Trop. 63(3-4), 77-82.

Labroue, F., Guillou, P., Marsac, H., Boisseau, C., Luquet, M., Arrayet, J., Martinat-Botte, F. and Terqui, M. 2000. Etude des performances de reproduction de 5 races locales porcines françaises. Journ. Rech. Porcine en France 32, 413-418.

Legault, C., Gauthier, M.C., Caritez, J.C. and Lagant, H. 1996. Analyse expérimentale de l'influence de l'âge à la première mise-bas et du type génétique sur la productivité de la truie. Ann. Zootech. 45, 63-73.

Lokossou, M.R. 1982. L'industrialisation de l'élevage, base de la production porcine en République Populaire du Bénin: étude du modèle AGROCAP au Sénégal. Thèse: Méd. Vét., Dakar.

Lougnon, J. and Picard, M. 1982. A propos du sex-ratio chez le porc. Journ. Rech. Porcine en France 14, 65-74.

Messi, J.M. 1982. Evaluation des performances de reproduction des types génétiques de porc à la station d'élevage de Kounden. Mémoire de fin d'étude. Faculté d'Agronomie et des Sciences agricoles, Université de Dschang, Cameroun, pp: 50.

MINEPIA, 2011. Amélioration quantitative et qualitative des animaux de commerce et de leurs produits, par la réduction des pertes dues aux maladies transfrontalières, pp: 46.

Missohou, A., Niang, M., Forcher, H. and Dieye, P.N. 2001. Les systèmes d'élevage porcin en Basse Casamance (Sénégal): note de recherche. Cahiers d'Agricultures 10, 405-408.

Mopate-Logtene, L., Koussou, M., Nguertoum, E., Ngo, T.A., Lakouetene, T., Awa, D. and MalMal, H.E. 2009. Caractéristiques et performances des élevages porcins urbains et périurbains des savanes d'Afrique Centrale: cas des villes de Garoua, Pala et Bangui. Savanes africaines en développement: innover pour durer, Garoua: Cameroun, pp: 9.

Mopate-Logtene, Y. and Kabore-Zoungrana, C.Y. 2010. Dynamique des élevages et caractéristiques des producteurs de porcs de la ville de N'Djaména, Tchad. In L. Seiny-Boukar, P. Boumard (éditeurs scientifiques), 2010 Actes du colloque «Savanes africaines en développement: innover pour durer», 20-23 avril 2009, Garoua, Cameroun. Prasac, N'Djamena, Tchad; Cirad, Montpellier, France, cédérom.

Nyabusore, J.B. 1982. Utilisation des drêches artisanales en alimentation porcine. Faculté des sciences agronomiques, Gembloux, Belgique (Mémoire de fin d'études), pp: 106.

Quiniou, N., Renaudeau, D., Collin, A. and Noblet, J. 2000. Effets de l'exposition au chaud sur les caractéristiques de la prise alimentaire du porc à différents stades physiologiques. Prod. Anim. 13, 233-245.

Razafimanantsoa, E. 1988. Note sur les performances d'élevage d'un troupeau de truies Large-White élevées dans le Moyen Ouest de Madagascar. Rev. Elev. Méd. Vét. Pays Trop. 41, 459-461.

Rozeboom, D., Pettidrew, J., Moser, R., Cornelius, S.G. and El Kandelgy, S.M. 1996. Influence of gilt age and body composition at first breeding on sow reproductive performance and longevity. J. Anim. Sci. 74, 138-150.

Sambou, G. 2010. Les éleveurs de porcs recycleurs des déchets organiques à Mbeubeuss: entre désespoir et quête d une vie meilleure. Cirad pig tropical, pp: 7.

Smith, O.B. 1982. Observations pendant six ans de la performance des porcs Large-white élevés dans un environnement tropical. Bulletin de la santé et reproduction animales en Afrique 30(5), 15-19.

Solignac, T., Castaing, J. and Le Foll, P. 1989. Etude de la croissance du porcelet: influence de la pathologie digestive et de quelques paramètres zootechniques et comportementaux. Journ. Rech. Porcine en France 21, 161-166.

Thorne, P. 1992. Developing the use of local feed

resources for pigs and poultry in Karibati. Rev. Mond. Zootech. 72, 20-25.

Youssao, A.K.I., Koutinhouin, G.B., Kpodekon, T.M., Yacoubou, A., Bonou, A.G., Adjakpa, A., Ahounou, S. and Taiwo, R. 2009. Amélioration génétique des performances zootechniques du porc local du Bénin par croisement avec le Large-white. Int.

J. Bio. Chem. Sci. 3(4), 653-662.

Youssao, A.K.I., Koutinhouin, G.B., Kpodekon, T.M., Bonou, A.G., Adjakpa, A., Dotcho, C.D.G. and Atodjinou, F.T.R. 2008. Pig Production and Indigenous Genetic Resources in Suburban Areas of Cotonou and Abomey-Calavi in Benin. Revue Élev. Méd. Vét. Pays Trop. 61(3-4), 235-243.

2

Prenatal transmission of scrapie in sheep and goats

D.B. Adams*

24 Noala Street, Aranda, ACT 2614, Australia

Abstract

Unsettled knowledge as to whether scrapie transmits prenatally in sheep and goats and transmits by semen and preimplantation embryos has a potential to compromise measures for controlling, preventing and eliminating the disease. The remedy may be analysis according to a systematic review, allowing comprehensive and accessible treatment of evidence and reasoning, clarifying the issue and specifying the uncertainties. Systematic reviews have clearly formulated questions, can identify relevant studies and appraise their quality and can summarise evidence and reasoning with an explicit methodology. The present venture lays a foundation for a possible systematic review and applies three lines of evidence and reasoning to two questions. The first question is whether scrapie transmits prenatally in sheep and goats. It leads to the second question, which concerns the sanitary safety of artificial breeding technologies, and is whether scrapie transmits in sheep and goats by means of semen and washed or unwashed *in vivo* derived embryos. The three lines of evidence derive from epidemiological, field and clinical studies, experimentation, and causal reasoning, where inferences are made from the body of scientific knowledge and an understanding of animal structure and function. Evidence from epidemiological studies allow a conclusion that scrapie transmits prenatally and that semen and embryos are presumptive hazards for the transmission of scrapie. Evidence from experimentation confirms that semen and washed or unwashed *in vivo* derived embryos are hazards for the transmission of scrapie. Evidence from causal reasoning, including experience from other prion diseases, shows that mechanisms exist for prenatal transmission and transmission by semen and embryos in both sheep and goats.

Keywords: Goat, Prenatal, Scrapie, Sheep, Transmission.

Introduction

Control and prevention of communicable diseases such as scrapie is beyond reach when knowledge about of pathways of transmission is absent, or when false knowledge is accepted or true knowledge is rejected. The demonstration of prenatal transmission of scrapie in sheep (Garza *et al.*, 2011; Rubenstein *et al.*, 2012; Foster *et al.*, 2013; Spiropoulos *et al.*, 2014) is of major importance in this regard because it establishes a firm basis for the control and possible elimination of scrapie. False rejection of prenatal transmission in these circumstances will deny benefits to animal health and welfare, preclude some analytical perspectives on atypical scrapie, and limit possibilities for understanding all neurodegenerative diseases in all species. Emerging concerns for scrapie and animal health are the conservation of rare breeds of sheep and goats, safeguards against incursions of scrapie into scrapie-free regions and the potential for an inter-species jump as occurred with bovine spongiform encephalopathy (BSE) and people (Ulvund, 2008). Past views about scrapie downplayed or rejected prenatal transmission. Parry (1983) claimed that transmission of an infectious agent played little part in the natural history of scrapie and that the disease

propagated from generation to generation through inheritance of the scrapie trait. Thirteen years later a review by Hoinville (1996) summarised scrapie as an infectious disease with a genetic influence on the incubation period and where horizontal transmission eclipsed maternal transmission; that is, transmission from dam to offspring *in utero* or in the immediate post-partum period. Later reviews (Detwiler and Baylis, 2003; Jeffrey and Gonzalez, 2007; Fast and Groschup, 2013) conclude that the available evidence supported scrapie transmission after birth and not before birth. These conclusions are reflected in influential operational guides such as those from the World Organisation for Animal Health (OIE, 2011) and Animal Health Australia (2009), which include explicit statements on transmission, and in current recommendations for the sanitary safety of artificial insemination and embryo transfer in sheep and goats (IETS, 2010).

Given the significance of matters mentioned above, the recent experimental demonstration of prenatal transmission of scrapie in sheep merits exposure to possible refutation by testing its agreement or not with evidence from (1) epidemiological, field and clinical studies; (2) experimentation, and (3) causal reasoning,

---
*Corresponding Author: David B. Adams. 24 Noala Street, Aranda, ACT 2614, Australia.
Email: *dadams@homemail.com.au*

which refers to inferences made from the body of scientific knowledge. This work investigates the three streams of evidence and the method employed follows that of a systematic review rather than an expert, narrative or other sort of review (Petticrew and Roberts, 2006). A review qualifies as systematic 'if it is based on a clearly formulated question, identifies relevant studies, appraises their quality and summarizes the evidence by use of explicit methodology' (Khan et al., 2003). A systematic review allows for scrutiny of arguments, encourages reasoned refutation, and facilitates the progressive refinement of knowledge.

Questions for review

Two explicit questions are addressed. The first question is: Does scrapie transmit prenatally in the sheep and goat? Prenatal refers to the period from oogenesis to parturition. The second question is tied to the definition of hazard in the Terrestrial Code of the World Organisation for Animal Health (OIE, 2015). The OIE defines a hazard as a biological, chemical or physical agent in, or a condition of, an animal or animal product with the potential to cause an adverse health effect. In the present case, the biological agent is the scrapie agent, the animal products are in vivo derived embryos and semen and the adverse health effect is scrapie that may be transmitted to sheep or goats by means of in vivo derived embryos or semen. So, the explicit question is: Does scrapie transmit in sheep and goats by means of semen and washed or unwashed in vivo derived embryos? Washing refers to the procedure recommended by the International Transfer Society (IETS, 2010).

The prion theory

Credence is given to the prion theory for causation of the transmissible spongiform encephalopathies or TSEs (Prusiner, 1998, 2013), which include scrapie in sheep and goats. The prion theory has explanatory and predictive power and has demonstrated its value for understanding scrapie in sheep (Hunter, 2007). For instance, scrapie disease can be controlled by selection of sheep carrying the variant of the prion gene that codes for resistance to scrapie (Goldmann, 2008). In addition, the presence of misfolded prion protein (designated as PrP^{Sc}), which reflects a fundamental event in prion diseases, underpins the immunochemical tests for diagnosing scrapie (Katz et al., 1992; Miller et al., 1993) and the more recent PMCA (protein misfolding cyclic amplification) tests (Saa et al., 2005). Prions are infectious agents consisting of a misfolded version of the cellular prion molecule (PrP^c) that is encoded by the prion gene sequence (PRNP). Misfolded prion molecules form aggregations and induce a chain reaction whereby malformed PrP^{Sc} 'seeds' impose their dysfunctional malformation on functional prion proteins (Caughey et al., 2009; Soto, 2012; Supattapone, 2015). A key consequence is

disruption to the nervous system, which eventually results in death.

Access to information

Relevant studies for review were sought through three Internet databases, which were interrogated with relevant keywords.

The Internet databases were Pubmed of the United States National Institutes of Health: http://www.ncbi.nlm.nih.gov/sites/entrez?db=pubmed, Agricola of the United States Department of Agriculture: http://agricola.nal.usda.gov, and Google Scholar: http://scholar.google.com.au.

A bibliography prepared by the US National Institute of Neurological Diseases (Gibbs et al., 1969) provided access to the literature on scrapie published before 1969 and was noteworthy for its coverage of papers in languages other than English. A monograph on scrapie by Parry (1983) also assisted with coverage of the earlier literature on scrapie. A published account of a seminar on scrapie held in Washington DC in 1964 (Agricultural Research Service, US Department of Agriculture, 1966) provided insights into thinking about scrapie at that point in time.

Procedures for identifying, marshalling and evaluating evidence

Three sources of evidence (Fig. 1) were applied to the explicit questions under review. These sources relate to experimentation (designed studies), the epidemiology of scrapie and to causal reasoning. Collectively, they can exhaust Hill's nine criteria for causation (Hill, 1977).

Experimentation refers to studies undertaken with a predetermined design and employing either deliberate infection of animals with the scrapie agent (manipulative studies) or the selection of cohorts of scrapie-infected animals (correlative or observational studies). The soundness of designed studies was evaluated according to a framework compiled from Oehlert (2000) and Ruxton and Colegrave (2006) (see online supporting material below).

Evidence from epidemiology refers to studies of the distribution and determinants of scrapie in sheep populations where systematic records exist. A particular issue is whether the relative risk of scrapie is higher in the offspring of scrapie-infected sires or dams when susceptible genotypes are accounted for. A higher relative risk of scrapie related to sires implicates direct transmission of the scrapie agent in semen. A higher relative risk related to dams implicates prenatal infection with scrapie including transmission of the scrapie agent before implantation. Another issue is that of the infectivity. Porta (2014) defines infectivity as a measure of the ability of a disease agent to establish itself in the host. Infectivity refers to the proportion of a cohort or group that become infected after exposure to an infectious agent such as the scrapie agent.

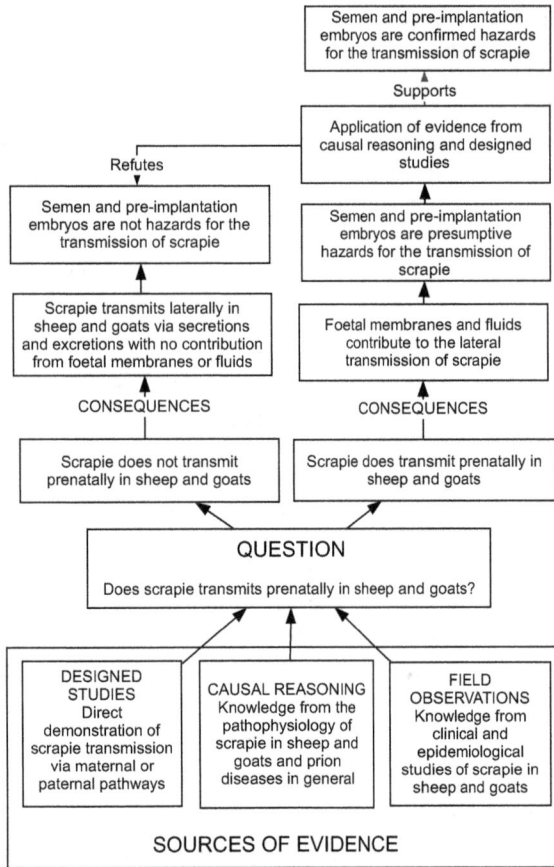

Fig. 1. Diagram showing the three sources of evidence for a systematic review on prenatal transmission of scrapie in sheep and goats.

Causal reasoning, the third source of evidence shown in Fig. 1, refers to inferences from the body of scientific knowledge and particularly knowledge about the aetiology and pathogenesis (i.e. the pathophysiology or disordered physiology) of scrapie in sheep and goats and the transmissible spongiform encephalopathies in general. Kassirer *et al.* (2009) explain causal reasoning as 'an aspect of the diagnostic process based on the cause-and-effect relations between clinical variables or chains of variables. It is a function of the anatomic, physiologic, and biochemical mechanisms that operate in the normal workings of the [human] body and the pathophysiologic behavior of these mechanisms in disease'.

Hypothesis testing and epistemic uncertainty

Hypothesis testing on the two explicit question under review involves four alternative conclusions or evaluations that cover the concepts of a type I error (false positive) and a type II error (false negative). The four possible conclusions for prenatal transmission of scrapie or transmission of scrapie via semen or *in vivo* derived embryos are shown in Table 1. Hansson (2013) points out that type I errors are considered more vexing than type II errors in the 'internal dealings of science'.

On the other hand, type II errors can have severe practical consequences when risks are being managed. A type I error in relation to scrapie may involve unnecessary actions, wasted energy and loss of opportunity. In contrast, a type II error may lead to outbreaks of scrapie, the possibility of propagating epidemics and all the adverse impacts of disease. Conclusions 1 and 2 proceed from the hypothetico-deductive method and refer to clear-cut decisions where a single significant finding can vindicate rejection or otherwise of a given hypothesis. In contrast, Conclusions 3 and 4 relate to assessments that are not clear-cut and depend upon the weight of evidence from multiple sources or the assessment of how the inevitable imperfections in scientific studies may affect the informative value of a given study. They represent epistemic uncertainty (uncertainty as to knowledge) and connect to the reality of clinical reasoning, which requires 'a dogged determination to make adequate decisions based on inadequate information' (Nardone, 1990). Assessments within Conclusions 3 and 4 will come from processes of clinical reasoning (Radostits *et al.*, 2000; Kassirer *et al.*, 2009), the Hill criteria for causality (Hill, 1977), and explanations from the core disciplines of veterinary science; anatomy, physiology and pathology (Hagan and Smithcors, 1964). Conclusions 1 and 2 classify as nominal scale variables that reflect epistemic certainty according to two categories, 'no' or 'yes' (Bonita *et al.*, 2006). In contrast, Conclusions 3 and 4 reflect epistemic uncertainty (imperfect knowledge) and the implied uncertainty can be considered as an ordinal scale variable. 'An ordinal-scale variable has values that can be ranked but are not necessarily evenly spaced, such as stages of cancer' (US Department of Health and Human Services, 2013). The ordinal scale used in this report for epistemic uncertainty within Conclusions 3 and 4 connects uncertainty to judgements about the strength of evidence for or against prenatal transmission of scrapie and for or against ovine and caprine germ plasm being a hazard for the transmission of scrapie. Grades within the ordinal scale refer to evidence of a strength that is deemed to be extremely weak, weak, marginal, strong or extremely strong.

Statistical analysis

Statistical analyses were conducted with Acastat™ Software (AcaStat Software, 43584 Merchant Mill Terrace, Leesburg, VA 20176) or StatPlus:Mac 2009 (AnalystSoft).

Table 1: Hypothesis testing on prenatal transmission of scrapie and transmission of scrapie via semen and *in vivo* derived embryos and the four conclusions possible.

Possible conclusion	Prenatal transmission	Transmission via semen or washed in vivo derived embryos	Nature of conclusion
1	Scrapie does not transmit prenatally and it is concluded correctly that it does not transmit in this way.	Scrapie does not transmit via semen or washed in vivo derived embryos and it is concluded correctly that it does not transmit in this way.	Categorical: Yes or no answer.
2	Scrapie does transmit prenatally it is concluded correctly that it does transmit in this way.	Scrapie does transmit via semen or washed in vivo derived embryos it is concluded correctly that it does transmit in this way.	Categorical: Yes or no answer.
3 – Possibility of Type I error (False Positive)	Scrapie does not transmit prenatally and it is concluded incorrectly that it does transmit in this way.	Scrapie does not transmit via semen or washed in vivo derived embryos and it is concluded incorrectly that it does transmit in this way.	Ordinal scale of evidence with grades 1-5. 1: Extremely weak. 2: Weak 3: Marginal 4: Strong 5: Extremely strong
4 - Possibility of Type II error (False Negative)	Scrapie does transmit prenatally and it is concluded incorrectly that it does not transmit in this way.	Scrapie does transmit via semen or washed in vivo derived embryos it is concluded incorrectly that it does not transmit in this way.	Ordinal scale of evidence with grades 1-5. 1: Extremely weak. 2: Weak 3: Marginal 4: Strong 5: Extremely strong

Evidence from epidemiological, clinical and field studies of scrapie

Relative risk of scrapie in offspring of scrapie-infected parents

Ten publications involving 14 populations of sheep were found with data relevant to the relative risk of scrapie in the offspring of scrapie-infected parents. Four of these publications have appeared since the pioneering epidemiological analysis by Hoinville (1996) of the incidence of scrapie in the offspring of affected and unaffected sheep. Results from these 14 populations are shown in Table 2. Four populations of sheep came from England, seven from Scotland, two from the United States and one from France. Estimates of relative risk in terms of risk ratios are given in one publication (Redman *et al.*, 2002) and did not require recalculation. Figures for incidence proportions in progeny groups (parents with scrapie versus parents without scrapie) were available in the remaining publications. Relative risks were calculated as risk ratios. Statistical significance is indicated by whether the lower 95% confidence limit of the risk ratio exceeds one.

The mean, median and range of the relative risk of scrapie in the offspring of scrapie-infected ewes for data collated in Table 2 was 4.0, 2.9, and 0.7 to 12.7 for 13 populations. The mean, median and range of the relative risk of scrapie in the offspring of scrapie-infected rams for data collated in Table 2 was 3.8, 2.4, and 1.2 to 11.3 for 11 populations. Table 2 covers a total of 49,614 sheep. With two exceptions, risk ratios in Table 2 were all above one and were statistically significant according to 95% confidence limits. The first exception relates to the offspring of scrapie-infected rams in the study of Dickinson *et al.* (1965). Here, scrapie occurred in two only out of the five rams in the key group. Low numbers of sheep and the use of flock rather than individual histories for the selection of parental groups detract from the power of the study by Dickinson *et al.* (1965). The other exception was in the study of Gonzalez *et al.* (2012), which gave a lower confidence limit of 0.7. However, the frequency of scrapie in the offspring of infected dams compared with uninfected dams was significantly higher in this instance according to the Pearson chi-square test (P<0.017).

Relative risks applying to the offspring of scrapie-infected ewes were significantly greater than those applying to the offspring of scrapie-infected rams, p<0.05 by Wilcoxon paired-sample test (Zar, 1996). This statistical significance may not translate to biological significance. Infection of the conceptus as a result of scrapie in the sire will be overshadowed when scrapie is already present in the dam.

Studies of scrapie transmission undertaken in the UK with scrapie free sheep from New Zealand and with scrapie susceptible genotypes confirm that the sufficient cause of scrapie disease is composed of two necessary causes (Houston *et al.*, 2002; Ryder *et al.*, 2004; Foster *et al.*, 2006).

Table 2. Relative risk of scrapie in offspring of parents with and without scrapie from 11 publications and 14 populations of sheep (IP = incidence proportion; RR = risk ratio; CI = confidence interval; n.a. = not available).

Population of sheep*		1	2	3	4	5	6	7	8	9	10	11	12	13	14
No scrapie in sire or dam	IP	26/334	5/27	5/165	53/153	18/311	26/105	111/342 for dam, 45/127 for sire	47/78	n.a.	n.a.	n.a.	n.a.	58/21,907 for dam, 447/17,150 for sire	57/71
Scrapie in dam only	RR (95% CI)	10.4 (2.7 – 39.5)	0.7 (0.1 – 2.1)	12.7 (7.0 – 23.0)	1.9 (1.5 – 2.4)	7.7 (7.7 – 34.4)	1.8 (1.0 – 3.3)	2.5 (1.7 – 3.8)	1.3 (1.1 – 1.6)	3.2 (>1.0)	2.9 (>1.0)	1.9 (>1.0)	3.5 (>1.0)	6.0 (4.7 – 7.5)	5.7 (0.8 – 38.6)
	IP	4/8	4/38	11/33	47/76	23/46	13/31	51/82	148/201	n.a.	n.a.	n.a.	n.a.	74/577	35/36
Scrapie in sire only	RR (95% CI)	3.8 (2.6 – 5.7)	2.6 (1.5 – 4.5)	6.0 (2.6 – 13.6)	1.2 (1.0 – 1.3)	11.3 (6.3 – 20.5)	1.3 (1.1 – 1.6)	1.5 (1.2 – 1.8)	n.a.	2.4 (>1.0)	7.8 (>1.0)	1.3 (>1.0)	2.1 (>1.0)	3.8 (2.5 – 5.8)	n.a.
	IP	24/68	22/32	32/70	24/65	57/124	50/129	76/170	n.a.	n.a.	n.a.	n.a.	n.a.	22/232	n.a.
Scrapie in sire and dam	RR (95% CI)	83.0 (20.4 – 337.4)	1.4 (1.0 – 2.0)	6.8 (3.0 – 15.4)	2.4 (1.8 – 3.2)	27.4 (13.6 – 55.1)	7.3 (2.5 – 20.7)	n.a.	n.a.	3.3 (>1.0)	6.1 (>1.0)	2.0 (>1.0)	2.8 (>1.0)	n.a.	n.a.
	IP	30/32	19/46	33/52	18/21	48/56	14/18	n.a.	n.a.	n.a.	n.a.	n.a.	n.a.	n.a.	n.a.

*Data published by – 1: Parry (1962); 2: Dickinson et al. (1965); 3: Gordon (1966); 4: Dickinson et al. (1974); 5: Parry (1983); 6 and 7: Hourrigan et al. (1979); 8: Elsen et al. (1999); 9 – 12: Redman et al. (2002); 13: Hoinville et al. (2010); 14: Gonzalez et al. (2012).
n.a.: Not available.

These necessary causes are the exposure to the scrapie agent and the possession of a scrapie-susceptible genotype in at-risk sheep. Hence, higher relative risks in the offspring of scrapie-infected parents will result from the action of both necessary causes.

The question is the degree to which prenatal transmission contributes to the overall incidence of infection and the nature of the biological relationship that allows for transmission. Conclusion 4 applies and higher relative risks of scrapie in the progeny of scrapie infected parents provide strong evidence that scrapie transmits prenatally.

Two publications were identified for sheep where estimates of relative risks of scrapie infection in the offspring of scrapie-infected parents take account of the transmission of genetic susceptibility as determined by laboratory testing of DNA for variants of the prion gene (Elsen *et al.*, 1999; Hoinville *et al.*, 2010). In doing so, the two publications weigh heavily towards prenatal transmission being a contributor to the relative risks in Table 2. Conclusion 4 can thus be upgraded. Higher relative risks of scrapie in progeny in this situation provide extremely strong evidence that scrapie transmits prenatally.

Elsen *et al.* (1999) investigated a scrapie outbreak in a flock of hyper-prolific Romanov sheep in southern France. In this outbreak, 1,015 animals were exposed to scrapie, and 304 died from the disease between April 1, 1993 and May 1, 1997. Susceptibility genotypes were determined from blood samples. Epidemiological analysis used survival times and the Cox or proportional hazards model, which is applicable to survival times when several possible causal factors of disease may operate simultaneously (Friedman, 2004). A significantly increased incidence of scrapie in the offspring of scrapie-affected ewes ($p= 0.021$ and $p=0.001$ for the susceptible genotypes of lambs) was observed when the confounding effect of transmitted susceptibility was controlled.

The second publication describing relative risks associated with scrapie-infected parents, and which used laboratory testing of DNA to account for the transmission of genetic susceptibility, is that of Hoinville *et al.* (2010). The study covers 38 flocks of sheep, a total of 981 cases of scrapie, and 32,580 at risk sheep in Great Britain between 1994 and 2003. Once again, genetic susceptibility was determined by laboratory testing of DNA for variants at codons 136, 154 and 171 of the prion gene.

The study had a case-control design and a suite of statistical tests including Cox proportional hazard regression was used for analysis. Hoinville *et al.* (2010) found a significantly ($p < 0.05$) increased incidence of scrapie in the offspring of scrapie affected ewes but not rams after the effect of PrP genotype was controlled.

Epidemiological observations on pathways for scrapie transmission in sheep

Publications on the epidemiology of scrapie mention paternal transmission, maternal transmission, vertical transmission and horizontal or lateral transmission. These terms refer to transmission during either the prenatal, neonatal or postnatal periods in the life of sheep. The relationships among possible transmission pathways and their boundaries are shown diagrammatically in Fig. 2.

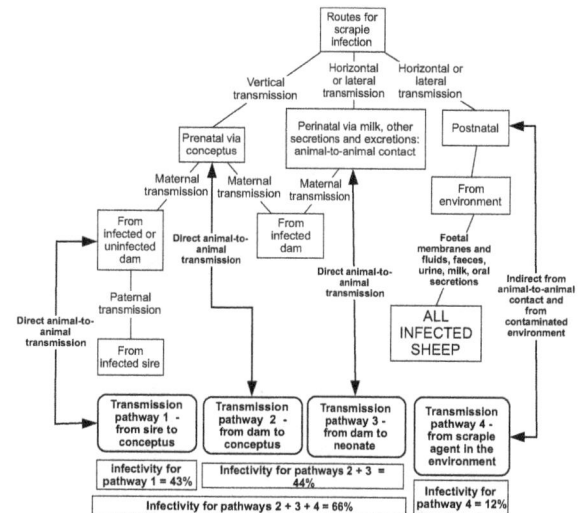

Fig. 2. Diagram showing relationships among possible transmission pathways for scrapie in the sheep and their connection the prenatal, neonatal and postnatal periods and the presence of the scrapie agent in sires, dams, the conceptus and the external environment.

Fig. 2 shows that the possible pathways for transmission of the scrapie agent are from parent to offspring directly or from non-parents, parents (that is, all members of a population) and fomites in the postnatal environment. Four transmission pathways are identified and these align with prenatal, neonatal (birth to weaning) and postnatal periods in the life of offspring and entail pathways from sire or dam to the conceptus (pathways 1 and 2), from dam to the neonate in the period from birth to weaning (pathway 3) and from all infected sheep postnatally (pathway 4). The prenatal period commences with oogenesis and terminates at parturition. All sheep will be exposed to the scrapie agent in the environment.

Populations 1-6 in Table 2 contain data from 2,060 offspring and 606 cases of scrapie that can be used to calculate infectivities (the proportion of exposures that result in infection) related to the four transmission pathways shown in Fig. 2. Lowest infectivity (12%) occurred from pathway 4; that is, lateral transmission from the scrapie agent in the environment.

Highest infectivity resulted when both sire and dam were scrapie infected. Infectivity from the paternal source (sire to conceptus, pathway1) was similar to that from the maternal source (pathways 2 and 3), implying that perinatal infection is overshadowed by infection occurring before birth.

Direct observation in sheep of prenatal transmission of scrapie

A single study in sheep has been identified where prenatal infection with the scrapie agent was demonstrated directly (Hourrigan *et al.*, 1979). Lambs were removed from exposure to natural scrapie at birth and at 4, 9 or 20 months after birth and placed in isolation pens for long-term observation.

Six out of 54 sheep removed from exposure at birth succumbed to scrapie according to the diagnostic criteria employed. Twenty-three more deaths from scrapie occurred in sheep that were removed from exposure at different times during postnatal life. These 23 deaths represent the results of exposure to the scrapie agent during the prenatal period plus various lengths of exposure during postnatal life. According to linear regression analysis, the trend line and correlation are statistically significant (y = 1.571x + 11.042, R^2 = 0.966, p<0.0172). Increasing periods of postnatal exposure acted additively to increase the burden of scrapie.

Clinical observations on prenatal transmission of scrapie

Couquet *et al.* (2005) report a pregnant ewe with suspected scrapie that was transferred to a veterinary diagnostic laboratory and gave birth to a ewe lamb 10 days later. The ewe was euthanased 16 days after the lamb was born and a post mortem diagnosis of scrapie was made by immunoblotting.

The lamb was separated from its mother as soon as it emerged from the birth canal, received no colostrum, was fed with milk replacers and was isolated to prevent horizontal transmission of scrapie. Six months later the lamb showed the first signs of scrapie and four months later it was euthanized when it could no longer stand. Scrapie was confirmed post mortem by immunoblotting and immunohistochemistry. This observation and that of Hourrigan *et al.* (1979) support the prenatal transmission of scrapie.

Evidence from experimentation
Scrapie infectivity in sheep semen

Before 2012, the possibility that sheep semen could transmit scrapie was investigated by two approaches. One approach sought to transmit scrapie by parenteral administration of semen in lambs (Palmer, 1959), outbred mice (Hourrigan *et al.*, 1979; Hadlow *et al.*, 1982) or transgenic mice expressing the highest susceptibility variant of the ovine prion gene (Sarradin *et al.*, 2008). The other approach applied methods such as immunohistochemistry or immunoblotting to identify the diseased form of the prion protein (PrP^{Sc}) (Gatti *et al.*, 2002).

Poor sensitivity of test methods can explain the failure of these early studies to detect scrapie infectivity in ovine semen. An additional consideration, namely statistical power, applies to the study by Sarradin *et al.* (2008). The study of Sarradin *et al.* (2008) sought to detect scrapie by means of intracerebral injections of semen from scrapie-affected Romanov rams into scrapie-susceptible transgenic mice overexpressing the high susceptibility allele of the sheep prion (*PRNP*) gene. None of the test mice developed scrapie, whereas control mice inoculated with preparations of brain from scrapie-affected sheep died from scrapie within 165 days. Three rams exposed to natural scrapie were used and provided single semen samples *via* an artificial vagina at one month, seven months or 13 months before death from scrapie. Sarradin *et al.* (2008) employed three experimental units in their overall study and single experimental units for three possible treatment levels that may correspond with the stage of scrapie disease. The power of the study is thus weak and provides weak evidence that scrapie *does not* transmit via germ plasm.

The most recent study on ovine semen (Rubenstein *et al.*, 2012) demonstrated scrapie infectivity in two ways. One was by a transmission test with transgenic mice; that is by a test similar to that employed by Sarradin *et al.* (2008). The other involved a process for detecting the scrapie agent that comprised serial protein misfolding cyclic amplification (PMCA) followed by an immunoassay method (SOFIA).

The study by Rubenstein *et al.* (2012) merges clinical findings, history and laboratory testing into a coherent whole and is consistent with standard diagnostic methods. It was prompted by the discovery of scrapie in seven of 24 ewes in a 'sentinel' flock of that had been free of scrapie for 13 years. These sheep had been physically separated from scrapie-infected animals. The crucial point from the case history is that scrapie-infected rams had been used for breeding four months before scrapie was detected in the ewes.

The detection of scrapie infectivity on the semen of sheep by means of transmission studies with transgenic mice and protein misfolding cyclic amplification (PMCA) overturns earlier negative findings. Semen from scrapie-infected sheep is thus confirmed as a hazard for the transmission of scrapie.

Scrapie infectivity in the ovine and caprine conceptus

Thirteen publications were found that demonstrate the scrapie agent in the conceptus of sheep and provide direct anatomical proof of prenatal transmission of scrapie in this species. Two publications provide similar findings for goats (O'Rourke *et al.*, 2011; Schneider *et al.*, 2015). Samples examined in these publications were obtained either post-partum or prepartum at various times during gestation. The scrapie agent was detected by various methods including test transmissions in sheep, goats and mice, Western blot analysis, immunohistochemistry, enzyme linked immunosorbent assays (ELISA), protein multiplication cyclic amplification (PMCA), and bioassay in transgenic tg388 mice that overexpress the ovine prion gene

Nine of the publications sought for and found the scrapie agent in extra-embryonic tissues only (Pattison et al., 1972, 1974; Onodera et al., 1993; Race et al., 1998; Caplazi et al., 2004; Alverson et al., 2006; Lacroux et al., 2007; Santucciu et al., 2010). Three of the publications examined both extra-embryonic membranes and the foetus proper by means of Western blot analysis or immunohistochemistry and detected the scrapie agent in extra-embryonic membranes only (Tuo et al., 2001, 2002: Andreoletti et al., 2002).

Garza et al. (2011) and Spiropoulos et al. (2014) found the scrapie agent in both extra-embryonic tissues and the foetus proper by means of PMCA or bioassay in tg388 mice. These last two findings are consistent with an anatomical view of the conceptus as a whole organism, made up of the extra-embryonic membranes and foetus. Extra-embryonic membranes are external organs of the foetus and share the same circulatory system. The cells of foetus and extra-embryonic membranes have the same genotype.

Precedents from commonplace causes of abortion in ewes argue against a barrier in the conceptus that protects the ovine foetus from pathogens. The causative organisms of campylobacteriosis, listeriosis, toxoplasmosis and Border disease are found in both foetal membranes and the foetus (Broadbent, 1972; Hedstrom et al., 1987; Nettleton et al., 1998; Dubey, 2009).

Coetzer et al. (1994) list the protozoa, rickettsias, chlamydias, viruses, and bacteria capable of prenatal infection in sheep.

Prenatal infection with scrapie is thus conceivable at any time from oogenesis to parturition and the scrapie infection seen in the cotyledonary chorioallantois may be the result of transmission either before or after implantation. A high concentration of PrP^{Sc} in the cotyledonary chorioallantois may reflect contiguity with maternal tissue and transplacental transmission. It may also indicate that the cotyledonary chorioallantois contains enough cellular prion protein (PrP^c) for conversion to the disease form (PrP^{Sc}) (Colby and Prusiner, 2013). In this connection, Tuo et al. (2001) found that the relative concentration of PrP^c in the ovine cotyledonary chorioallantois was about four times and eight times that found in foetal bladder and kidney and similar to that found in foetal brain. Thumdee et al. (2007) report similar findings. Johnson et al. (2014) found that estrogen stimulation increases in PrP^c

expression in uteroplacental tissues, including the chorioallantois. In consequence, the high concentration of PrP^{Sc} in the cotyledonary chorioallantois may simply reflect the relatively high tissue expression of PrP^c.

It is conceivable that the scrapie agent may arrive in the conceptus before implantation and infect oocytes or early embryos. Thumdee et al. (2007) found that the ovine prion gene is expressed in immature and mature ovine oocytes and ovine morulas. Similarly, Peralta et al. (2012) have identified relatively high expression of the mRNA that codes for PrP in bovine conceptuses at day 4 of gestation. These findings signify the very early availability of normal prion protein (PrP^c) for conversion to the abnormal misfolded form (PrP^{Sc}), a hallmark of prion disease (Prusiner, 1998). Prenatal infection with the scrapie agent as early as the oocyte stage is plausible.

To sum up, observations of the scrapie agent in foetal membranes and the foetus itself provide definitive anatomical evidence for the prenatal transmission of scrapie in both sheep and goats.

Scrapie infectivity in washed or unwashed in vivo derived embryos

Seven studies were identified that relate to the explicit question of whether scrapie can transmit in sheep by means of washed or unwashed in vivo derived embryos (Foster et al., 1992; Foote et al., 1993; Foster et al., 1996; Wang et al., 2001, 2002; Foster et al., 2006; Low et al., 2009; Foster et al., 2013). These are discussed in reverse chronological order. Table 3 shows results of analysis. The study of Foster et al. (2013) builds on an understanding of the importance of the prion protein gene (PRNP) and codons 136, 154 and 171 gene in genetic resistance to scrapie in sheep. In Cheviot sheep, PRNP genotypes of VRQ/VRQ and VRQ/ARQ are at risk from both local endemic scrapie and the SSBP/1 strain of the scrapie agent whereas the PRNP genotypes of VRQ/AHQ and VRQ/ARR are at risk only from the SSBP/1 strain. The clear-cut differences in the expression of disease that distinguish the SSBP/1 strain from the local endemic strain of scrapie were utilized in analysis.

Foster et al. (2013) studied Cheviot sheep at a site in Scotland and asked whether scrapie developed in embryo-derived offspring that were exposed to the SSBP/1 agent in surrogate dams and whether or not this exposure required genetic susceptibility in these dams. Accordingly, there were three exposure groups. The first group consisted of offspring derived from embryos that were gestated in ewes with a range of PRNP genotypes and which were not exposed to SSBP/1 scrapie ('infection controls' or 'unexposed group). The second group consisted of offspring derived from embryos that were gestated in ewes with scrapie resistant PRNP genotypes, which were challenged with SSBP/1.

Table 3. Evidential value of studies on the transmission of scrapie in sheep by *in vivo* derived embryos.

Studies by	Breed of sheep and source of scrapie agent	Evidence for or against transmission of scrapie by embryos
Foster *et al.* (2103)	Cheviot sheep with designed exposure to SSBP/1 strain of scrapie and adventitious exposure to local endemic strain of scrapie.	Definitive for washed and unwashed embryos
Low *et al.* (2009)	Embryos from sheep with natural scrapie gestated in scrapie free Suffolk ewes from New Zealand.	Weak against washed embryos
Foster *et al.* (2006)	Cheviot sheep but embryo donors had no exposure to scrapie.	Ruled out as evidence
Wang *et al.* (2001, 2002)	Suffolk sheep with a high incidence of natural scrapie.	Ruled out as evidence (see text)
Foster *et al.* (1996)	Cheviot sheep with designed exposure to SSBP/1 strain. Adventitious exposure to local endemic strain of scrapie *via* semen from infected rams.	Definitive for washed and unwashed embryos
Foote *et al.* (1993)	Suffolk sheep infected with third to fourth passage strain of Suffolk scrapie agent. Cheviot sheep with SSBP/1 strain of scrapie.	Ruled out as evidence
Foster *et al.* (1992); additional data from EFSA (2010)	Cheviot sheep. SSBP/1 strain.	Strong for unwashed embryos.

This exposure group can demonstrate prenatal transfer or of SSBP/1 scrapie from ewes with *PRNP* genotypes coding for scrapie resistance. The third group consisted of offspring derived from embryos that were gestated in ewes with scrapie susceptible *PRNP* genotypes, which were challenged with SSBP/1. This exposure group can demonstrate or not prenatal transfer of SSBP/1 scrapie from ewes with *PRNP* genotypes coding for scrapie susceptibility.

Embryos came from a panel of 15 donors with *PRNP* genotypes encoding for at least one VRQ allele and which were inseminated by semen from three rams, one of which had the *PRNP* genotype of VRQ/ARQ and the other two had the *PRNP* genotype of VRQ/ARR. Some embryos were washed according to IETS recommendations and others were not. Three of the embryo donors developed endemic scrapie after embryo collection. The remaining embryo donors and the three rams died with illnesses other than endemic scrapie in its expected form.

Sixteen cases of scrapie attributable to either the SSBP/1 or the endemic strain of scrapie were diagnosed in the 59 sheep that originated from transferred embryos. The distribution of these cases within exposure groups and according to *PRNP* genotypes permits three significant conclusions. First, embryo washing according to the recommendations of the IETS did not protect lambs from scrapie and can be regarded as an ineffective secondary protective measure. Second, prenatal transmission of scrapie occurs in sheep and is possible when dams have *PRNP* genotypes that code for susceptibility to scrapie. The observation that SSBP/1 scrapie transmitted from susceptible but not resistant dams inoculated with SSBP/1 scrapie indicates that genetically resistant dams provide an

effective barrier against prenatal transmission. Third, scrapie is transmissible by *in vivo* derived embryos in sheep. Conclusion 2 of the hypothesis-testing protocol applies to the study of Foster *et al.* (2013): *Scrapie transmits in sheep by means of unwashed or washed in vitro derived embryos and it is concluded correctly that it does so.*

Low *et al.* (2009) report a correlative experiment in which embryos transferred from naturally infected ewes were used to investigate whether *in vivo* derived embryos can carry the agent of classic scrapie. The study was conducted on quarantined premises with Suffolk sheep that were homozygous for the ARQ allele of the *PRNP* gene.

In Suffolks, ARQ/ARQ homozygotes and ARQ/ARH heterozygotes have the greatest susceptibility to natural scrapie infection (Baylis *et al.*, 2004). Thirty-nine experimental lambs were produced from embryos out of naturally infected donor ewes. Since the use of natural scrapie necessitated null treatment controls, 17 unexposed lambs were produced from embryos collected from New Zealand–derived Suffolk ewes.

Twenty-eight sheep derived from scrapie-exposed embryos survived to an end point of five years of age and 12 of the 17 sheep derived from unexposed embryos survived to the same endpoint.

No histopathological or immunohistochemical evidence of scrapie was found at *post mortem* in any of the embryo-derived sheep. From this, Low *et al.* (2009) concluded that their study provided no evidence for transmission of scrapie and reinforced published evidence that vertical transmission of scrapie may be circumvented by embryo transfer procedures. Estimates of statistical power provided by Low *et al.* (2009) set the likelihood of scrapie transmission by *in vivo* derived embryos as high as one in 11 or 9.1%, with 95% confidence limits.

The method for estimating statistical power is not described and it is unclear whether calculations are based on 28 embryo-derived sheep or eight scrapie affected ewes that donated embryos. Calculations on embryo-derived offspring would be confounded by pseudoreplication (Ruxton and Colgrave, 2006). Embryos are dependent variables and units for measurement whereas ewes donating embryos are the independent variables and units for experiment. The stated 9.1% risk cannot be determined from eight experimental units. The results of Low *et al.* (2009) thus provide weak evidence against the transmission of scrapie in sheep by means of washed *in vitro* derived embryos.

Foster *et al.* (2006) describe a project that employed embryo transfer to generate scrapie-free flocks of sheep containing individuals with PrP genotypes known to confer high susceptibility. The findings are crucially significant for understanding the aetiology of scrapie. They confirm that scrapie disease has two necessary causes: susceptibility of hosts and the presence of the scrapie agent. However, none of the semen donors, embryo donors or embryo recipients in the study of Foster *et al.* (2006) exhibited scrapie. As a consequence, there was no testable exposure to the scrapie agent that could be linked to embryos. In short, the scrapie agent did not transmit via *in vivo* derived embryos because it was absent from the donors of germ plasm in the first place and the study is not relevant to the explicit question of this review.

The study by Wang *et al.* (2001) was a correlative experiment to investigate the potential for scrapie to transmit by embryo transfer in flocks where the disease is endemic. A supplementary paper (Wang *et al.*, 2002) provided information on the scrapie-resistance genotypes of the sheep that were used. The experiment consisted of obtaining embryos from donor ewes out of six different scrapie-infected flocks of Suffolk sheep, transferring these embryos to scrapie-free recipients and monitoring the occurrence of scrapie in embryo-derived offspring, embryo donors and embryo recipients. Embryos from 38 donor ewes were transferred to 58 recipients and resulted in 94 viable lambs, which were monitored until they were 60 months old.

Scrapie according to an unstated definition was not observed in the response units (the offspring). However, the study of Wang *et al.* (2001, 2002) has insufficient power for accepting its stated hypothesis that 'the transmission of scrapie may be circumvented by embryo transfer'. The timing of embryo collection in relation to the stage of scrapie infection is not described and an important dimension in scrapie exposure is unknown. The mortality rate of embryo-

derived sheep in the first year of life was an exceptional 21.3%. Causes of death are not reported and mortalities could have assorted differentially according to the scrapie status of embryo donors. Deaths before 12 months of age could well have been due to scrapie. Scrapie can be exhibited in lambs as young as six months (Brotherston *et al.*, 1968; Couquet *et al.*, 2005). Other issues that affect the evidential value of the study by Wang *et al.* (2001, 2002) regarding the transmission of scrapie in sheep by *in vivo* derived embryos are detailed in the online supporting material.

Foster *et al.* (1996) investigated the progeny of embryos with genotypes that were homozygous or heterozygous for scrapie susceptibility, which were obtained from scrapie-susceptible or scrapie-resistant ewes injected or not with the SSBP/1 strain of the scrapie agent 246 days before embryos were harvested and which were washed or not according the protocols of the IETS. Donor ewes were inseminated with semen from two homozygous scrapie-susceptible rams to ensure that both homozygous and heterozygous-susceptible lambs were in the treatment groups. Scrapie disease, referable to the field strain, was diagnosed in these two rams at 236 and 287 days after semen collection:

Scrapie, referable to the field strain and not the SSBP/1 strain, appeared in homozygous and heterozygous-susceptible lambs derived from donor ewes that were exposed or not to the SSBP/1 strain of scrapie and from ova that were washed or not according to the IETS protocol. Scrapie disease did not appear in the heterozygous susceptible lambs derived from scrapie resistant ewes. Abductive reasoning (inference to the best explanation) attributes the appearance of scrapie in the treatment groups of Foster *et al.* (1996) to transmission of the scrapie agent from infected semen to embryos. The washing of embryos according to IETS requirements did not prevent transmission.

Foster *et al.* (1996) were hesitant in incriminating the scrapie-infected rams as the source of scrapie seen in their treatment groups: the argument being the absence of sound case for scrapie infectivity in semen at that time. Scrapie infectivity in ram semen has now been demonstrated (Rubenstein *et al.*, 2012). The results of Foster *et al.* (1996) can thus be attributed to the transmission of scrapie by semen. The infection pathway from ram to embryo donor and thence to embryo recipients entails transmission by embryos. As a consequence, the results of Foster *et al.* (1996) show the transmission of scrapie by *in vivo* derived embryos treated according to the requirements of the IETS.

Foote *et al.* (1993) describe two experiments on the transmission of scrapie by *in vivo* derived embryos. The first experiment was conducted at a site in Texas and involved Suffolk sheep, a Suffolk-passaged strain of scrapie and four treatments: (1) embryos from scrapie-infected donor ewes were gestated in scrapie-free recipients ('via embryo'); (2) embryos from scrapie free donors were gestated in scrapie-infected recipients ('via uterus'); (3) embryos derived from scrapie-free donors were gestated in scrapie-free recipients ('negative controls'); and, (4) embryos derived from scrapie-infected ewes were gestated in scrapie-infected recipients ('positive controls'). The second experiment was conducted at a site in Utah and involved Cheviot sheep, the SSBP/1 strain of scrapie and two treatments: (1) embryos from scrapie-infected donor ewes were gestated in scrapie-free recipients and (2) embryos derived from scrapie-infected ewes were gestated in scrapie-infected recipients ('positive controls').

The proposition examined by Foote et al. (1993) was that the appearance of their conception of scrapie demonstrates scrapie transmission or not by means of in vivo derived embryos. No such scrapie was observed. However, the large and unexplained mortalities observed in the study merit examination. In particular, mortality to 23 months of age was distributed disproportionately among the four treatment groups and may point to an unexpected consequence of exposure to the scrapie agent.

When data from the two experiments are pooled mortalities rates were 32% for the 'via embryo' group, 52% for the 'via uterus' group, 45% for the group exposed both 'via embryo' and 'via uterus' and 23% for the scrapie unexposed group. These percentages are significantly different ($P<0.0158$ by Pearson Chi-square) and indicate an impact of prenatal exposure to the scrapie agent. Mortalities calculated from numbers of Suffolk offspring alive at 24 months and 60 months were 24.4% for the 'via embryo' group and 6.1% for the negative controls ($P < 0.031$). These results indicate an impact of the scrapie agent on unwashed in vivo derived embryos in sheep and deserve further consideration. The study of Foote et al. (1993) is ruled out as evidence on whether scrapie transmits via pre-implantation embryos.

The earliest study of scrapie infectivity in in vivo derived embryos (Foster et al., 1992; EFSA, 2010) involved Cheviot sheep and the SSBP/1 strain of scrapie at the National Pathogenesis Unit in Edinburgh. It investigated whether scrapie can be transferred early in gestation or in the ovary and it used embryos from scrapie-infected ewes as the experimental manipulation. Genetic susceptibility to scrapie was determined according to information on the Sip (scrapie incubation period) and prion protein genotype and was obtained from pedigrees and restriction fragment length analysis (RFLP). Subsequent analysis of the Sip genotype identified three dominant codons in the ovine prion gene (136, 154 and 171) that control susceptibility to scrapie (Hunter et al., 1996). Six donor ewes were injected subcutaneously with an extract from brains of sheep containing the SSBP/1 isolate of the scrapie agent six months before hormonally induced superovulation, intrauterine insemination and the collection of embryos. Scrapie appeared at 40, 70, 82 and 95 days after embryo collection in the homozygous susceptible donors and at 146 and 180 days in the heterozygous susceptible donors. The single ram used as a semen donor was heterozygous for the susceptibility gene. The ram was subsequently injected with the SSBP/1 isolate of the scrapie agent and showed signs of scrapie 309 days later. Sixteen ewes homozygous for scrapie resistance were used as surrogate dams for 37 embryos and gave birth to 26 lambs. Lambing occurred indoors in premises disinfected with a 20% sodium hypochlorite solution. Lambs were weaned at four months of age, were strictly isolated from other sheep and were grazed on pasture that had never been exposed to scrapie-infected or parturient sheep. The success rate of embryo transfer was 26 lambs from 37 embryos or 70%. Six of the 26 embryo-derived lambs died within the first year of life and as a result of 'diseases unrelated to scrapie'. All six homozygous susceptibles developed scrapie. Two of the 11 heterozygotes developed scrapie and a further six were put down because of what was stated to be metabolic illness (EFSA, 2010). Two of these six sheep with metabolic illness were scrapie-positive according to immunoblots. In other words, four of the 11 heterozygotes were diagnosed with scrapie and another four died from 'metabolic illness' during the period of experimental observations. None of the three homozygous resistant sheep died during the period of experimental observations.

In summary, of the 26 sheep derived from 37 transferred embryos, 10 or 38% died from scrapie. A further 10 or 38% of the 26 embryo-derived sheep died from other diseases, including four from 'metabolic illness'. Six of these died before the age of 12 months. The total mortality to about three years of age was 20 out of 26 sheep or 77%. Deaths from causes other than classically expressed scrapie arouse interest given that scrapie infection was the experimental treatment. A thought experiment can be used to calculate a prior probability for testing significance. The question is how many cases of scrapie could be expected in 20 identical sheep in identical circumstances except for exposure to SBPP/1 scrapie in embryo donors. An incidence of up to four cases allows for statistical significance by the Pearson Chi-square test. The incidence of scrapie recorded by Foster et al. (1992) far exceeds an estimate of prior probability. Scrapie due to the endemic strain in the Cheviot flock at the National Pathogenesis Unit had a maximum annual incidence of 1% and a maximum incidence of 5.4% in birth cohorts recorded (Redman et al., 2002). Accordingly, the study of Foster et al. (1992) is judged as strong evidence that scrapie transmits prenatally in sheep (see online supporting material).

Evidence from causal reasoning

A set of pathophysiological observations line up to prevent rejection and allow acceptance of prenatal transmission of scrapie in sheep. These observations constitute the case around causal reasoning derived from knowledge of scrapie in sheep and goats. They relate to preconditions for prenatal transmission that affirm biological plausibility, an important criterion of causation (Hill, 1977). Key preconditions are: (1) The scrapie agent is able to disperse throughout the body and to the reproductive organs. (2) Exposure to the scrapie agent is possible at any point during the prenatal period from oogenesis to the zygote/blastocyst, embryogenesis and foetal stages. (3) The conceptus is susceptible to infection with the scrapie agent. The pertinent pathophysiological observations occur in sequence starting from the fact that scrapie is a contagious disease and can be spread from animal to animal by direct or indirect contact (Greig, 1940; Gordon, 1957; Dickinson et al., 1965; Brotherston et al., 1968; Hourrigan et al., 1979; Hoinville, 1996; Detwiler and Baylis, 2003; Ryder et al., 2004; Foster et al., 2006; Gough et al., 2015; Hawkins et al., 2015). The property of contagiousness requires that the scrapie agent operate portals of exit from infected animals and portals of entry into uninfected animals and has capacity to pass the usual barriers against infection. Demonstrated portals of exit for the scrapie agent in sheep include excretions and ejecta (faeces, urine and foetal membranes) and secretions (milk, oral secretions and semen) (Table 4). These various portals of exit demonstrate that the scrapie agent is able to traverse biological membranes and disperses through the body. The presence of the scrapie agent in foetal membranes shows that the scrapie agent can pass across cell and tissue barriers within the reproductive tract of sheep. As to dispersal of the scrapie agent through the body, the presence of the scrapie agent in blood, prionaemia, carries the same consequences for the pathogenesis of scrapie as those applying to viraemia and bacteraemia in viral and bacterial diseases. Prionaemia signifies (1) that the scrapie agent can be distributed throughout the body, including the reproductive tract and (2) that mechanisms exist for passage of the scrapie agent across the endothelial cell sheet and into interstitial fluid and the lymphatic system, where the known functions of the lymphoreticular system in the pathogenesis of scrapie (Jeffrey and González, 2007; van Keulen et al., 2008) can come into play. Haematogenous carriage was reported for scrapie in sheep in 2002 and has been corroborated repeatedly with different detection methods. Hunter et al. (2002) showed that transfusions of blood from BSE or scrapie-infected sheep transmitted these two diseases to

uninfected sheep. Thorne and Terry (2008) demonstrated the presence of the scrapie agent in the blood of scrapie-infected sheep by means of PMCA. Houston et al. (2008) corroborated earlier findings of the research group (Hunter et al., 2002) and showed transmission rates by blood transfusion of 36% for BSE and 43% for scrapie. Terry et al. (2009) found PrP^{Sc} in cells isolated from the blood of 55% of sheep infected with scrapie and 71% of sheep infected with BSE. PrP^{Sc} was found in blood cells several months before the onset of clinical signs in scrapie-infected sheep. Rubenstein et al. (2010) used PMCA and found the disease-associated form of the prion protein (PrP^{Sc}) in blood plasma from sheep at both the preclinical and clinical stages of scrapie. Edwards et al. (2010) used immunoassays to investigate the nature of the blood cells of scrapie-infected sheep that carried PrP^{Sc}, the surrogate marker for prion disease. The mononuclear cells in blood carrying PrP^{Sc} during the preclinical and clinical stages of scrapie had a cell surface phenotype that defined them as a subpopulation of B lymphocytes. Dassanayake et al. (2011) used similar methods to associate the scrapie agent in the blood of sheep with a sub-population of B lymphocytes and also with platelet rich plasma. Subsequently, Dassanayake et al. (2012) identified the scrapie agent in both B and T lymphocytes in the blood of scrapie-infected sheep and the blood of scrapie-infected goats. Other demonstrations of the scrapie agent in the blood of sheep come from Bannach et al. (2012), Andreoletti et al. (2012) and Lacroux et al. (2012). Bannach et al. (2012) employed a method for based on surface-FIDA (fluorescence intensity distribution analysis) and showed that disease-specific aggregates of prion protein could be detected in the blood plasma of scrapie-infected sheep. Andreoletti et al. (2012) used bioassays in genetically susceptible sheep and transgenic mice overexpressing the ovine prion gene for scrapie susceptibility to investigate scrapie transmission by blood. They showed that the efficacy for transmitting the PG127 strain of scrapie depended more on the viability of transfused white blood cells than upon the degree of infectivity that was measured by intracerebral inoculation in transgenic mice. As a consequence, bioassays that use non-living material, including highly sensitive versions with transgenic mice, are inherently limited as to the information they can provide on infectivity of the scrapie agent. The scrapie agent can be found in the lymphoreticular system of both sheep (van Keulen et al., 1996; Schreuder et al., 1998; Andreoletti et al., 2000; O'Rourke et al., 2000, 2002; Press et al., 2004; Gonzalez et al., 2008; Dennis et al., 2009; Ryder et al., 2009; Jeffrey et al., 2011; Toppets et al., 2011), and goats (Monleon et al., 2001; Gonzalez et al., 2009, 2010).

Table 4. Evidence for scrapie infectivity in tissues and excretions of sheep and goats.

Tissue	References	Methods of detection
Faeces, gut, liver	Sheep: Everest et al. (2011); Terry et al. (2011).	sPMCA, IHC, immunoblotting
Urine and kidneys	Sheep: Ligios et al. (2007); Rubenstein et al. (2012).	
Foetal membranes and fluids	Sheep: Pattison et al. (1972, 1974); Onodera et al. (1993); Race et al. (1998); Tuo et al. (2001, 2002); Andreoletti et al. (2002); Alverson et al. (2006); Lacroux et al. (2007). Goats: O'Rourke et al. (2011); Schneider et al. (2015).	sPMCA, IHC, transmission to tg388 mice, SAF detection, immunoblotting, transmission to sheep
Lochia	Not examined	
Secretions		
Milk	Sheep: Konold et al. (2008); Lacroux et al. (2008); Maddison et al. (2009); Ligios et al. (2011); Konold et al. (2013a). Goats: Konold et al. (2013b).	sPMCA, IHC, transmission to tg388 mice
Oral secretions and salivary glands	Sheep: Vascellari et al. (2007); Maddison et al. (2010); Gough et al. (2012).	sPMCA; IHC
Semen	Sheep: Rubenstein et al. (2012).	sPMCA, transmission to tg388 mice

In both sheep and goats, the scrapie agent is present in cells of the lymphocyte lineage (T cell and B cells) and the mononuclear phagocyte lineage (macrophages and dendritic cells) and in discrete and diffuse lymphoid organs where it is used to diagnose scrapie during the preclinical stage of infection. These observations indicate correspondence between the pathogenesis of scrapie in sheep and goats and imply a similar status for their germplasm as hazards for scrapie.

The general migratory and circulatory activities of lymphocytes and mononuclear phagocytes, which allow concerted function of the lymphoreticular and immune systems and immunosurveillance, are known to operate in the female and male reproductive tracts of sheep and goats. Transit of PrPSc-bearing lymphocytes and mononuclear phagocytes through reproductive tissues and organs will enable exposure of germplasm to the scrapie agent. In this connection, Smith et al. (1970) investigated the nature of the cells present in afferent or peripheral lymph draining the ovary and uterus of six sheep. They recorded a cell concentration of 200-700 cells per μl in lymph from a lymphatic in the mesovarium and in the drainage field of the ovary. The cell population was comprised of comprising 90-95% lymphocytes and 5-10% mononuclear phagocytes. Staples et al. (1982) used dyes to identify lymphatics within the mesometrium and along the utero-ovarian pedicle in sheep and goats. Lymph from these lymphatics in both sheep and goats contained up to 200 cells per μl and consisted of more than 94% lymphocytes and less than 6% mononuclear phagocytes.

Alders and Shelton (1990) extended findings about cells in ovarian uterine by looking at subsets according to some cluster of differentiation (CD) surface markers.

A relatively higher proportion of T cells occurred in utero-ovarian lymph (approx. 80% CD5+, 50% CD4+ and 23% CD8+) compared with peripheral blood (approx. 55% CD5+, 18% CD4+ and 12% CD8+). A relatively lower proportion of B cells occurred in lymph (approx. 10%) compared to blood (approx. 30%).

Smith et al. (1970) also investigated cells in peripheral lymph draining from the testis of five sheep. They found a cell concentration of 100–300 cells per μl that was composed of 75-82% lymphocytes, 5-20% mononuclear phagocytes and 0-8% other cells (polymorphonuclear neutrophils, eosinophils, large basophilic cells and cells of the plasma cell series). In other words, cells able to carry the scrapie agent transit through testicular tissue in the sheep.

Knowledge of the cellular content in peripheral lymph draining from the female reproductive tract of both sheep and goats attests to a pathway for entry of the scrapie agent into the ovarian/oviductal/uterine environment. Cells with a known potential for carrying the scrapie agent migrate through tissues of the female reproductive tract of the two species. In sheep, at least, the same considerations about exposure to the scrapie agent apply in the male reproductive tract.

Immune responses in early pregnancy in the sheep involve traffic to the reproductive tissues of lymphoid cells known to carry the scrapie agent: for example, CD68 positive dendritic cells (Scott et al., 2006, 2009). CD68 detects the molecule macrosialin and is useful for identifying cells of the mononuclear phagocyte system (Janeway et al., 2001; Galli et al., 2011), which functions in the antigen-presentation step of the immune response (Paul, 2013).

The CD68 marker stimulates additional interest because it has been employed in studies of the pathogenesis of scrapie in sheep and because studies in mice assign a role to dendritic cells (CD68-positive) in spreading the scrapie agent within the body (Beringue *et al.*, 2000; Huang *et al.*, 2002).

Andreoletti *et al.* (2002) identified CD68 positive cells in the endometrium of ewes with scrapie-infected placentas but it was unclear whether the misfolded prion protein in these cells implicated a scrapie transmission pathway from the dam to the foetus, the foetus to the dam or transmission in both directions. Åkesson *et al.* (2011) highlighted the participation of CD68 bearing cells in the transit of experimentally introduced prion protein from the gut of lambs. They undertook a study where recombinant ovine prion protein (rPrP) was inoculated into gut loops of young lambs and its transportation across the intestinal wall was tracked. This inoculated rPrP was associated with macrophages expressing the CD68 molecule. Accordingly, adjustments to the maternal immune system during pregnancy that allow for the presence of non-self or foreign tissue, the conceptus, in the uterine tubes and uterus (Robertson, 2000; Ott and Gifford, 2010) can open pathways for transmission of the scrapie agent.

Passage of the scrapie agent across biological membranes will involve the processes of endocytosis, exocytosis and transcytosis by which macromolecules and particles are taken into cells, expelled from cells and transported across cellular sheets (Alberts *et al.*, 2002). These processes apply to prions (including the scrapie agent) because prions are proteins (Colby and Prusiner, 2013).

Exosomes are essential to endocytosis, exocytosis and transcytosis. Exosomes are small membranous vesicles that are secreted by cells of various sorts and found in body fluids such as urine and plasma and cell culture media. Exosomes may function in communication between cells, removing unwanted protein from cells and transferring pathogens, such as prions, and toxic proteins, such as the amyloid precursor protein involved in Alzheimer's disease, between cells (Bellingham *et al.*, 2012).

Transport of scrapie prions by means of exosomes was suggested by observations that supernatants from long-term cells cultures of scrapie-infected ovine brain transmitted scrapie by intracerebral inoculation of mice (Gustafson and Kanitz, 1966).

Jeffrey *et al.* (2009) found that accumulations of PrP[Sc] at the ultrastructural level corresponded with abnormal endocytosis, increased endo-lysosomes, microfolding of plasma membranes and was associated with the release and transfer of PrP[Sc] among neurons and glial cells. McGovern and Jeffrey (2013) investigated abnormal prion protein in chromaffin cells of the adrenal gland of sheep infected with scrapie and showed that accumulations of PrP[Sc] was associated

with changes in cell membranes. They suggested that PrP[Sc] released from chromaffin cells in exosomes was a source of the scrapie agent in blood. Finally, Åkesson *et al.* (2011) found prominent transcytotic activity and exosome release from the follicle associates epithelium of ileal Peyer's patches but this could not be associated with transportation of PrP[Sc] across the mucosal barrier. In short, exosomes and the processes of endocytosis and exocytosis provide a means by which the scrapie agent can enter cells and depart from cells. The known portals of entry and exit for the scrapie are thus explainable at the cellular and sub-cellular level of biological organisation. Furthermore, the transmission of scrapie by means of exosomes demonstrates that cells do not have to be in direct contact to allow transfer of the scrapie agent. Relevance for prenatal transmission is that the scrapie agent can transmit at any site in the reproductive tract.

Extension of findings to goats

Correspondence between key aspects of pathophysiology of scrapie in sheep and goats argues for prenatal transmission in both species and by extension is extremely strong presumptive evidence that semen and unwashed embryos from goats are hazards for the transmission of scrapie.

(1) The scrapie agent is found in the conceptus of infected goats (O'Rourke *et al.*, 2011; Schneider *et al.*, 2015) and infected sheep (Race, 1998; Tuo *et al*, 2001, 2002: Andreoletti *et al.*, 2002; Alverson *et al.*, 2006; Lacroux *et al.*, 2007).

(2) The scrapie agent occurs in the blood of infected sheep (Hunter *et al.*, 2002; Houston *et al.*, 2008; Thorne and Terry, 2008; Edwards *et al.*, 2010; Rubenstein *et al.*, 2010; Andreoletti *et al.*, 2012; Bannach *et al.*, 2012; Lacroux *et al* ., 2012) and in the blood of infected goats (Dassanayake *et al.*, 2011, 2012).

(3) The milk of infected sheep and infected goats (Konold *et al.*, 2013a, 2013b) can carry the scrapie agent.

(4) The lymphoreticular system of infected sheep (van Keulen *et al.*, 1996; Schreuder *et al.*, 1998; Andreoletti *et al.*, 2000; O'Rourke *et al.*, 2000, 2002; Gonzalez *et al.*, 2008; Dennis *et al.*, 2009; Ryder *et al.*, 2009; Toppets *et al.*, 2011), and infected goats (Gonzalez *et al.*, 2009, 2010; Monleon *et al.*, 2011). In both sheep and goats, the scrapie agent is present in cells of the lymphocyte lineage (T cell and B cells) and the mononuclear phagocyte lineage (macrophages and dendritic cells) and in discrete and diffuse lymphoid organs, where it is used to diagnose scrapie during the preclinical stage of infection.

Concluding remarks

Evidence from each of three sources (epidemiological and clinical observation, experiment and causal reasoning) demonstrates that scrapie transmits prenatally in sheep and goats. Their convergence allows a firm decision. One line of evidence, causal reasoning, was useful for detecting unstated and untenable premises and is suggested more deliberate use biosecurity. For example, it raised the possibility that prenatal transmission of scrapie in sheep formed a possible basis for action from the time that scrapie infectivity was identified in foetal membranes (Pattison *et al.*, 1972). The definitive argument comes from anatomy and precludes uncertainty.

Prenatal transmission characterises semen and *in vivo* derived embryos as presumptive hazards for the transmission of scrapie in sheep and goats, bearing in mind the OIE's definition of a hazard: 'a biological, chemical or physical agent in, or a condition of, an animal or animal product with the potential to cause an adverse health effect' (OIE, 2015). The second line of evidence, experimentation, confirms that semen (Rubenstein *et al.*, 2012) and *in vivo* derived embryos from sheep are hazards for the transmission of scrapie. Two studies (Foster *et al.*, 1996; Foster *et al.*, 2013) confirm that *in vivo* derived embryos from scrapie infected sheep, whether washed or unwashed according to the recommendations of the International Embryo Transfer Society (2010), can transmit scrapie. Studies of Foote *et al.* (1993) and Foster *et al.* (1992) point to transmission of scrapie by unwashed *in vivo* derived embryos from scrapie infected sheep transmit scrapie. The study of Low *et al.* (2009) provides weak evidence that washed *in vivo* derived embryos from scrapie infected sheep do not transmit scrapie.

Causal reasoning, the third line of evidence pursued in the systematic review, shows that conclusions from epidemiology and experimentation are biologically plausible, an important criterion of causation (Hill, 1977). Key pathophysiological preconditions for scrapie transmission by semen and *in vivo* derived embryos operate in the sheep and goat. The scrapie agent is able to disperse throughout the body and to the reproductive organs. Carriage of the scrapie agent by lymphocytes and mononuclear phagocytes combine with the phenomenon of lymphocyte recirculation to allow exposure to the scrapie agent throughout the male and female reproductive systems. There are no privileged sites. Exposure to the scrapie agent is possible at any point during the prenatal period from spermatogenesis or oogenesis to the zygote/blastocyst, embryogenesis and foetal stages. Exosomes containing the scrapie agent occur in tissue fluids and can expedite transmission. The cellular prion protein is expressed in immature and mature ovine oocytes and this marks the onset of susceptibility to scrapie infection. Causal reasoning provides definitive evidence that scrapie transmits prenatally in goats and extremely strong presumptive evidence that semen and unwashed embryos from goats are hazards for the transmission of scrapie.

References

Agricultural Research Service, US Department of Agriculture. 1966. Report of Scrapie Seminar Held At Washington, D.C., January 27-30, 1964. Agricultural Research Service, US Department of Agriculture.

Åkesson, C.P., McGovern, G., Dagleish, M.P., Espenes, A., Press, C. McL., Landsverk, T. and Jeffrey, M. 2011. Exosome-producing follicle associated epithelium is not involved in uptake of PrPd from the gut of sheep (Ovis aries): an ultrastructural study. PLoS One. 6, e22180.

Alberts, B., Johnson, A., Lewis, J., Raff, M., Roberts, K. and Walter, P. 2002. Molecular Biology of the Cell, 4th Ed. Garland Science, New York.

Alders, R.G. and Shelton, J.N. 1990. Lymphocyte subpopulations in lymph and blood draining from the uterus and ovary in sheep. Reprod. Fertil. Dev. 17, 27-40.

Alverson, J., O'Rourke, K.I. and Baszler, T.V. 2006. PrP^{Sc} accumulation in fetal cotyledons of scrapie-resistant lambs is influenced by fetus location in the uterus. J. Gen. Virol. 87, 1035-1041.

Andreoletti, O., Berthon, P., Marc, D., Sarradin, P., Grosclaude, J., van Keulen, L., Schelcher, F., Elsen, J.M. and Lantier F. 2000. Early accumulation of PrP^{Sc} in gut-associated lymphoid and nervous tissues of susceptible sheep from a Romanov flock with natural scrapie. J. Gen. Virol. 81, 3115-3126.

Andreoletti, O., Lacroux, C., Chabert, A., Monnereau, L., Tabouret, G., Lantier, F., Berthon, P., Eychenne, F., Lafond-Benestad, S., Elsen, J.M. and Schelcher, F. 2002. PrP^{Sc} accumulation in placentas of ewes exposed to natural scrapie: influence of foetal PrP genotype and effect on ewe-to-lamb transmission. J. Gen. Virol. 83, 2607-2616.

Andreoletti, O., Litaise, C., Simmons, H., Corbiere, F., Lugan, S., Costes, P., Schelcher, F., Vilette, D., Grassi, J. and Lacroux, C. 2012. Highly efficient prion transmission by blood transfusion. PLoS Pathogens. 8, e 002782.

Animal Health Australia. 2009. Australian Veterinary Emergency Plan. Ausvetplan Disease Strategy, Scrapie, Version 3.0, 2009. Anonymous. https://www.animalhealthaustralia.com.au/our-publications/ausvetplan-manuals-and-documents/accessed on 26 January 2016.

Bannach, O., Birkmann, E., Reinartz, E., Jaeger, K.E., Langeveld, J. P., Rohwer, R. G., Gregori, L., Terry, L.A., Willbold, D. and Riesner, D. 2012. Detection of prion protein particles in blood plasma of scrapie infected sheep. PLoS One. 7, e36620.

Baylis, M., Chihota, C., Stevenson, E., Goldmann, W., Smith, A., Sivam, K., Tongue, S. and Gravenor, M.B. 2004. Risk of scrapie in British sheep of different prion protein genotypes. J. Gen. Virol. 85,

2735-2740.

Bellingham, S.A., Guo, B.B., Coleman, B.M. and Hill, A.F. 2012. Exosomes: vehicles for the transfer of toxic proteins associated with neurodegenerative diseases? Front. Physiol. 3, 124.

Beringue, V., Demoy, M., Lasmezas, C. I., Gouritin, B., Weingarten, C., Deslys, J. P., Andreux, J. P., Couvreur, P. and Dormont, D. 2000. Role of spleen macrophages in the clearance of scrapie agent early in pathogenesis. J. Pathol. 190, 495-502.

Bonita, R., Beaglehole, R. and Kjellström, T. 2006. Basic Epidemiology, 2nd Ed. World Health Organization, Geneva.

Broadbent, D.W. 1972. Listeria as a cause of abortion in sheep. Aust. Vet. J. 48, 391-394.

Brotherston, J.G., Renwick, C.C., Stamp, J.T., Zlotnik, I. and Pattison, I.H. 1968. Spread of scrapie by contact to goats and sheep. J. Comp. Pathol. 78, 9-17.

Caplazi, P., O'Rourke, K., Wolf, C., Shaw, D. and Baszler, T. V. 2004. Biology of PrP^Sc accumulation in two natural scrapie-infected sheep flocks. J. Vet. Diagn. Invest. 16, 489-496.

Caughey, B., Baron, G.S., Chesebro, B. and Jeffrey, M. 2009. Getting a grip on prions: oligomers, amyloids, and pathological membrane interactions. Ann. Rev. Biochem. 78, 177-204.

Coetzer, J.A.W., Thomson, G.R. and Tustin, R.C. Eds. 1994. Infectious Diseases of Livestock with Special Reference to Southern Africa. Oxford University Press, Cape Town.

Colby, D.W. and Prusiner, S.B. 2011. De novo generation of prion strains. Nat. Rev. Microbiol. 9, 771-777.

Couquet, C., Cornuejols, M.J., Fremont, A., Allix, S., El Hachimi, K.H., Adjou K.T., Ouidja, M.O., Brugere, H. and Brugere-Picoux, J. 2005. Observation d'un cas de transmission maternelle de la tremblante chez le mouton. B. Acad. Vet. France 158, 25-28.

Dassanayake, R.P., Schneider, D.A., Truscott, T.C., Young, A.J., Zhuang, D. and O'Rourke, K.I. 2011. Classical scrapie prions in ovine blood are associated with B lymphocytes and platelet-rich plasma. BMC Vet. Res. 7, 75.

Dassanayake, R.P., Schneider, D.A., Herrmann-Hoesing, L.M., Truscott, T.C., Davis, W.C. and O'Rourke, K.I. 2012. Cell-surface expression of PrP^c and the presence of scrapie prions in the blood of goats. J. Gen. Virol. 93, 1127-1131.

Dennis, M.M., Thomsen, B.V., Marshall, K.L., Hall, S.M., Wagner, B.A., Salman, M.D., Norden, D.K., Gaiser, C. and Sutton, D.L. 2009. Evaluation of immunohistochemical detection of prion protein in rectoanal mucosa-associated lymphoid tissue for

diagnosis of scrapie in sheep. Am. J. Vet. Res. 70, 63-72.

Detwiler, L.A. and Baylis, M. 2003. The epidemiology of scrapie. Rev. Sci. Tech. OIE. 22, 121-143.

Dickinson, A.G., Young, G.B., Stamp, J.T. and Renwick, C.C. 1965. An analysis of natural scrapie in Suffolk sheep. Heredity. 20, 485-503.

Dickinson, A.G., Stamp, J.T. and Renwick, C.C. 1974. Maternal and lateral transmission of scrapie in sheep. J. Comp. Pathol. 84, 19-25.

Dubey, J.P. 2009. Toxoplasmosis in sheep – the last 20 years. Vet. Parasitol. 163, 1-14.

Edwards, J.C., Moore, S.J., Hawthorn, J.A., Neale, M.H. and Terry, L.A. 2010. PrP(Sc) is associated with B cells in the blood of scrapie-infected sheep. Virology 405, 110-119.

EFSA. 2010. EFSA Panel on Biological Hazards (BIOHAZ); Scientific Opinion on Risk of transmission of TSEs via semen and embryo transfer in small ruminants (sheep and goats). EFSA J. 8, 1429-1448.

Elsen, J.M., Amigues, Y., Schelcher, F., Ducrocq, V., Andreoletti, O., Eychenne, F., Khang, J.V., Poivey, J.P., Lantier, F. and Laplanche, J.L. 1999. Genetic susceptibility and transmission factors in scrapie: detailed analysis of an epidemic in a closed flock of Romanov. Arch. Virol. 144, 431-445.

Everest, S.J., Ramsay, A.M., Chaplin, M.J., Everitt, S., Stack, M.J., Neale, M.H., Jeffrey, M.S., Moore, J.S., Bellworthy, J. and Terry, L.A. 2011. Detection and localisation of PrP in the liver of sheep infected with scrapie and bovine spongiform encephalopathy. PLoS One. 6, e19737.

Fast, C. and Groschup, M.H. 2013. Classical and atypical scrapie in sheep and goats. In Prions and Diseases, Volume 2, Animals, Humans and the Environment. Eds. Zou, W-Q. and Gambetti. P. New York: Springer, pp: 15-44.

Foote, W.C., Clark, W., Maciulis, A., Call, J.W., Hourrigan, J., Evans, R.C., Marshall, M.R. and de Camp, M. 1993. Prevention of scrapie transmission in sheep, using embryo transfer. Am. J. Vet. Res. 54, 1863-1868.

Foster, J.D., McKelvey, W.A., Mylne, M.J., Williams, A., Hunter, N., Hope, J. and Fraser, H. 1992. Studies on maternal transmission of scrapie in sheep by embryo transfer. Vet. Rec.130, 341-343.

Foster, J.D., Hunter, N., Williams, A., Mylne, M.J., McKelvey, W.A., Hope, J., Fraser, H. and Bostock, C. 1996. Observations on the transmission of scrapie in experiments using embryo transfer. Vet. Rec.138, 559-562.

Foster, J., McKenzie, C., Parnham, D., Drummond, D., Chong, A., Goldman, W. and Hunter, N. 2006. Lateral transmission of natural scrapie to scrapie-free New Zealand sheep placed in an endemically infected UK flock. Vet. Rec. 159, 633-634.

Foster, J.D., Goldmann, W. and Hunter, N. 2013. Evidence in sheep for pre-natal transmission of scrapie to lambs from infected mothers. PLoS One. 8, e79433.

Friedman, G.D. 2004. A Primer of Epidemiology, Fifth Edition. McGraw-Hill Professional, New York.

Galli, S.J., Borregaard, N. and Wynn, T.A. 2011. Phenotypic and functional plasticity of cells of innate immunity: macrophages, mast cells and neutrophils. Nature Immunol. 12, 1035-1044.

Garza, M.C., Fernandez-Borges, N., Bolea, R., Badiola, J.J., Castilla, J. and Monleon, E. 2011. Detection of PrPres in genetically susceptible fetuses from sheep with natural scrapie. PLoS One. 6, e27525.

Gatti, J. L., Metayer, S., Moudjou, M., Andreoletti, O., Lantier, F., Dacheux, J. L. and Sarradin, P. 2002. Prion protein is secreted in soluble forms in the epididymal fluid and proteolytically processed and transported in seminal plasma. Biol. Reprod. 67, 393-400.

Gibbs, C.J.Jr., Gajdusek, D.C. and Harvey, J. 1969. Bibliography on Scrapie. National Institute of Neurological Diseases and Stroke, Bethesda, Maryland.

Goldmann, W. 2008. PrP genetics in ruminant transmissible spongiform encephalopathies. Vet. Res. 39, 30.

Gonzalez, L., Horton, R., Ramsay, D., Toomik, R., Leathers, V., Tonelli, Q., Dagleish, M. P., Jeffrey, M. and Terry, L. 2008. Adaptation and evaluation of a rapid test for the diagnosis of sheep scrapie in samples of rectal mucosa. J. Vet. Diagn. Invest. 20, 203-208.

Gonzalez, L., Martin, S., Siso, S., Konold, T., Ortiz-Pelaez, A., Phelan, L., Goldmann, W., Stewart, P., Saunders, G., Windl, O., Jeffrey, M., Hawkins, S. A., Dawson, M. and Hope, J. 2009. High prevalence of scrapie in a dairy goat herd: tissue distribution of disease-associated PrP and effect of PRNP genotype and age. Vet. Res. 40, 65.

Gonzalez, L., Martin, S., Hawkins, S.A., Goldmann, W., Jeffrey, M. and Siso, S. 2010. Pathogenesis of natural goat scrapie: modulation by host PRNP genotype and effect of co-existent conditions. Vet. Res. 41, 48.

Gonzalez, L., Dagleish, M.P., Martin, S., Finlayson, J., Siso, S., Eaton, S.L., Goldmann, W., Witz, J., Hamilton, S., Stewart, P., Pang, Y., Steele, P., Reid, H.W., Chianini, F. and Jeffrey, M. 2012. Factors influencing temporal variation of scrapie incidence within a closed Suffolk sheep flock. J. Gen. Virol. 93, 203-211.

Gordon, W.S. 1957. Scrapie. Vet. Rec. 69, 1324-1328.

Gordon, W.S. 1966. Variation in susceptibility of sheep to scrapie and genetic implications. In Report of Scrapie Seminar Held At Washington, D.C., January 27-30, 1964. Agricultural Research Service, US Department of Agriculture, 53-68. https://archive.org/stream/report9153scra/report9153scra_djvu.txt/accessed on 3 August 2015.

Gough, K.C., Baker, C.A., Rees, H.C., Terry, L.A., Spiropoulos, J., Thorne, L. and Maddison, B.C. 2012. The oral secretion of infectious scrapie prions occurs in preclinical sheep with a range of PRNP genotypes. J. Virol. 86, 566-571.

Gough, K.C., Baker, C.A., Simmons, H.A., Hawkins, S.A. and Maddison, B.C. 2015. Circulation of prions within dust on a scrapie affected farm. Vet. Res. 46, 40.

Greig, J.R. 1940. Scrapie: observations on the transmission of the disease by mediate contact. Vet. J. 6, 203-206.

Gustafson, D.P. and Kanitz, C.L. 1966. Long-term cell cultures from brain of sheep affected with scrapie. In Report of Scrapie Seminar Held At Washington, D.C., January 27-30, 1964. Agricultural Research Service, US Department of Agriculture, 69-88. https://archive.org/stream/report9153scra/report9153scra_djvu.txt/accessed on 3 August 2015.

Hadlow, W.J., Kennedy, R.C. and Race, R.E. 1982. Natural infection of Suffolk sheep with scrapie virus. J. Inf. Dis.146, 657-664.

Hagan, W.H. and Smithcors, J.F. 1964. Veterinary Science. In Encyclopaedia Britannica, Volume 23. Chicago: William Benton, pp: 117-118.

Hansson, S.O. 2013. The Ethics of Risk: Ethical Analysis in an Uncertain World. Palgrave MacMillan.

Hawkins, S.A., Simmons, H.A., Gough, K.C. and Maddison, B.C. 2015. Persistence of ovine scrapie infectivity in a farm environment following cleaning and decontamination. Vet. Rec. 176, 99.

Hedstrom, O.O., Sona, R.J., Lassen, E.D., Hultgren, B.D., Crisman, R.O., Smith, B.B. and Snyder, S.P. 1987. Pathology of Campylobacter jejuni in sheep. Vet. Pathol. 24, 419-426.

Hill, A.B. 1977. A Short Textbook of Medical Statistics. Hodder and Stoughton, London.

Hoinville, L.J. 1996. A review of the epidemiology of scrapie in sheep. Rev. Sci. Tech. OIE. 15, 827-852.

Hoinville, L.J., Tongue, S.C. and Wilesmith, J.W. 2010. Evidence for maternal transmission of scrapie in naturally affected flocks. Prev. Vet. Med. 93, 121-128.

Hourrigan, J., Klingsporn, A. and Clark, W.W. 1979. Epidemiology of Scrapie in the United States. In Slow Transmissible Diseases of the Nervous System, Volume 1. Eds., S.B. Prusiner and W.J. Hadlow. Academic Press, New York, 331-356.

Houston, E.F., Halliday, S.I., Jeffrey, M., Goldmann, W. and Hunter, N. 2002. New Zealand sheep with scrapie-susceptible PrP genotypes succumb to experimental challenge with a sheep-passaged scrapie isolate (SSBP/1). J. Gen. Virol. 83, 1247-1250.

Houston, F., McCutcheon, S., Goldmann, W., Chong, A., Foster, J., Siso, S., Gonzalez, L., Jeffrey, M. and Hunter, N. 2008. Prion diseases are efficiently transmitted by blood transfusion in sheep. Blood. 112, 4739-4745.

Huang, F.P., Farquhar, C.F., Mabbott, N.A., Bruce, M.E. and MacPherson, G.G. 2002. Migrating intestinal dendritic cells transport PrP^{Sc} from the gut. J. Gen. Virol. 83, 267-271.

Hunter, N., Foster, J.D., Goldmann, W., Stear, M.J., Hope, J. and Bostock, C. 1996. Natural scrapie in a closed flock of Cheviot sheep occurs only in specific PrP genotypes. Arch. Virol. 141, 809-824.

Hunter, N., Foster, J., Chong, A., McCutcheon, S., Parnham, D., Eaton, S., MacKenzie, C. and Houston, F. 2002. Transmission of prion diseases by blood transfusion. J. Gen. Virol. 83, 2897-2905.

Hunter, N. 2007. Scrapie: uncertainties, biology and molecular approaches. Biochim. Biophys. Acta 1772, 619-628.

IETS. 2010. Manual of the International Embryo Transfer Society. International Embryo Transfer Society, Inc. 2441 Village Green Place Champaign, IL 61822.

Janeway, C.A.Jr, Travers, P., Walport, M. and Shlomchik, M.J. 2001. Immunobiology, 5th Ed. Garland Science, New York.

Jeffrey, M. and Gonzalez, L. 2007. Classical sheep transmissible spongiform encephalopathies: pathogenesis, pathological phenotypes and clinical disease. Neuropath. Appl. Neuro. 33, 373-394.

Jeffrey, M., McGovern, G., Goodsir, C. M., Siso, S. and Gonzalez, L. 2009. Strain-associated variations in abnormal PrP trafficking of sheep scrapie. Brain Pathol. 19, 1-11.

Jeffrey, M., McGovern, G., Siso, S. and Gonzalez, L. 2011. Cellular and sub-cellular pathology of animal prion diseases: relationship between morphological changes, accumulation of abnormal prion protein and clinical disease. Acta Neuropathol. 121, 113-134.

Johnson, M.L., Grazul-Bilska, A.T., Reynolds, L.P. and Redmer, D.A. 2014. Prion (PrP^c) expression in ovine uteroplacental tissues increases after estrogen treatment of ovariectomized ewes and during early pregnancy. Reproduction. 148, 1-10.

Kassirer, J.P., Wong, J.B. and Kopelman, R.I. 2009. Learning Clinical Reasoning 2nd Ed. Wolters Kluwer/Lippincott, Williams and Wilkins.

Katz, J.B., Pedersen, J.C., Jenny, A.L. and Taylor, W.D. 1992. Assessment of western immunoblotting for the confirmatory diagnosis of ovine scrapie and bovine spongiform encephalopathy (BSE). J. Vet. Diagn. Invest. 4, 447-449.

Khan, K.S., Kunz, R., Kleijnen, J. and Antes, G. 2003. Five steps to conducting a systematic review. J. Roy. Soc. Med. 96, 118-121.

Konold, T., Moore, S.J., Bellworthy, S.J. and Simmons, H.A. 2008. Evidence of scrapie transmission via milk. BMC Vet. Res. 4, 14.

Konold, T., Moore, S.J., Bellworthy, S.J., Terry, L.A., Thorne, L., Ramsay, A., Salguero, F.J., Simmons, M.M. and Simmons, H.A. 2013a. Evidence of effective scrapie transmission via colostrum and milk in sheep. BMC Vet. Res. 9, 99.

Konold, T., Simmons, H.A., Webb, P.R., Bellerby, P.J., Hawkins, S.A. and González, L. 2013b. Transmission of classical scrapie via goat milk. Vet. Rec. 172, 455.

Lacroux, C., Corbiere, F., Tabouret, G., Lugan, S., Costes, P., Mathey, J., Delmas, J.M., Weisbecker, J.L., Foucras, G., Cassard, H., Elsen, J.M., Schelcher, F. and Andreoletti, O. 2007. Dynamics and genetics of PrP^{Sc} placental accumulation in sheep. J. Gen. Virol. 88, 1056-1061.

Lacroux, C., Simon, S., Benestad, S.L., Maillet, S., Mathey, J., Lugan, S., Corbiere, F., Cassard, H., Costes, P., Bergonier, D., Weisbecker, J.L., Moldal, T., Simmons, H., Lantier, F., Feraudet-Tarisse, C., Morel, N., Schelcher, F., Grassi, J. and Andreoletti, O. 2008. Prions in milk from ewes incubating natural scrapie. PLoS Pathog, 4, e1000238.

Lacroux, C., Vilette, D., Fernandez-Borges, N., Litaise, C., Lugan, S., Morel, N., Corbiere, F., Simon, S., Simmons, H., Costes, P., Weisbecker, J. L., Lantier, I., Lantier, F., Schelcher, F., Grassi, J., Castilla, J. and Andreoletti, O. 2012. Prionemia and leukocyte-platelet-associated infectivity in sheep transmissible spongiform encephalopathy models. J. Virol. 86, 2056-2066.

Ligios, C., Cancedda, G.M., Margalith, I., Santucciu, C., Madau, L., Maestrale, Basagni, C., Saba, M. and Heikenwalder, M. 2007. Intraepithelial and interstitial deposition of pathological prion protein in kidneys of scrapie-infected sheep. PLoS One. 2, e859.

Ligios, C., Cancedda, M.G., Carta, A., Santucciu, C., Maestrale, C., Demontis, F., Saba, M., Patta, C., DeMartini, J.C., Aguzzi, A. and Sigurdson, C.J. 2011. Sheep with scrapie and mastitis transmit infectious prions through the milk. J. Virol. 85, 1136-1139.

Low, J.C., Chambers, J., McKelvey, W.A., McKendrick, I.J. and Jeffrey, M. 2009. Failure to transmit scrapie infection by transferring preimplantation embryos from naturally infected donor sheep. Theriogenology. 72, 809-816.

Maddison, B.C., Baker, C.A., Rees, H.C., Terry, L.A., Thorne, L., Bellworthy, S.J., Whitelam, G.C. and Gough, K.C. 2009. Prions are secreted in milk from clinically normal scrapie-exposed sheep. J. Virol. 83, 8293-8296.

Maddison, B.C., Rees, H.C., Baker, C.A., Taema, M., Bellworthy, S.J., Thorne, L., Terry, L.A. and Gough, K.C. 2010. Prions are secreted into the oral cavity in sheep with preclinical scrapie. J. Infect. Dis. 201, 1672-1676.

McGovern, G. and Jeffrey, M. 2013. Membrane toxicity of abnormal prion protein in adrenal chromaffin cells of scrapie infected sheep. PLoS One. 8, e58620

Miller, J.M., Jenny, A.L., Taylor, W.D., Marsh, R.F., Rubenstein, R. and Race, R.E. 1993. Immunohistochemical detection of prion protein in sheep with scrapie. J. Vet. Diagn. Invest. 5, 309-316.

Monleon, E., Garza, M.C., Sarasa, R., Alvarez-Rodriguez, J., Bolea, R., Monzon, M., Vargas, M.A., Badiola, J.J. and Acin, C. 2011. An assessment of the efficiency of PrP^{Sc} detection in rectal mucosa and third-eyelid biopsies from animals infected with scrapie. Vet. Microbiol. 147, 237-243.

Nardone, D.A. 1990. Collecting and Analyzing Data: Doing and Thinking. In Clinical Methods, The History, Physical, and Laboratory Examination, 3rd edition. Eds. Walker, H.K., Hall, W.D. and Hurst, J.W. Butterworths, http://www.ncbi.nlm.nih.gov/books/NBK201/.

Nettleton, P.F., Gilray, J.A., Russo, P. and Dlissi, E. 1998. Border disease of sheep and goats. Vet. Res. 27, 327-340.

Oehlert, G.W. 2000. A First Course in the Design and Analysis of Experiments. W.H. Freeman and Company, New York.

OIE. 2011. Scrapie, Chapter 2.7.13. In OIE Terrestrial Manual. World Organisation for Animal Health, Paris. http://www.oie.int/en./ accessed on 3 June 2015.

OIE. 2015. OIE Terrestrial Animal Code. World Organisation for Animal Health, Paris. http://www.oie.int/en./ accessed on 3 June 2015.

Onodera, T., Ikeda, T., Muramatsu, Y. and Shinagawa, M. 1993. Isolation of scrapie agent from the placenta of sheep with natural scrapie in Japan. Microbiol. Immunol. 37, 311-316.

O'Rourke, K.I., Baszler, T.V., Besser, T.E., Miller, J.M., Cutlip, R.C., Wells, G.A., Ryder, S.J., Parish, S.M., Hamir, A.N., Cockett, N.E., Jenny, A. and Knowles, D.P. 2000. Preclinical diagnosis of scrapie by immunohistochemistry of third eyelid lymphoid tissue. J. Clin. Microbiol. 38, 3254-3259.

O'Rourke, K.I., Duncan, J.V., Logan, J.R., Anderson, A.K., Norden, D.K., Williams, E.S., Combs, B.A., Stobart, R.H., Moss, G.E. and Sutton, D.L. 2002. Active surveillance for scrapie by third eyelid biopsy and genetic susceptibility testing of flocks of sheep in Wyoming. Clin. Diagn. Lab. Immunol. 9, 966-971.

O'Rourke, K., Zhuang, D., Truscott, T., Yan, H. and Schneider, D. 2011. Sparse PrP^{Sc} accumulation in the placentas of goats with naturally acquired scrapie. BMC Vet. Res. 7, 7.

Ott, T.L. and Gifford, C.A. 2010. Effects of early conceptus signals on circulating immune cells: lessons from domestic ruminants. Am. J. Reprod. Immunol. 64, 245-254.

Palmer, A.C. 1959. Attempt to transmit scrapie by injection of semen from an affected ram. Vet. Rec. 71, 664.

Parry, H.B. 1962. Scrapie: a transmissible and hereditary disease of sheep. Heredity. 17, 75-105.

Parry, H.B. 1983. Scrapie Disease in Sheep: Historical, Epidemiological, Pathological and Practical Aspects of the Natural Disease. Ed. D.R. Oppenheimer. Academic Press, London.

Pattison, I.H., Hoare, M.N., Jebbett, J.N. and Watson, W.A. 1972. Spread of scrapie to sheep and goats by oral dosing with foetal membranes from scrapie-affected sheep. Vet. Rec. 90, 465-468.

Pattison, I.H., Hoare, M.N., Jebbett, J.N. and Watson, W.A. 1974. Further observations on the production of scrapie in sheep by oral dosing with foetal membranes from scrapie-affected sheep. Brit. Vet. J. 130, lxv-lxvii.

Paul, W.E. 2013. Fundamental Immunology 7th Ed. Wolters Kluwer Health/Lippincott Williams and Wilkins, Philadelphia.

Peralta, O.A., Huckle, W.R. and Eyestone, W.H. 2012. Developmental expression of the cellular prion protein (PrP^c) in bovine embryos. Mol. Reprod. Dev. 79, 488-498.

Petticrew, M. and Roberts, H. 2006. Systematic reviews in the social sciences: a practical guide. Blackwell Publishing, Oxford.

Porta, M. 2014. A Dictionary of Epidemiology. Oxford University Press, Oxford.

Press, C.M., Heggebo, R. and Espenes, A. 2004. Involvement of gut-associated lymphoid tissue of ruminants in the spread of transmissible spongiform encephalopathies. Adv. Drug Deliv. Rev. 56, 885-899.

Prusiner, S.B. 1998, Prions. Proc. Natl. Acad. Sci. U S A. 95, 13363-13383.

Prusiner, S.B. 2013. Biology and genetics of prions causing neurodegeneration. Ann. Rev. Genet. 47, 601-623.

Race, R., Jenny, A. and Sutton, D. 1998. Scrapie infectivity and proteinase K-resistant prion protein in sheep placenta, brain, spleen, and lymph node: implications for transmission and antemortem diagnosis. J. Infect. Dis. 178, 949-953.

Radostits, O.M., Tyler, J.W. and Mayhew, I.G. 2000. Making a diagnosis. In Veterinary Clinical Examination and Diagnosis. Eds. Radostits, O.M., Mayhew, I.G. and Houston, D.M. London: W.B. Saunders, pp: 11-49.

Redman, C.A., Coen, P.G., Matthews, L., Lewis, R.M., Dingwall, W.S., Foster, J.D., Chase-Topping, M.E., Hunter, N. and Woolhouse, M.E. 2002. Comparative epidemiology of scrapie outbreaks in individual sheep flocks. Epidemiol. Infect. 128, 513-521.

Robertson, S.A. 2000. Control of the immunological environment of the uterus. Rev. Reprod. 5, 164-174.

Rubenstein, R., Chang, B., Gray, P., Piltch, M., Bulgin, M. S., Sorensen-Melson, S. and Miller, M. W. 2010. A novel method for preclinical detection of PrP^{Sc} in blood. J. Gen. Virol. 91, 1883-1892.

Rubenstein, R., Bulgin, M.S, Chang, B., Sorensen-Melson, S., Petersen, R.B. and Lafauci, G. 2012. PrP^{Sc} detection and infectivity in semen from scrapie-infected sheep. J. Gen. Virol. 93, 1375-1383.

Ruxton, G.D. and Colegrave, N. 2006. Experimental Design for the Life Sciences, Second Edition, Oxford University Press, Oxford.

Ryder, S., Dexter, G., Bellworthy, S. and Tongue, S. 2004. Demonstration of lateral transmission of scrapie between sheep kept under natural conditions using lymphoid tissue biopsy. Res. Vet. Sci. 76, 211-217.

Ryder, S.J., Dexter, G.E., Heasman, L., Warner, R. and Moore, S.J. 2009. Accumulation and dissemination of prion protein in experimental sheep scrapie in the natural host. BMC Vet. Res. 5, 9.

Saa, P., Castilla, J. and Soto, C. 2005. Cyclic amplification of protein misfolding and aggregation. Methods Mol. Biol. 299, 53-65.

Santucciu, C., Maestrale, C., Madau, L., Attene, S., Cancedda, M.G., Demontis, F. Tilocca, M.G., Saba, M., Macciocu, S., Carta, A. and Ligios, C. 2010. Association of N176K and L141F dimorphisms of the PRNP gene with lack of pathological prion protein deposition in placentas of naturally and experimentally scrapie-affected ARQ/ARQ sheep. J. Gen. Virol. 91, 2402-2407.

Sarradin, P., Melo, S., Barc, C., Lecomte, C., Andreoletti, O., Lantier, F., Dacheux, J.L. and Gatti, J.L. 2008. Semen from scrapie-infected rams does not transmit prion infection to transgenic mice. Reproduction. 135, 415-418.

Schneider, D.A., Madsen-Bouterse, S.A., Zhuang, D., Truscott, T.C., Dassanayake, R.P. and O'Rourke, K.I. 2015. The placenta shed from goats with classical scrapie is infectious to goat kids and lambs. J. Gen. Virol. 96, 2464-2469.

Schreuder, B.E., van Keulen, L.J., Vromans, M.E., Langeveld, J.P. and Smits, M.A. 1998. Tonsillar biopsy and PrP^{Sc} detection in the preclinical diagnosis of scrapie. Vet. Rec. 142, 564-568.

Scott, J.L., Ketheesan, N. and Summers, P.M. 2006. Leucocyte population changes in the reproductive tract of the ewe in response to insemination Reprod. Fertil. Dev.18, 627-634.

Scott, J.L., Ketheesan, N. and Summers, P.M. 2009. Spermatozoa and seminal plasma induce a greater inflammatory response in the ovine uterus at oestrus than dioestrus. Reprod. Fertil. Dev., 21, 817-826.

Smith, J.B., McIntosh, G.H. and Morris, B. 1970. The traffic of cells through tissues: a study of peripheral lymph in sheep. J. Anat. 107. 87-100.

Soto, C. 2012. Transmissible proteins: expanding the prion heresy. Cell 149, 968-977.

Spiropoulos, J., Hawkins, S.A.C., Simmons, M.M. and Bellworthy, S.J. 2014. Evidence of in utero transmission of classical scrapie in sheep. J. Virol. 88, 4591-4594.

Staples, L.D., Fleet, I.R. and Heap, R.B. 1982. Anatomy of the utero-ovarian lymphatic network and the composition of afferent lymph in relation to the establishment of pregnancy in the sheep and goat. J. Reprod. Fertil. 64, 409-420.

Supattapone, S. 2015. Expanding the prion disease repertoire. Proc. Natl. Acad. Sci. U S A. 112, 11748-11749.

Terry, L.A., Howells, L., Hawthorn, J., Edwards, J.C., Moore, S.J., Bellworthy, S.J., Simmons, H., Lizano, S., Estey, L., Leathers, V. and Everest, S.J. 2009. Detection of PrP^{Sc} in blood from sheep infected with the scrapie and bovine spongiform encephalopathy agents. J. Virol. 83, 12552-12558.

Terry, L.A., Howells, L., Bishop, K., Baker, C.A., Everest, S., Thorne, L., Maddison, B.C. and Gough, K.C. 2011. Detection of prions in the faeces of sheep naturally infected with classical scrapie. Vet. Res. 42, 65.

Thorne, L. and Terry, L. A. 2008. In vitro amplification of PrP^{Sc} derived from the brain and blood of sheep infected with scrapie. J. Gen. Virol. 89, 3177-3184.

Thumdee, P., Ponsuksili, S., Murani, E., Nganvongpanit, K., Gehrig, B., Tesfaye, D., Gilles, M., Hoelker, M., Jennen, D., Griese, J., Schellander, K. and Wimmers, K. 2007. Expression of the prion protein gene (PRNP) and cellular prion protein (PrP^c) in cattle and sheep fetuses and maternal tissues during pregnancy. Gene Expr. 13, 283-297.

Toppets, V., Defaweux, V., Piret, J., Kirschvink, N., Grobet, L. and Antoine, N. 2011. Features of follicular dendritic cells in ovine pharyngeal tonsil: an in vivo and in vitro study in the context of scrapie pathogenesis. Vet. Immunol. Immunopathol. 141, 26-32.

Tuo, W., Zhuang, D., Knowles, D.P., Cheevers, W.P., Sy, M.S. and O'Rourke, K.I. 2001. Prp^c and Prp^{Sc} at the fetal-maternal interface. J. Biol. Chem. 276, 18229-18234.

Tuo, W., O'Rourke, K.I., Zhuang, D., Cheevers, W.P., Spraker, T.R. and Knowles, D.P. 2002. Pregnancy status and fetal prion genetics determine PrP^{Sc} accumulation in placentomes of scrapie-infected sheep. Proc. Natl. Acad. Sci. USA. 99, 6310-6315.

Ulvund, M.J. 2008. Ovine scrapie disease: Do we have to live with it? Small Ruminant Res. 76, 131-140.

US Department of Health and Human Services. 2013. Self-Study Course SS1000, Principles of Epidemiology in Public Health Practice, Third Edition. www.cdc.gov/ophss/csels/dsepd/ss1978/ss1978.pdf.

van Keulen, L.J., Schreuder, B.E., Meloen, R.H., Mooij-Harkes, G., Vromans, M.E. and Langeveld, J. P. 1996. Immunohistochemical detection of prion protein in lymphoid tissues of sheep with natural scrapie. J. Clin. Microbiol. 34, 1228-1231.

van Keulen, L.J., Bossers, A. and van Zijderveld, F. 2008. TSE pathogenesis in cattle and sheep. Vet. Res. 39, 24.

Vascellari, M., Nonno, R., Mutinelli, F., Bigolaro, M., Di Bari, M.A., Melchiotti, E., Marcon, S., D'Agostino, C., Vaccari, G., Conte, M., De Grossi, L., Rosone, F., Giordani, F. and Agrimi, U. 2007. PrP^{Sc} in salivary glands of scrapie-infected sheep. J. Virol. 81, 4872-4876.

Wang, S., Foote, W.C., Sutton, D.L., Maciulis, A., Miller, J.M., Evans, R.C., Holyoak, G.R., Call, J.W., Bunch, T.D., Taylor, W.D. and Marshall, M.R. 2001. Preventing experimental vertical transmission of scrapie by embryo transfer. Theriogenology 56, 315-327.

Wang, S., Cockett, N.E., Miller, J.M., Shay, T.L., Maciulis, A., Sutton, D.L., Foote, W.C., Holyoak, G.R., Evans, R.C., Bunch, T.D., Beever, J.E., Call, J.W., Taylor, W.D. and Marshall, M.R. 2002. Polymorphic distribution of the ovine prion protein (PrP) gene in scrapie-infected sheep flocks in which embryo transfer was used to circumvent the transmissions of scrapie. Theriogenology. 57, 1865-1875.

Zar, J.H. 1996. Biostatistical Analysis 3rd Ed. Prentice-Hall, Upper Saddle River, New Jersey.

3

Ovarian teratoma displaying a wide variety of tissue components in a broiler chicken (*Gallus Domesticus*): morphological heterogeneity of pluripotential germ cell during tumorigenesis

S. Ohfuji*

Department of Histopathology, Diagnostic Animal Pathology Office, Hokkaido, Japan

Abstract

Spontaneous ovarian teratoma was found in a seven-week-old female Chunky broiler chicken that was slaughtered for food. On *post-mortem* inspection, a spherical tumor mass attaching to a juvenile ovary was found in the abdominal cavity. Histopathologically, the tumor was comprised of immature mesenchymal stroma and a variety of mature tissue elements of mesodermal and ectodermal origin. In addition, there were multiple indistinguishable tissue elements, which showed no malignant cytological features but were unidentifiable as to corresponding embryological layer of origin. These heterogeneous teratoma tissues consisted of a variety of glandular, cystic, duct-like, and tubular structures, some of which exhibited a lining by a mixture of both keratinizing/non-keratinizing stratified squamous epithelial cells and cuboidal/columnar epithelial cells. The ovarian tetatoma was considered a benign and congenital one. The highly diverse differentiation of the teratoma might have manifested a morphological aspect of intrinsic character of the pluripotential germ cells during tumorigenesis.

Keywords: Chicken, Heterogeneous differentiation, Ovary, Teratoma.

Introduction

Although uncommon, ovarian teratomas that are classified into a category of the germ cell tumors have been previously described in human beings (Kraus, 1977; Outwater *et al.*, 2001; Kuno *et al.*, 2004; Schanmughapriya *et al.*, 2011), nonhuman primates (Baskin *et al.*, 1982), experimental rats (Tsubota *et al.*, 2004), and domestic animals, including horses, pigs, dogs, and cattle (Dehner *et al.*, 1970; Gruys *et al.*, 1976; Rodríguez *et al.*, 1994; Basaraba *et al.*, 1998; MacLachlan and Kennedy, 2002; Sato *et al.*, 2003; Lefebvre *et al.*, 2005; Schlafer and Miller, 2007; Gamba *et al.*, 2014). Spontaneous ovarian or intra-abdominal teratomas have been reported in the avian species, including chickens (Campbell and Appleby, 1966; Helmboldt *et al.*, 1974; Gupta, 1976; Mohamed *et al.*, 2006), ducks (Cullen *et al.*, 1991; Bolte and Burkhardt, 2000), a goose (Reece and Lister, 1993), and a bald eagle (Ford *et al.*, 2006). It appears that ovarian teratomas are rare in broiler chickens possibly due to their young age; a short life span.

Most ovarian teratomas are benign in domestic animals, with the exception of their malignant counterparts that have rarely been reported in the bitch and mare (Gruys *et al.*, 1976; McEntee, 1990). Unlike most of other tumor types, ovarian teratomas certainly differentiate to produce a wide variety of tissue components which are composed of well-differentiated mature tissues, and this phenomenon is explained by the fact that the tumors arise from pluripotential germ cells that

have undergone somatic differentiation (Dahl *et al.*, 1990; MacLachlan and Kennedy, 2002; Schlafer and Miller, 2007). Although ovarian teratomas commonly show variable tissue components, the occurrence of heterogeneous components which are difficult to give appropriate anatomical designation may be uncommon in the tumor. Therefore, the purpose of the present study was to describe the histopathological features of a spontaneously occurring benign ovarian teratoma in a broiler chicken, which presented with not only well-differentiated mature tissues of mesodermal and ectodermal origin, but also remarkably diverse differentiation of teratoma components unidentifiable as to corresponding embryological layer of origin.

Materials and Methods

A flock of seven-week-old Chunky chickens (*Gallus domesticus*) were slaughtered at an abattoir. These chickens had been managed for meat production by a commercial company where there were no epidemiological or other serious problems. The flock was composed of approximately 150 chickens derived from a similar genetic background. Physical examination prior to slaughter revealed no significant clinical signs in all these chickens. At *post-mortem* examination, a female broiler chicken exhibited a tumor mass in the abdominal cavity. The remaining chickens from the same flock, which were processed on the same day, were reported by the veterinary meat inspectors to be unaffected with neoplastic lesions in the ovary or other visceral organs. For

*****Corresponding Author:** Susumu Ohfuji. Department of Histopathology, Diagnostic Animal Pathology Office, Hokkaido, Japan. E-mail: *tksohfuji@juno.ocn.ne.jp*

histopathological diagnosis of the ovarian tumor, tissue samples were taken immediately after slaughter from the tumor. Additional samples were collected from major visceral organs, including the liver, spleen, kidney, heart, lung, and intestine. These tissue samples were fixed in 10% formalin. After fixation, a whole ovarian tumor was cut into many portions that were prepared for histopathology. All tissue blocks were embedded in paraffin wax, processed routinely, sectioned at 4 µm, and stained with hematoxylin and eosin (HE).

Results

On *post-mortem* examination, the broiler chicken under study exhibited a spherical tumor mass, approximately 9.0 cm in diameter (Fig. 1a). The tumor mass was loosely attached to a juvenile ovary. It was soft as a whole, except for some areas gritty to feel on sectioning, and its cut surface showed a mottled gray and tan appearance with occasional cystic areas. Other organs, such as the heart, lung, kidney, spleen, liver, and bowel, were unremarkable.

On histopathology, the tumor was covered by single layer of cuboidal epithelial cells. The tumor comprised a haphazard arrangement of immature mesenchymal stroma and a variety of disorganized, different, somatic tissue elements, enabling a diagnosis of teratoma to be made. Immature mesenchymal cells exhibited round or ellipsoidal pale nuclei with small nucleoli, a small amount of basophilic cytoplasm, and rare mitotic figures (<1 per 200 x field). Many teratoma elements were mature, including extensive areas of the central nervous gray matter, which either contained polygonal neurons and oligodendroglia (Fig. 1b) or had rarely cuboidal-lined small rosettes; large cavities reminiscent of the cerebral ventricles

which were lined by a single layer of spherical cells; nerve fiber bundles of the peripheral nervous system (Fig. 1c); varying-sized groups of striated myofibers (Fig. 1d); bone trabeculae accompanied by osteoblasts, multinucleated osteoclasts, and hematopoietic (erythropoietic and leukopoietic) bone marrow (Fig. 1e); scattered islands of hyaline cartilage enclosed with a membrane of many collagen fibers (Fig. 1f); scattered areas of adipose tissue; and a few encapsulated lymphoid follicles.

Other teratoma elements consisted of a variety of aberrant tissue types, which exhibited no characteristics to a sufficiently distinctive degree to allow identification of intrinsic somatic organs or tissues. Apparent malignant features, such as anisokaryosis, anisocytosis, substantial mitotic figures indicative of rapid growth, and metastatic or invasive behavior, were not recognized in these tissue types. Such aberrant teratoma elements included secretory glands with or without duct-like lumens (Figs. 2a and 2b); glandular structures lined by a layer of cuboidal or columnar epithelial cells (Fig. 2c); duct-like structures lined by a single to multilayered pale cuboidal or columnar epithelial cells (Fig. 2d); cystic structures lined by a single layer of squamous epithelial cells, which were surrounded by immature mesenchymal cells and collagen fibers (Fig. 2e); and variably-sized cystic structures similar to epidermoid cysts or feather follicles devoid of feathers, which were lined by keratinizing stratified squamous epithelial cells (Fig. 2f). In addition, the most unique teratoma elements were comprised of a triad of epithelial-lined cystic, tubular, and duct-like structures. First, cystic structures were composed of a partial lining by multilayered cuboidal epithelial cells, the other

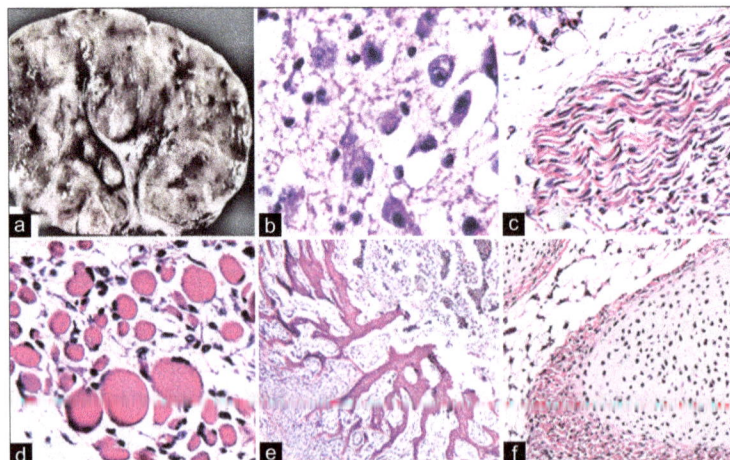

Fig. 1. (a) Teratoma after fixation shows a cavitary appearance on cut section. (b) Polygonal neurons in the neuropil-like area of teratoma (HE x 200). (c) Nerve bundle similar to peripheral nerve (HE x 100). (d) A group of varying sized striated myofibers (HE x 100). (e) Bone trabeculae accompanied by hematopoietic bone marrow (HE x 100). (f) Insular hyaline cartilage surrounded by a membrane of collagen fibers (HE x 100).

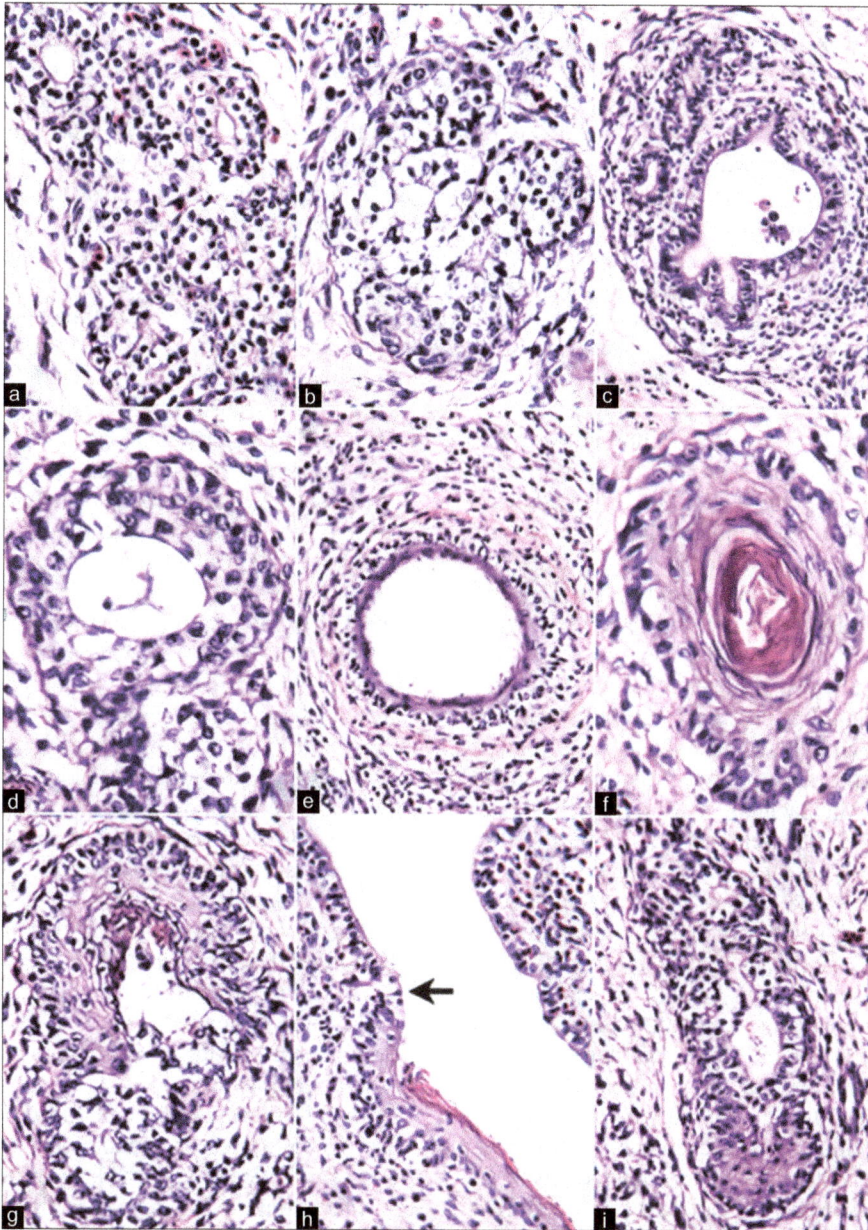

Fig. 2. (a) Teratoma represents secretory gland composed of cuboidal-lined acinar structure which has duct-like lumens (HE x 100). (b) Secretory gland composed of cuboidal-lined acinar structure without ducts (HE x 100). (c) Glandular structure lined by a layer of cuboidal or columnar epithelial cells (HE x 100). (d) Tubular structure lined by a single to multilayered, pale, cuboidal or columnar epithelial cells (HE x 200). (e) Cystic structure lined by a single layer of squamous epithelial cells, which is surrounded by immature mesenchymal cells and collagen fibers (HE x 100). (f) Cystic structure similar to epidermoid cyst or feather follicle lacking feathers which is lined by keratinizing stratified squamous epithelial cells (HE x 200). (g) Cystic structure composed of a partial lining of both multilayered cuboidal epithelial cells and keratinizing stratified squamous epithelial cells (HE x 100). (h) Tubular structure is lined by both columnar epithelial cells and keratinizing stratified squamous epithelial cells, with sharp transition boundary (arrow) between the two types of epithelial cells (HE x 200). (i) Duct-like structure lined by cuboidal epithelial cells which are connected with stratified squamous epithelial cells (HE x 200).

half being lined by keratinizing stratified squamous epithelial cells (Fig. 2g). Second, tubular structures were lined by both a layer of columnar epithelial cells and keratinizing stratified squamous epithelial cells (Fig. 2h). Third, duct-like structures, which consisted of pale cuboidal epithelial cells constituting duct-like lumens of secretory glands, were connected with non-keratinizing stratified squamous epithelial cells (Fig. 2i). Other than various teratoma components described above, relatively poor capillary networks were present throughout the tumor. Tissues that can determine or suggest the origin of the tumor were not recognized elsewhere in the tumor. Other visceral organs did not exhibit metastatic tumor lesions or any other significant lesions.

Discussion

Teratoma of the avian species has been recognized in the ovary, testes, kidney, adrenal gland, cerebrum, spinal cord, pineal body, and eye (Hooper, 2008; Reece, 2008; Paździor et al., 2012). In the current broiler chicken, the normal appearance of every other abdominal visceral organ, and the anatomical location of the tumor, (which was closely associated with intact ovary and covered by a single layer of cuboidal epithelial cells, as seen in normal ovaries), indicated that this teratoma was most likely a primary tumor originating from the ovary. Low mitotic rate of mesenchymal stromal cells indicating slow growth of the tumor, which was recognized in a seven-week-old chicken, and the absence of metastasis and invasion suggested this ovarian teratoma to be a benign and congenital one.

Ovarian teratoma, which has been reported previously in domestic animal species, such as the bitch, cat, sow, mare, and cow, may generally contain mature rather than undifferentiated somatic tissues (Basaraba et al., 1998; MacLachlan and Kennedy, 2002; Lefebvre et al., 2005; Schlafer and Miller, 2007). Likewise, tissue types of ovarian teratoma reported previously in the avian species may usually display well-differentiated adult morphology, even if they vary from teratoma to teratoma. In this species, teratoma tissues consist of keratinized epithelium-lined sac containing feathers, epithelial pearls formed by squamous epithelium, bone, cartilage, smooth muscle, nerve, fat, trachea, or melanocytes (Reece and Lister, 1993; Bolte and Burkhardt, 2000; Reece, 2008), and individual teratoma component shows a built-in mature anatomical feature characteristic of each somatic tissue, which can be easily identified as such. Ovarian teratoma described in the current chicken was composed of not only a variety of well-differentiated mature tissue components of mesodermal and ectodermal origin, but also multiple aberrant and heterogeneous components, particularly a variety of glandular, cystic, duct-like, and tubular structures. These heterogeneous teratoma components were unidentifiable as to corresponding embryological layer of origin. Some of these unusual structures exhibited a lining by a mixture of both keratinizing/non-keratinizing stratified squamous epithelial cells and cuboidal/columnar epithelial cells, showing simultaneous differentiation of tumor cells into two different types of epithelial cells within a single teratoma component. Although ectodermal origin was suggested by the presence of partial lining by squamous

epithelium (Berman, 2009), this notion could not be established because of the participation of cuboidal/columnar epithelial lining. All such epithelial-lined structures did not exhibit cytologically malignant features, namely anisokaryosis, anisocytosis, and frequent mitotic figures, and therefore were regarded as mature rather than anaplastic teratoma components. In the present ovarian teratoma, histological features of those aberrant teratoma components, which were lined by a combination of two different types of epithelial cells (keratinizing/non-keratinizing stratified squamous epithelial cells and cuboidal/columnar epithelial cells) were reminiscent of those in transdifferentiation, dedifferentiation, or simple squamous metaplasia. The phenomenon of transdifferentiation is suggested to have played a role in sacrococcygeal teratoma in human beings (Jurić-Lekić et al., 1993). Identification of dedifferentiation is documented in an ovarian teratoma (Yasunaga et al., 2011) and other teratomas involving internal visceral organs or tissues in human beings (Game et al., 2001; Kim et al., 2012). Although ovarian carcinoma associated with squamous metaplasia is described in the bovine species (McEntee, 1990) and human beings (Kay, 1961), and even if the stratified squamous epithelium is commonly seen in ovarian teratoma, there are no reports of ovarian teratoma displaying features of ongoing squamous metaplasia in either the medical or veterinary literature. In this chicken's ovarian teratoma, the epithelia-lined structures did not show any changes associated with metaplasia. Therefore, it was not possible to accurately determine which event (transdifferentiation, dedifferentiation, or squamous metaplasia) was implicated in the development of the aberrant teratoma components during tumorigenesis.

Even if the pluripotential cell lineage can differentiate to produce a variety of somatic tissues, it seems unusual that ovarian teratoma of the broiler chicken described in this report exhibited so many morphologically diverse tissue elements. In conclusion, it may be thought that such a highly heterogeneous variant of ovarian teratoma might have indicated a curious morphological aspect of the pluripotential germ cells during tumorigenesis. This morphological expression would be largely attributable to intrinsic character of the pluripotential germ cell lineage. The present study was limited to the histopathological investigation. Thus, further cytogenetic, ultrastructural, and immunohistochemical investigations appear warranted to better understand the highly heterogeneous differentiation of tissue components in the ovarian teratoma such as that described in this report.

Conflict of interest
Author declares that he has no conflict of interest.

References

Basaraba, R.J., Kraft, S.L., Andrews, G.A., Leipold, H.W. and Small, D. 1998. An ovarian teratoma in a cat. Vet. Pathol. 35, 141-144.

Baskin, G.B., Soike, K., Jirge, S.K. and Wolf, R.W. 1982. Ovarian teratoma in an African green monkey (Cercopithecus aethiops). Vet. Pathol. 19, 219-221.

Berman, J.J. 2009. Neoplasms: Principles of development and diversity, Sudbury, Jones and Bartlett Publishers, pp: 198-210.

Bolte, A.L. and Burkhardt, E. 2000. A teratoma in a Muscovy duck (Cairina moschata). Avian Pathol. 29, 237-239.

Campbell, J.G. and Appleby, E.C. 1966. Tumours in young chickens bred for rapid body growth (broiler chickens): A study of 351 cases. J. Pathol. Bacteriol. 92, 77-90.

Cullen, J.M., Newbold, J.E. and Sherman, G.J. 1991. A teratoma in a duck infected congenitally with duck hepatitis B virus. Avian Dis. 35, 638-641.

Dahl, N., Gustavson, K.H., Rune, C., Gustavsson, I. and Pettersson, U. 1990. Benign ovarian teratoma. An analysis of their cellular origin. Cancer Genet. Cytogenet. 46, 115-123.

Dehner, L.P., Norris, H.J., Garner, F.M. and Taylor, H.B. 1970. Comparative pathology of ovarian neoplasms. III. Germ cell tumours of canine, bovine, feline, rodent, and human species. J. Comp. Pathol. 80, 299-306.

Ford, S.L., Wentz, S. and Garner, M. 2006. Intracoelomic teratoma in a juvenile bald eagle (Haliaeetus leucocephalus). J. Avian Med. Surg. 20, 175-179.

Gamba, C.O., Damasceno, K.A., Rocha, Jr., S. S., Mendes, H.M., Faleiros, R.R. and Cassali, G.D. 2014. Ovarian teratoma in an equine fetus: A case report. Vet. Q. 34, 164-166.

Game, X., Houlgatte, A., Fournier, R., Duhamel, P., Baranger, B. and Khoury, S. 2001. Dedifferentiation of mature teratomas secondary to testicular cancer: Report of 2 cases. Prog. Urol.11, 73-76.

Gruys, E., van Dijk, J.E., Elsinghorst, T.A.M. and van der Gaag, I. 1976. Four canine ovarian teratomas and a nonovarian feline teratoma. Vet. Pathol. 13, 455-459.

Gupta, B.N. 1976. Teratoma in a chicken (Gallus domesticus). Avian Dis. 20, 761-768.

Helmboldt, C.F., Migaki, G., Langheinrich, J.A. and Jakowski, R.M. 1974. Teratoma in domestic fowl (Gallus gallus). Avian Dis. 18, 142-148.

Hooper, C.C. 2008. Teratoma in the cerebrum of a fantail pigeon. Avian Pathol. 37, 141-143.

Jurić-Lekić, G., Trosić, A. and Svajger, A. 1993. Lentoids within sacrococcygeal teratoma: Origin by transdifferentiation?. Hum. Pathol. 24, 227-229.

Kay, S. 1961. Carcinoma with squamous metaplasia of the ovary (so-called adenoacanthoma). Am. J.

Obestet. Gynecol. 81, 763-772.

Kim, J.Y., Lee, C.H., Park, W.Y., Kim, J.Y., Kim, A.R., Shin, N., Park, D.Y. and Huh, G.Y. 2012. Adenocarcinoma with sarcomatous dedifferentiation arising from mature cystic teratoma of the anterior mediastinum. Pathol. Res. Pract. 15, 741-745.

Kraus, F.T. 1977. Female genitalia. In Pathology, Eds., Anderson, W. A. D. and Kissane, J.M. Saint Louis, CV Mosby, pp: 1680-1775.

Kuno, N., Kadomatsu, K., Nakamura, M., Miwa-Fukuchi, T., Hirabayashi, N. and Ishizuka, T. 2004. Mature ovarian cystic teratoma with a highly differentiated homunculus: A case report. Birth Defects Res. A. Clin. Mol. Teratol. 70, 40-46.

Lefebvre, R., Theoret, C., Doré., M., Girard, C., Laverty, S. and Vaillancourt, D. 2005. Ovarian teratoma and endometritis in a mare. Can. Vet. J. 46, 1029-1033.

MacLachlan, N. J. and Kennedy, P. C. 2002. Tumors of the genital systems. In Tumors in domestic animals, Edt., Meuten, D. J. Ames, Iowa State Press, pp: 547-574.

McEntee, K. 1990. Ovarian neoplasms. In Reproductive pathology of domestic animals, San Diego, Academic Press, pp: 69-93.

Mohamed, Z. A., Hassan, E. I. and Salim, A.I. 2006. Malignant teratoma in a domestic fowl (Gallus gallus domesticus). Sudan. J. Vet. Res. 21, 75-80.

Outwater, E. K., Siegelman, E. S. and Hunt, J. L. 2001. Ovarian teratoma: Tumor types and imaging characteristics. Radiography 21, 475-490.

Paździor, K., Szweda, M., Otrocka-Domagala, I. and Rotkiewicz, T. 2012. Extragonadal teratoma in a domestic turkey (Meleagris gallopavo domestica). Avian Pathol. 41, 285-289.

Reece, R. L. 2008. Other tumors of unknown etiology. In Diseases of poultry, Edt., Saif, Y.M, Ames, Blackwell, pp: 593-616.

Reece, R. L. and Lister, S. A. 1993. An abdominal teratoma in a domestic goose (Anseriformes, Anser anser domesticus). Avian Pathol. 22, 193-196.

Rodríguez, J. L., de las Mulas, J. M. and de los Monteros, A. E. 1994. Ovarian teratoma in a ferret (Mustela putorius furo): A morphological and immunohistochemical study. J. Zoo Wildlife Med. 25, 294-299.

Sato, T., Hontake, S., Shibuya, H., Shirai, W. and Yamaguchi, T. 2003. A solid mature teratoma of a feline ovary. J. Feline Med. Surg. 5, 349-351.

Schanmughapriya, S., Senthilkurnar, G., Balakrishnan, K., Vasanthi, N., Vinodhini, K. and Natarajaseenivasan, K. 2011. Bilateral ovarian teratoma complicated with carcinosarcoma in a 68 year old woman: A case report. BMC Cancer 11, 218-220.

Schlafer, D. H. and Miller, R. B. 2007. Neoplastic diseases of the ovary. In Maxie MG (ed) Jubb,

Kennedy, and Palmer's pathology of domestic animals. Edt., Maxie, M. G. Edinburgh, Elsevier Saunders, pp: 450-456.

Tsubota, K., Yoshizawa, K., Fujihira, S., Okazaki, Y., Matsumoto, M., Nakatsuji, S. and Oishi, Y. 2004. A spontaneous ovarian immature teratoma in a juvenile rat. J. Toxicol. Pathol. 17, 211-218.

Yasunaga, M., Saito, T., Eto, T., Okadome, M., Ariyoshi, K., Nishiyama, K. and Oda, Y. 2011. Dedifferentiated chondrosarcoma in a mature cystic teratoma of the ovary: A case report and review of the literature. Int. Gynecol. Pathol. 30, 391-394.

4

Isolation and molecular identification of *Vibrio* spp. by sequencing of 16S rDNA from seafood, meat and meat products in Libya

S.M. Azwai[1], E.A. Alfallani[1], S.K. Abolghait[2], A.M. Garbaj[3], H.T. Naas[3], A.A. Moawad[4], F.T. Gammoudi[1], H.M. Rayes[1], I. Barbieri[5] and I.M. Eldaghayes[1],*

[1]*Department of Microbiology and Parasitology, Faculty of Veterinary Medicine, University of Tripoli, P.O. Box 13662, Tripoli, Libya*

[2]*Department of Food Hygiene and Control, Faculty of Veterinary Medicine, Suez Canal University, 41522 Ismailia, Egypt*

[3]*Department of Food Hygiene and Control, Faculty of Veterinary Medicine, University of Tripoli, P.O. Box 13662, Tripoli, Libya*

[4]*Department of Food Hygiene and Control, Faculty of Veterinary Medicine, Cairo University, 12211 Giza, Egypt*

[5]*Istituto Zooprofilattico Sperimentale della Lombardia e dell'Emilia Romagna, Via Bianchi, 9 - 25124 Brescia, Italy*

Abstract

The genus *Vibrio* includes several food-borne pathogens that cause a spectrum of clinical conditions including septicemia, cholera and milder forms of gastroenteritis. Several *Vibrio* spp. are commonly associated with food-borne transmission including *Vibrio cholerae*, *Vibrio parahemolyticus*, and *Vibrio vulnificus*. Microbiological analysis for enumeration and isolation of *Vibrio* spp. were carried out for a total of 93 samples of seafood, meat and meat products from different geographic localities in Libya (Tripoli, Regdalin, Janzour and Tobruk). *Vibrio* spp. were detected by conventional cultural and molecular method using PCR and sequencing of 16S rDNA. Out of the 93 cultured samples only 48 (51.6%) yielded colonies on Thiosulfate Citrate Bile Salt agar (TCBS) with culture characteristics of *Vibrio* spp. More than half (n=27) of processed seafood samples (n=46) yielded colonies on TCBS, while only 44.6% of samples of meat and meat products showed colonies on TCBS. Among cultured seafood samples, the highest bacterial count was recorded in clam with a count of 3.8 x10⁴ CFU\g. Chicken burger samples showed the highest bacterial count with 6.5 x10⁴ CFU\g. Molecular analysis of the isolates obtained in this study, showed that 11 samples out of 48 (22.9%) were *Vibrio* spp. *Vibrio parahemolyticus* was isolated from camel meat for the first time. This study is an initial step to provide a baseline for future molecular research targeting *Vibrio* spp. foodborne illnesses. This data will be used to provide information on the magnitude of such pathogens in Libyan seafood, meat and meat products.

Keywords: 16S rDNA, Libya, Meat, Seafood, *Vibrio*.

Introduction

Libya enjoys one of the longest coastlines (1800 km) on the southern Mediterranean basin; this makes seafood an important item for consumers. In general, the overall consumption of meat and meat products in Libya is increasing with the consumption of camel meat being higher than beef. This increase in meat consumption is including as well various traditional meat products that have long been known in the country and prepared by families at home or during religious feasts.

Improperly handled seafood, meat and meat products could pose a great source of infectious agents that are transmissible to humans. *Vibrio* spp. are among the infectious agents that can result in deterioration of meat or represent a potential disease source for humans. The risk of disease from ingesting pathogens found in raw meat is significantly higher than cooked meat, although both can be contaminated (Newell *et al.*, 2010). Meat can be incorrectly or insufficiently cooked, allowing disease-carrying pathogens to be ingested. In addition, meat can be contaminated during the production

process at any time, from the slicing of prepared meats to cross-contamination of food in a refrigerator. All of these situations may lead to a greater risk of disease.

From public health point of view, *Vibrio* spp. represents a greater portion of the food borne illnesses across the coast cities worldwide (Rebaudet *et al.*, 2013). This could be due to food contamination with *Vibrio* spp. shed from seafood or prevalent usage of undercooked seafood/meat or surface contamination during marine shipping of such foods. Despite the vast majority of environmental *V. parahemolyticus* isolates are avirulent, it is leading cause of gastroenteritis linked to seafood consumption in the United States (Iwamoto *et al.*, 2010). Some *Vibrio* spp. poses a significant health threat to humans who suffer from immune disorders and liver diseases. It enters human hosts via wound infections or consumption of raw shellfish (primarily oysters), and infections frequently progresses to septicemia and death in susceptible individuals (Harwood *et al.*, 2004). The cosmopolitan distribution of *Vibrio* spp. and the lack of abattoirs for proper meat inspection, prompted us

Corresponding Author: Dr. Ibrahim Eldaghayes. Department of Microbiology and Parasitology, Faculty of Veterinary Medicine, University of Tripoli, P.O. Box 13662, Tripoli, Libya. E-mail: ibrahim.eldaghayes@vetmed.edu.ly

to carry out this study. The main objective of this study was to characterize bacteria isolated from seafood, meat and meat products that may cause foodborne illnesses. We plan to use this data to help create a baseline for future research into foodborne illness in Libya.

Materials and Methods

Collection of samples

A total of 93 samples (Table 1) of seafood, meat and meat products that includes 21 of shrimps; 5 of clam; 20 of fish; 34 samples of raw meat (10 beef, 9 camel meat, 6 mutton and 9 chickens) and 13 samples of meat products (2 beef sausages, 5 beef burgers, 5 chicken burgers and 1 kebab) were randomly collected from different geographic localities in Libya [Tripoli, Regdalin (120 km west of Tripoli), Janzour (30 km west of Tripoli) and Tobruk (1400 km east of Tripoli)]. Each sample was 250 g in weight. The Samples were packed in sterile plastic bags and stored in an insulated box containing crushed ice. The samples were transferred as quickly as possible to Food Hygiene and Control Laboratory at the Faculty of Veterinary Medicine, University of Tripoli. All samples were subjected to *Vibrio* spp. microbiological enumeration and isolation.

Samples processing

Preparation of samples, decimal dilutions, culturing and enumeration techniques of bacteria were performed according to the methods described previously (Downes

and Ito, 2001). Briefly, 25 g from each sample was aseptically transferred into a sterile polyethylene stomacher bag and blended with 225 ml of sterile alkaline peptone water (Catalogue #610098, LIOFILCHEM, Italy) in a stomacher homogenizer (Stomacher 400, Seaward medicals, UK.) at 230 rpm for 60 s. Serial dilutions were made using sterile 0.1% peptone water.

Isolation, cultural characteristics and enumeration of Vibrio spp.

Determination of the *Vibrio* spp. count was performed using *Vibrio* spp. selective Thiosulfate Citrate Bile Salt agar plates (TCBS: catalogue #611010, LIOFILCHEM, Italy). TCBS agar plates were inoculated by spreading 0.1 ml of the serial dilutions and incubated at 37°C for 48 h. TCBS plates were examined for the presence of either yellow, round, 2-3 mm diameter colonies (suspect: *V. cholera*, *V. fluvialis* or *V. alginolyticus*) or green, round, 2-3 mm diameter colonies (suspect: *V. parahemolyticus* or *V. vulnificus*). Countable plates are those containing 25 to 250 colonies (Kaysner and DePaola, 2001).

Purification of Vibrio spp.

For purification, single colony from each grown type of *Vibrio* suspect colonies was streaked onto another TCBS agar and incubated overnight at 37°C. This process has been performed until obtaining pure consistent colonies.

Table 1. Total number, enumeration and molecular identification of suspected *Vibrio* spp. in processed samples.

Type of sample	No. of samples	No. of suspected Vibrio spp. growth on TCBS (%)	No. of positive Vibrio spp. by 16S r DNA sequencing	Average CFU/g
Shrimp	21	11 (52.3)	1	6.25×10^2
Clam	5	4 (80)	1	3.8×10^4
Sardine	8	7 (87.5)	3	3.7×10^3
Mackerel	4	3 (75)	3	3.8×10^3
Annular sea bream	2	1 (50)	1	4.5×10^3
Amberjack	1	None	None	-
Common dentex	1	1 (100)	1	3.7×10^3
Shark	1	None	None	-
Dusky grouper	2	None	None	-
Sea needle	1	None	None	-
Beef	10	5 (50)	None	2.9×10^3
Camel meat	9	3 (33.33)	1	5.3×10^2
Chicken	9	5 (55.55)	None	7.2×10^3
Mutton	6	None	None	-
Beef burger	5	4 (80)	None	1.2×10^4
Chicken burger	5	4 (80)	None	6.5×10^4
Beef kebab	1	None	None	-
Beef sausage	2	None	None	-
Total	93	48 (51.6)	11	

Identification of Vibrio spp. by PCR and sequencing of 16S rDNA

DNA extraction of Vibrio isolates

The procedure of DNA extraction of *Vibrio* isolates was done using the GF-1 bacterial DNA extraction kit (Cat# GF-BA-100, Vivantis, Malaysia). Briefly, a single colony of pure isolate was picked up from TCBS agar and inoculated into 5 ml nutrient broth then incubated at 37°C. A total volume of 1-3 ml of bacterial culture was centrifuged at 10000 rpm for 2 min then supernatant was discarded. The pellet was then re-suspended by adding 100 μl of buffer R1 (Cat. # GF-BA-100, Vivantis, Malaysia).

The re-suspended cells were centrifuged at 10000 rpm for 5 min then the supernatant was decanted completely. The protein of the pellet was denaturized by re-suspension in 180 μl of Buffer R2 (Cat. # GF-BA-100, Vivantis, Malaysia) and 20μl of proteinase K, then incubated at 65°C for 20 min with shaking every 5 min. Homogenization was achieved by adding 400 μl of Buffer BG (Cat. # GF-BA-100, Vivantis, Malaysia) and mix by inverting tube and incubation at 65°C for 10 min. 200 μl of absolute ethanol was added with immediate mixing to prevent precipitation of DNA due to high ethanol concentration. The sample was transferred (maximum volume 650 μl) into the column and centrifuged at 10000 rpm for 1 min. The flow was discarded and the column was washed by 750 μl of wash buffer (Cat. # GF-BA-100, Vivantis, Malaysia) by centrifugation at 10000 rpm for 1 min. The flow was discarded the DNA was eluted in 50 μl of elution buffer, which left for 5 min at room temperature and then centrifuged at 1500 rpm 1 min.

Amplification of 16S rDNA

Partial 16S rDNA was amplified using the universal oligonucleotides primers Forward S-D-Bact-0341-b-S-17 and Reverse S-D-Bact-0785-a-A-21 adopted from (Herlemann *et al.*, 2011). Briefly, 0.2 μg of genomic DNA was added to 25 μl Maximo Dry PCR Master Mix (Cat. # S295, GeneON, UK). The mixture was then amplified in a DNA Thermal Cycler (TECHNE TC-512) using the following program: one denaturation step at 94 °C for 5 min; 35 cycles of denaturation, 92 °C for 30 s, annealing temperature for 30 s at 55°C, extension at 68 °C for 60 s; and a final extension at 72 °C for 10 min.

The PCR products were electrophoresed in 2% agarose gel (Cat. # 604-005, GeneON, UK) incorporated with nucleic acid gel stain – 10000X (Gel RED, Cat. # S420, GeneON, UK) at voltage 100 volt for one hour (SCIE-PLAS, UK). The sizes of the amplified fragments were determined by comparison with the GelPilot 100 bp increment Ladder (Qiagen, Cat. No. 239035, Melbourne Australia) a ready-to-use 6 fragments (100–600 bp) DNA marker. The gel was photographed with gel-documentation system micro DOC with UV-trans-illuminator (CSLUVTS312, Cleaver Scientific, UK).

DNA sequencing and analysis

The amplified 16S rDNA PCR fragment (464 bp) was excised from the gel and the DNA was extracted from the gel using GF-1 Ambi Clean kit (Cat. # GF-GC-100, Vivantis, Malaysia). Briefly, the net weight of gel slice was determined and 1 volume of Buffer DB was added to 1 volume of gel (A gel slice of mass 0.1g will have a volume of 100 μl). Then the gel was incubated at 50°C until gel has melted completely. The sample was transferred into a column assembled in a clean collection tube. Centrifuge at 10000 rpm for 1 min. The flow was discarded and the column was washed with 750 μl buffer and centrifuged at 10000 rpm for 1 min. The flow was discarded t and the column was dried by centrifugation at 10000 rpm for 1 min to remove residual ethanol. DNA was then eluted by adding 30 μl of elution buffer and mixture was left for 2 min.

The purified 16S rDNA amplicons underwent cycle sequencing by Big Dye® Terminator v1.1 kit (AB Applied Biosystems) and sequence reactions were separated on a four capillary ABI PRISM® 3130 Genetic Analyzer at IZSLER (Istituto Zooprofilattico Sperimentale della Lombardia e dell 'Emilia Romagna, Bianchi, 9 - 25124 Brescia, Italy). Sequences were assembled and edited using SeqMan module within Lasergene package, (DNAStar Inc., Madison, WI, USA) The obtained consensus sequences were subjected to BLAST search both at NCBI (http://www.ncbi.nlm.nih.gov/pubmed) and at 16S bacterial cultures Blast Server for the identification of prokaryotes (http://bioinfo.unice.fr/blast/).

Results

Isolation, cultural characteristics and enumeration of Vibrio spp.

The results from culture, enumeration and molecular identification of suspected *Vibrio* spp. in processed samples are shown in Table 1. Out of the 93 cultured samples, only 48 (51.6%) yielded colonies on TCBS with culture characteristics suggestive of *Vibrio* spp. (Fig. 1; Fig. 2a and 2b). More than half (27) of processed seafood samples (46) yielded colonies on TCBS, while only 21 out of 47 (44.6%) cultures of meat and meat products samples resulted in colonies on TCBS. No bacterial growth was revealed from the cultured samples of amberjack, shark, dusky grouper and sea needle, in addition to those from mutton, beef kebab and beef sausage (Table 1).

The highest bacterial count was recorded in a clam with a count of 3.8 x10⁴ CFU\g from the seafood samples. The highest bacterial count in meat products was from chicken burger samples with 6.5 x10⁴ CFU\g (Table 1 and Fig. 3).

Identification of Vibrio spp. by amplification and sequencing of 16S rDNA

All suspected isolates on TCBS were further analyzed molecularly by extraction of their DNA followed by sequencing of a portion of their 16S rDNA. Sequence

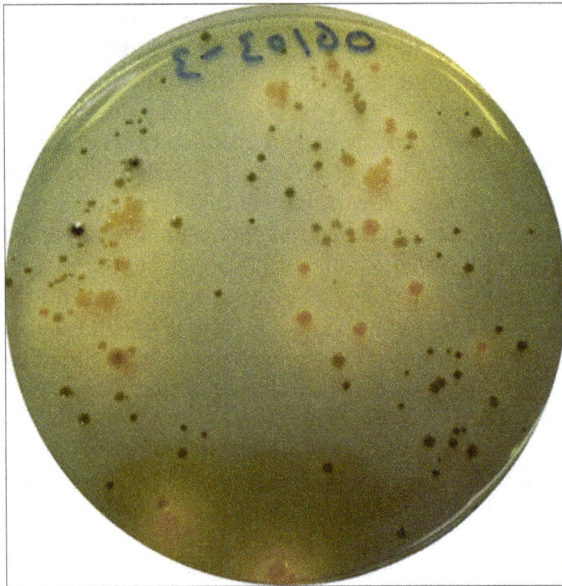

Fig. 1. TCBS plate showing the characteristic *Vibrio* spp. colonies (Green and yellow) during enumeration procedures.

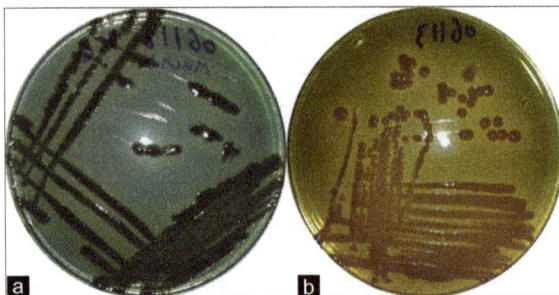

Fig. 2. Showing the pure consistent colonies of *Vibrio parahemolyticus* (a) and *Vibrio alginolyticus* colonies (b).

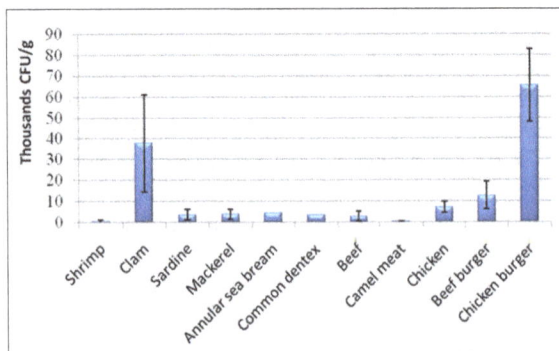

Fig. 3. Mean counts of *Vibrio* spp. in seafood, meat, and meat products samples. Error bar represents SD.

analysis showed that only 11 (22.9%) of these isolates were *Vibrio* spp. (Fig. 4 and Table 2).

Four out of the 11 *Vibrio* isolates were found to be *Photobacterium damselae* subsp. *Damselae* using the PCR-16S rDNA technique with 99 % nucleotide identity (Table 2). Moreover, the molecular test has revealed the presence of *Vibrio parahemolyticus* in a camel meat sample, which is the first report of the isolation of *Vibrio* from camel meat.

Discussion

Our results represent the first report of isolation and identification of *Vibrio* spp. by sequencing of 16S rDNA from seafood, meat and meat products samples in Libya. Only 11 samples out of 48 suspected *Vibrio* isolates (22.9%) in this study were identified to be *Vibrio* spp. by 16S rDNA sequencing. *V. parahemolyticus* and *V. alginolyticus* were the most frequently detected making up 27% of the isolates and the least frequently species was *V. owensii* 9%. A previous study, which examined the occurrence of *Vibrio* in mussels harvested from Adriatic Sea, found 48.4% of samples were positive for *Vibrio* spp., among which *V. alginolyticus* was most frequently found (32.2%) while *V. parahaemolyticus* was the least frequent (1.6%) (Ripabelli *et al.*, 1999). Another study determined the incidence of food borne pathogens in some European fish (France, Britain, Greece and Portugal) found *V. parahaemolyticus* was recorded in 35% of samples from Portugal and 14% from Greece but not in those from Britain or France (Davies *et al.*, 2001).

Using conventional cultivation on TCBS, Jakšić *et al.* (2002) determined the occurrence of *Vibrio* spp. in fish and shrimps harvested from Adriatic Sea. They were able to isolate *Vibrio* spp. from 19.65% of samples. The most frequently found were *V. parahemolyticus* (9.4%), *V. vulnificus* (6.8%) and *V. alginolyticus* (3.4%). Das *et al.* (2009) examined the occurrence of *Vibrio parahaemolyticus* in samples of finfish and *Penaeus monodon* from wholesale fish markets in Kolkata, India, by standard culture technique. The bacterium was isolated from 45.8% of shellfish and 16.7% of finfish samples. Xu *et al.* (2014) have investigated

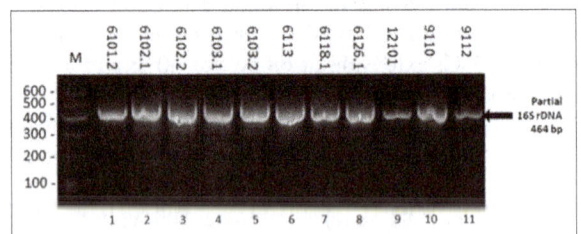

Fig. 4. Amplification of partial 16S rDNA (464 bp) of isolated *Vibrio* strains using the universal oligonucleotides primers (FOR S-D-Bact-0341-b-S-17 and REV S-D-Bact-0785-a-A-21). Lane (M) contains the 6 fragments (100–600 bp) DNA marker. Lanes 1-11 contains isolated *Vibrio* spp.

Table 2. Identification of suspected *Vibrio* spp. by PCR and sequencing of 16S rDNA.

Blast NCBI search results	Nucleotide identity %	Isolates code	Type of sample	Sampling area
Vibrio owensii	99	6101.2	Chub mackerel (Scomber japonicas)	Tripoli
Vibrio harveyi/Vibrio alginolyticus	99	6102.2	Chub mackerel (Scomber japonicas)	Tripoli
Vibrio harveyi/Vibrio alginolyticus	99	6113	Clam shellfish	Tripoli
Vibrio harveyi/Vibrio alginolyticus	99	12101	Shrimp	Tripoli
Vibrio parahaemolyticus	99	6118.1	Camel meat	Regdalin
Vibrio parahaemolyticus	99	9110	Common dentex	Tobruk
Vibrio parahaemolyticus	99	9112	Annular sea bream	Tobruk
Photobacterium damselae subsp. *Damselae*; 99% *Vibrio*	99	6102.1	Chub mackerel (Scomber japonicas)	Tripoli
Photobacterium damselae subsp. *Damselae*; 99% *Vibrio* sp.	99	6103.1	Sardine	Tripoli
Photobacterium damselae subsp. *Damselae*; 99% *Vibrio* sp.	99	6103.2	Sardine	Tripoli
Photobacterium damselae subsp. *damselae*; *Vibrio olivaceus*	99	6126.1	Sardine	Tripoli

the prevalence, pathogenicity, and serotypes of *V. parahaemolyticus* in shrimp from Chinese retail markets. *V. parahaemolyticus* was detected in (37.7%) of samples by the most probable number method.

V. owensii, which has been isolated from cultured crustaceous in Australia and recognized as a novel *Vibrio* spp. (Cano-Gómez *et al.*, 2010) was among the suspected isolates in our study from samples of mackerel, a case which have not been reported earlier.

From the results obtained in the present study, *Photobacterium damselae* subsp. *damselae* (formerly *V. damsela*) was the most frequently bacterium isolated (36%) from the processed samples. This microorganism has been recognized as a pathogen for a wide variety of aquatic animals, such as crustaceans, molluscs, fish and cetaceans. In addition, this bacterial pathogen has been reported to cause diseases in humans and, for this reason, it may be considered as an agent of zoonoses (Austin, 2010). According to Bergey's Manual of Systematic Bacteriology (Thyssen and Oliver, 2005), *P. damselae* subsp. *damselae* belongs to the genus *Photobacterium* included in the family *Vibrionaceae*, displaying morphological characteristics typical of members of the family.

Occurrence of *Vibrio* spp. in meat and meat products is not widely reported. However, Zakhariev *et al.* (1976) has investigated *V. parahaemolyticus* in pork sausage. Gardner (1980) have associated *V. costicola* with the spoilage of cured meats. Garcia-Lopez *et al.* (1998) had indicated the association of *Vibrio* spp. among other Gram-negative bacteria associated with spoilage of meat and meat products. Similarly, Doulgeraki *et al.* (2012) had concluded that *V. parahemolyticus* are among those organisms which are responsible for spoilage of raw meat during storage at different conditions. An interesting finding in this study was the isolation of *V. parahemolyticus* from camel meat, which has never been reported previously. On the other hand, none of the bacteria isolated from all the processed samples (beef, chicken, mutton, beef burger, chicken burger, beef kebab and beef sausage) belonged to *Vibrio* spp. Further, the mixed selling of chicken meats, beef and camel meat together with seafood products at the retail markets could have allowed the cross contamination from contaminated seafood/water directly to meat (Herrera *et al.*, 2006; Nyachuba, 2010). The irresponsible and unhygienic act of washing chicken, beef and camel meats with sewage contaminated water/seawater could explain the reported *Vibrio* incidences (especially *V. cholera* and *V. parahemolyticus*) among these types of fresh meats (Maheshwari *et al.*, 2011). This may also explain the isolation of *V. parahemolyticus* from camel meat in this study.

No *Vibrio* detection from mutton meat samples. This may be related to the low pH (acidic), associated with high conjugated linolenic and free fatty acids intermingling the mutton meat. This assumption ideally coincides with the relative bacterial inhibitory effect of sheep meat (mutton) fat reported by several studies (Reineccius, 1979; Sofos, 1994; Garcia-Lopez *et al.*, 1998). However, lack of detection of *Vibrio* spp. in beef kebab and beef sausage samples may be attributed to the excessive dressing in spice, lemon/vinegar, garlic and onions that possess inhibitory effects on *Vibrio* growth (Beuchat, 1976).

In Libya, there is a lack of data concerning actual causes of food borne infections in general. So it is difficult to find a link between *Vibrio* spp. isolations and any of the reported food poisoning outbreaks in the country. However, correlations between *V. parahemolyticus* and food borne infections have been described in Taiwan (Pan *et al.*, 1997), USA (Fyfe *et al.*, 1997), France (Geneste *et al.*, 2000), Mexico (Velazquez-Roman *et al.*, 2012) and China (Ma *et al.*, 2014).

One of the major risks involves the consumption of raw or undercooked seafood, meat and meat products that may be contaminated by food borne pathogens present in the marine/retail markets (Genigeorgis, 1985; Jay *et al.*, 2005). Such risks are further increased if the food is mishandled during handling, slaughter, transportation, and processing where pathogens could multiply exponentially under favorable conditions (Oliver and Kaper, 1997).

In contrast to most other food borne pathogens, *Vibrio* spp. utilize aquatic habitats as their natural niche (Oliver and Kaper, 1997; Reidl and Klose, 2002). As a result, *Vibrio* spp. are commonly associated with polluted water, seafood, and other aquatic animals as the main source of contamination (Sutherland and Varnam, 2002). Food borne infections with *Vibrio* spp. are common in coastal cities where retail markets are close to the sea basin (Rebaudet *et al.*, 2013). The close vicinity of seafood, meat and meat products retail markets as well as processing facilities to the sea basin amplifies the potentials of *Vibrio* spp. contamination to such foods (Jackson *et al.*, 1997; Feldhusen, 2000; Sofos, 2008).

Finally, it is empirical to mention that the identity of the retrieved *Vibrio parahemolyticus* and *V. harveyi* were presumptively identified using morphological characteristics extracted from morphological cultural characteristics on the selective TCBS agar media. All isolates matched the standard morphological criteria previously established (Alsina and Blanch, 1994; Perilla *et al.*, 2003; Austin and Austin, 2012). Molecular confirmation of the retrieved *Vibrio* isolates was done using partial amplification of 16S rDNA using the universal oligo-nucleotides primers (FOR S-D-Bact-0341-b-S-17 and REV S-D-Bact-0785-a-A-21) where the specific 464 bp amplicon has been documented coinciding with that reported by (Herlemann *et al.*, 2011) for the same *Vibrio* spp. using the same specific primers and 16S rDNA PCR protocol.

Acknowledgements

This study was part of a project titled "Genetic authentication of bacterial isolates from meat and milk products in Libya and establishing the Food-borne Libyan-type Bacterial Collection (FLBC)" that was supported by a grant provided by the Libyan Authority for Research, Science and Technology (LARST). Authors are grateful to Veronica Papini, a technician in Istituto Zooprofilattico Sperimentale della Lombardia e dell'Emilia Romagna, Brescia, Italy, who performed the sequencing of the Partial 16S rDNA.

References

Alsina, M. and Blanch, A.R. 1994. A set of keys for biochemical identification of environmental Vibrio species. J. Appl. Bacteriol. 76, 79-85.

Austin, B. 2010. Vibrios as causal agents of zoonoses. Vet. Microbiol. 140, 310-317.

Austin, B. and Austin, D.A. 2012. Vibrionaceae representatives. In Bacterial fish pathogens (Springer), The Netherlands, pp: 357-411.

Beuchat, L. 1976. Sensitivity of Vibrio parahaemolyticus to spices and organic acids. J. Food Sci. 41, 899-902.

Cano-Gómez, A., Goulden, E.F., Owens, L. and Høj, L. 2010. Vibrio owensii sp. nov., isolated from cultured crustaceans in Australia. FEMS Microbiol. Lett. 302, 175-181.

Das, B., Manna, S., Sarkar, P. and Batabyal, K. 2009. Occurrence of Vibrio parahaemolyticus in different finfish and shellfish species. J. Food Saf. 29, 118-125.

Davies, A.R., Capell, C., Jehanno, D., Nychas, G.J. and Kirby, R.M. 2001. Incidence of foodborne pathogens on European fish. Food Control 12, 67-71.

Doulgeraki, A.I., Ercolini, D., Villani, F. and Nychas, G.J. 2012. Spoilage microbiota associated to the storage of raw meat in different conditions. Int. J. Food Microbiol. 157, 130-141.

Downes, F.P. and Ito, K. 2001. In Compendium of Methods for the Microbiological Examination of Foods. 4th Ed. American Public Health Association, Washington DC, pp: 473-481.

Feldhusen, F. 2000. The role of seafood in bacterialfoodborne diseases. Microbes Infect. 2, 1651-1660.

Fyfe, M., Yeung, S., Daly, P., Schallie, K., Kelly, M. and Buchanan, S. 1997. Outbreak of Vibrio parahaemolyticus related to raw oysters in British Columbia. Can. Commun. Dis. Rep. 23, 145-148.

Garcia-Lopez, M., Prieto, M. and Otero, A. 1998. The physiological attributes of Gram-negative bacteria associated with spoilage of meat and meat products. Microbiol. Meat Poult. 1-34.

Gardner, G.A. 1980. Identification and ecology of salt-requiring Vibrio associated with cured meats. Meat sci. 5(1), 71-81.

Geneste, C., Dab, W., Cabanes, P., Vaillant, V., Quilici, M. and Fournier, J. 2000. Les vibrioses non cho99
liques en France: cas identifiés de 1995 à 1998 par le Centre National de Référence. Bull. Épidemiologie Hebdomadaire 9, 38-40.

Genigeorgis, C.A. 1985. Microbial and safety implications of the use of modified atmospheres to extend the storage life of fresh meat and fish. Int. J. Food Microbiol. 1, 237-251.

Harwood, V.J., Gandhi, J.P. and Wright, A.C. 2004.

Methods for isolation and confirmation of Vibrio vulnificus from oysters and environmental sources: a review. J. Microbiol. Methods 59(3), 301-316.

Herlemann, D.P., Labrenz, M., Jürgens, K., Bertilsson, S., Waniek, J.J. and Andersson, A.F. 2011. Transitions in bacterial communities along the 2000 km salinity gradient of the Baltic Sea. ISME J. 5, 1571-1579.

Herrera, F., Santos, J., Otero, A. and García-López, M.L. 2006. Occurrence of foodborne pathogenic bacteria in retail prepackaged portions of marine fish in Spain. J. Appl. Microbiol. 100, 527-536.

Iwamoto, M., Ayers, T., Mahon, B.E. and Swerdlow, D.L. 2010. Epidemiology of seafood-associated infections in the United States. Clin. Microbiol. Rev. 23, 399-411.

Jackson, T.C., Acuff, G. and Dickson, J. 1997. Meat, poultry, and seafood. Food microbiology fundamentals and frontiers ASM Press, Washington, DC, pp: 83-100.

Jakšić, S., Uhitil, S., Petrak, T., Bažulić, D. and Gumhalter Karolyi, L. 2002. Occurrence of Vibrio spp. in sea fish, shrimps and bivalve molluscs harvested from Adriatic sea. Food Control 13, 491-493.

Jay, J.M., Loessner, M.J. and Golden, D.A. 2005. Modern food microbiology. 7th ed. Springer Science + Business Media. New York.

Kaysner, C.A. and DePaola, A. 2001. *Vibrio*. In Compendium of Methods for The Microbiological Examination of Foods. F.P. Downes and K. Ito, eds. Washington, DC, American Public Health Association, pp: 405-420.

Ma, C., Deng, X., Ke, C., He, D., Liang, Z., Li, W., Ke, B., Li, B., Zhang, Y., Ng, L. and Cui, Z. 2014. Epidemiology and etiology characteristics of foodborne outbreaks caused by Vibrio parahaemolyticus during 2008–2010 in Guangdong Province, China. Foodborne Pathog. Dis. 11, 21-29.

Maheshwari, M., Krishnaiah, N. and Ramana, D. 2011. Evaluation of Polymerase Chain Reaction for the detection of Vibrio cholerae in Contaminants. Ann. Biol. Res. 2, 212-217.

Newell, D.G., Koopmans, M., Verhoef, L., Duizer, E., Aidara-Kane, A., Sprong, H., Opsteegh, M., Langelaar, M., Threfall, J., Scheutz, F., van der Giessen, J. and Kruse, H. 2010. Food-borne diseases - the challenges of 20 years ago still persist while new ones continue to emerge. Int. J. Food Microbiol. 139 Suppl. 1:S3-15.

Nyachuba, D.G. 2010. Foodborne illness: is it on the rise? Nutr. Rev. 68, 257-269.

Oliver, J.D. and Kaper, J.B. 1997. *Vibrio* species. In: Doyle, M.P., Beuchat, L.R. and Montville, T.J. (eds) Food Microbiology. Fundamentals and Frontiers.

ASM Press, Washington DC, USA, pp: 228-264.

Pan, T.-M., Wang, T.-K., Lee, C.-L., Chien, S.-W. and Horng, C.-B. 1997. Food-borne disease outbreaks due to bacteria in Taiwan, 1986 to 1995. J. Clin. Microbiol. 35, 1260-1262.

Perilla, M., Ajello, G., Bopp, C., Elliott, J. and Facklam, R. 2003. Manual for the laboratory identification and antimicrobial susceptibility testing of bacterial pathogens of public health importance in the developing world. Haemophilus influenzae Neisseria meningitidis Streptococcus pneumoniae Neisseria gonorrhoeae Salmonella serotype Typhi Shigella and Vibrio cholerae. WHO: Geneva, Switzerland.

Rebaudet, S., Sudre, B., Faucher, B. and Piarroux, R. 2013. Cholera in coastal Africa: a systematic review of its heterogeneous environmental determinants. J. Infect. Dis. 208 Suppl. 1:S98-106.

Reidl, J. and Klose, K.E. 2002. Vibrio cholerae and cholera out of the water and into the host. FEMS Microbiol. Rev. 26, 125-139.

Reineccius, G. 1979. Symposium on meat flavor off-flavors in meat and fish-A review. J. Food Sci. 44, 12-24.

Ripabelli, G., Sammarco, M.L., Grasso, G.M., Fanelli, I., Caprioli, A. and Luzzi, I. 1999. Occurrence of Vibrio and other pathogenic bacteria in Mytilus galloprovincialis (mussels) harvested from Adriatic Sea, Italy. Int. J. Food Microbiol. 49, 43-48.

Sofos, J.N. 1994. Microbial growth and its control in meat, poultry and fish. In: Quality Attributes and Their Measurement in Meat, Poultry, and Fish Products. A.M. Pearson and T.R. Dutson (Eds.). Blackie Academic and Professional, Glasgow, U.K, pp: 359-403.

Sofos, J.N. 2008. Challenges to meat safety in the 21st century. Meat Sci. 78, 3-13.

Sutherland, J. and Varnam, A. 2002. de, W., Blackburn, C., McClure, P.J., editors. Enterotoxin-producing *Staphylococcus, Shigella, Yersinia, Vibrio, Aeromonas* and *Plesiomonas*. Foodborne pathogens hazards, risk analysis and control. Cambridge: Woodhead Publishing, pp: 385-415.

Thyssen, A. and Oliver, F. 2005. "Genus II. *Photobacterium*". Bergey's manual of systematic bacteriology, 2nd ed., Vol. 2, The *Proteobacteria*, Part B, The *Gammaproteobacteria*, Brenner, D.J., Krieg, N.R., Staley, J.T., Garrity, G.M., eds. New York, USA, Springer, pp 546-552.

Velazquez-Roman, J., León-Sicairos, N., Flores-Villaseñor, H., Villafaña-Rauda, S. and Canizalez-Roman, A. 2012. Association of pandemic Vibrio parahaemolyticus O3: K6 present in the coastal environment of Northwest Mexico with cases of recurrent diarrhea between 2004 and 2010. Appl.

Environ. Microbiol. 78, 1794-1803.

Xu, X., Wu, Q., Zhang, J., Cheng, J., Zhang, S. and Wu, K. 2014. Prevalence, pathogenicity, and serotypes of Vibrio parahaemolyticus in shrimp from Chinese retail markets. Food Control 46, 81-85.

Zakhariev, Z., Tyufekchiev, T., Valkov, V. and Todeva, M. 1976. Food poisoning caused by parahaemolytic and NAG vibrios after eating meat products. J. Hyg. Epidemiol. Microbiol. Immunol. 20, 150-156.

5

Review on mechanisms of dairy summer infertility and implications for hormonal intervention

B.U. Wakayo[1,*], P.S. Brar[2] and S. Prabhakar[2]

[1]*College of Veterinary Medicine-Jigjiga University, P.O.Box 1020, Jigjiga Ethiopian Somali Regional State, Ethiopia*
[2]*Deptartment of Veterinary Gynaecology and Obstetrics, Guru Angad Dev Veterinary and Animal Sciences University, Ludhiana-141 004, India*

Abstract

In dairy cows and buffaloes, summer heat stress (HS) reduces milk yield and delays return to pregnancy leading to financial loss. Clues for effective interventions against summer infertility (SI) lie in understanding the underlying mechanisms. This article reviews current knowledge on the mechanisms of bovine SI and their implication for hormonal management. Under HS dairy animals encounter anestrous, silent cycles and repeat breeding which extend their open period. These effects are attributed mainly to HS induced disturbances in luteinizing hormone (LH) secretion, follicular dominance and estrogen secretion, ovulation and oocyte competence, luteal development and progesterone secretion, utero-placental function and embryo-fetal development. Hormonal timed artificial insemination protocols and LH support around estrous improved summer pregnancy rates by avoiding need for estrus detection, assisting follicular development and ovulation, enhancing quality oocytes and stimulating luteal function. Progesterone supplementation to enhance embryonic development did not produce significant improvement in summer pregnancy rates. There is need for evaluating integrated approaches combining hormones, metabolic modifier and cyto-protective agents.

Keywords: Bovines, Heat stress, Hormones, Infertility.

Introduction

Cows and buffaloes under summer heat stress (HS) face depressed reproductive activity. Summer infertility (SI) is characterized by anestrous, poor estrus expression and reduced fertility on breeding (Nardone *et al.*, 2010). SI is more important in tropical and sub-tropical areas, and in high yielding animals (Hansen, 2004). With current trends of rising global temperature, negative impact of SI on dairy production is expected to increase.

Current evidence indicates that HS and associated physiological changes hold immediate and delayed negative effects on: gonadotrophins secretion, follicular dynamics, ovulation, corpus luteum (CL) development, steroidogenesis, oocyte developmental competence, embryonic survival, utero-placental function, lactation and post-natal development (Wolfenson *et al.*, 1997; Bilby *et al.*, 2008; Hansen, 2009).

Knowledge that major SI mechanisms involve endocrine disturbance led to the development of hormone based interventions. Along with proper husbandry, hormonal supplementation and synchronization protocols demonstrate promise in enabling quick return to pregnancy (Hansen, 2012). Integration with supportive and protective interventions to address other physiological disturbances and cell injury could further improve response to hormonal SI management strategies.

This review aimed to summarize the current knowledge on the mechanisms of bovine SI and examine their implication for successful hormonal intervention strategies.

Bovine Heat Stress

The bovine Thermoneutral Zone (TNZ) is between 16°C to 25°C. Within this range, animals maintain a physiological body temperature of 38.4°C to 39.1°C (Yousef, 1985). Ambient temperatures above 20°C to 25°C enhance heat gain beyond that lost from the body inducing a state of HS with elevated internal body temperature (Yousef, 1985; Kennedy, 1999; Vale, 2007; Sunil Kumar *et al.*, 2011).

Animals try to restore thermal balance through mechanisms which reduce heat production - gain (reduced food intake, metabolism and activity; shade seeking; etc) and/or enhance heat loss (increasing water intake; bathing in ponds or mud; increased sweating respiration and salivation; redistributing blood flow towards peripheral integuments; etc). Cellular response to HS involves increased production of heat shock proteins (HSP) like HSP-70 and antioxidants to limit protein damage (Basiricò *et al.*, 2011). Physiological adjustments in HS pose negative consequences on energy availability, water and ionic

*Corresponding Author: B.U. Wakayo. College of Veterinary Medicine-Jigjiga University, P.O.Box 1020, Jigjiga Ethiopian Somali Regional State, Ethiopia. Email: fikeurga@gmail.com

balance, milk production and fertility (Kennedy, 1999; Sunil Kumar *et al.*, 2011).

Reproductive Impact of Summer Heat Stress

The major impact of HS on reproduction involves delaying a return to gestation due to decreased submission rate and low conception / pregnancy rates (Nardone *et al.*, 2010). In heat stressed cows, duration and intensity of estrus decreases and incidence of anoestrous and silent ovulation increases (Hansen and Aréchiga, 1999; Lucy, 2002).

Cold season conception rates of 40% to 60% declines to 10% or 20% during hot summer months (Cavestany *et al.*, 1985). HS during gestation can compromise fetal development, lactation and neonatal development as well as postpartum ovarian activity (Bilby *et al.*, 2008). Buffaloes are more prone to HS and assume a seasonal calving avoiding summer breeding (Vale, 2007; Singh *et al.*, 2013).

Mechanisms of Summer Infertility

Summer heat stress disrupts reproduction in two general ways i.e. physiological adjustments such as redistribution of blood flow and energy deficits compromise reproductive activity indirectly and elevated internal body temperature directly disrupts endocrine mechanisms and cellular physiology (ovarian cells, germ cells, embryo or other) (Wolfenson *et al.*, 2000). Following sections attempt to summarize impacts of HS at various stages of the reproductive process, examine relationships between such effects and outline implications on key fertility indicators.

Effect on gonadotropin secretion

Both tonic and surge luteinizing hormone (LH) levels were depressed by HS in cows with low circulating estradiol concentrations (Gilad *et al.*, 1993). Poor LH surge interferes with maturation and ovulation of dominant follicles whereas low tonic LH levels hinder lutenization (luteal development) (Wolfenson *et al.*, 2000) and inhibit follicular growth and turnover in cyclic cows (Sirard, 2001).

Gonadotropin releasing hormone (GnRH) induced follicle stimulating hormone (FSH) secretion was similarly depressed during HS. However, tonic FSH secretion in HS is elevated due probably to reduced inhibition of negative feedback from small follicles (Wolfenson *et al.*, 1993; Khodaei-Motlagh *et al.*, 2011). FSH change related fertility effects are considered less relevant (Wolfenson *et al.*, 1993; Edwards and Hansen, 1996). Increased circulating prolactin level was reported during HS which could lead to acyclicity and infertility (Alamer, 2011; Singh *et al.*, 2013).

Effect on ovarian activity

HS reduced follicular dominance by inducing multiple large (> 10 mm) follicles as well as prolonged dominance of ovulatory follicles (Hansen, 2009).

Normal follicular selection and dominance could be disturbed by high tonic FSH availability. LH and negative energy balance (NEB) during HS can prevent maturation and ovulation of dominant follicles. Multiple dominant follicles can increase the rates of double ovulation and twin conceptions (Hansen, 2009). Prolonged follicular dominance disrupts normal oocyte maturation (Eg. premature meiosis) and reduces developmental competence (Mihm *et al.*, 1994).

Follicular estradiol secretion is depressed under HS primarily due to reduced theca cell androstenedione production associated with low 17a-hydroxylase expression. Reduced granulosa cells aromatase activity and viability also contribute to poor estradiol secretion (Badinga *et al.*, 1993; Wolfenson *et al.*, 2000; Khodaei-Motlagh *et al.*, 2011). Low estrogen secretion disrupts expression of estrus, gonadotropin surge, ovulation, transport of gametes and fertilization (Wolfeson *et al.*, 2000).

In case dominant follicle/s ovulate, subsequent plasma progesterone concentrations are reduced during HS (Khodaei-Motlagh *et al.*, 2011). This could be attributed to small size of ovulatory follicle/s and low tonic LH stimulation of luteinization and steroidogenesis. Moreover, *in vitro* studies have indicated that HS compromised the viability of small luteal cells which represent a major source of progesterone (Wolfeson *et al.*, 2000). Low progesterone secretion limits endometrial function and embryo development (Wolfeson *et al.*, 2000; Khodaei-Motlagh *et al.*, 2011).

Effect on oocyte competence

Summer HS reduces oocyte developmental competence by affecting growth and maturation (Ju, 2005; Hansen, 2009). This could reflect a direct effect on the oocyte or an indirect consequence to supportive follicular cell changes. Direct effects on oocytes include: increased oxidative damage and apoptotic cell death (Paula-Lopes and Hansen, 2002), irreversible changes on cytoskeleton and meiotic spindle which interferes with cell division (Hansen, 2002; Ju, 2005), reduced mRNA and protein reserves for early embryonic development and altered membrane integrity which affects signal transduction and protein transport (Zeron *et al.*, 2001; Hansen, 2002).

On the other hand, tangible differences in important gene transcript levels (progesterone and prostaglandin receptors, transcription factors Egr-1 and DNA binding protein, etc) were detected between follicles with competent vs. incompetent oocytes (Robert *et al.*, 2001). Moreover, prolonged follicular dominance leads to premature meiosis and aged oocytes having poor developmental prospect (Hansen, 2002).

Reduced oocyte competence results in poor fertility rate after service. Stress capable of inducing oocyte lesions in early stages of follicular growth could impair fertility even long after its removal meaning that depressed summer fertility persists even to autumn months (Wolfenson *et al.*, 2000; Hansen, 2002; Ju, 2005).

Effect on embryo and fetus

HS is a recognized cause of embryonic mortality. Embryonic loss in HS may result from poor oocyte quality. Moreover, peri-implantation embryos in early cleavage are highly sensitive to direct deleterious effects of HS (Ealy *et al.*, 1993; Bilby *et al.*, 2008; Hansen, 2009). HS causes embryonic death by interfering with protein synthesis (Edwards and Hansen, 1996), causing widespread apoptosis (Paula-Lopes and Hansen, 2002) and oxidative cell damage (Wolfenson *et al.*, 2000; Hansen, 2009) and reducing interferon-tau production for signaling pregnancy recognition (Wolfensen *et al.*, 1993; Bilby *et al.*, 2008).

Exposure of post-implantation embryos (early organogenesis) and fetus to HS leads to various teratologies (Wolfenson *et al.*, 2000; Hansen, 2009). Genotype, stage of development and presence of cytoprotective molecules in female reproductive tract determine embryonic response to elevated temperature (Hansen, 2007). Embryonic susceptibility to HS declines in late cleavage (8 cells to morula stages). This was attributed to developmentally regulated protective mechanisms like: increasing expression of heat shock proteins (recently questioned by Sakatani *et al.* (2012)), declining oxidant production, increasing cytoplasmic antioxidant (glutathione) concentration and improving capacity for regulated apoptosis (Hansen, 2002; Paula-Lopes and Hansen, 2002; Ju, 2005; Hansen, 2009). The principle gave basis for successful application of embryo transfer advanced stage embryos to avoid pregnancy losses in summer (Hansen, 2012).

Effect on uterus and placenta

Rise in internal body temperature causes re-distribution of blood flow away from uterus which hampers supply of nutrients and hormones to the conceptus. Endometrial PGF-2α secretion tends to increase in HS thereby threatening pregnancy maintenance (Vale, 2007; Bilby *et al.*, 2008). Placental weight and hormone secretion are reduced whereas vascular resistance is increased during HS. These effects further reduce perfusion of nutrients to the fetus and impair lactation (Hansen, 2009). Retarded fetal development due to inadequate nutrition can manifest as physiological and performance problems long after birth (Wolfenson *et al.*, 2000; Hansen, 2009).

Hormonal Intervention to Summer Infertility

Considering the role of endocrine disturbances in delaying service and hampering conception, hormonal intervention presents a logical response for management of SI (Khodaei-Motlagh *et al.*, 2011). Multiple principles and protocols have been tried.

• Timed artificial insemination (TAI) protocols like OvSynch (GnRH – PGF-2α - GnRH) help to circumvent estrus detection, resolve anestrous and silent cycle constraints, facilitate LH support to follicular and oocyte development. Such protocols helped to increase pregnancy rates and reduce open periods in HS. Replacing GnRH with human Chorionic Gonadotropin (hCG) (Hansen and Aréchiga, 1999) and simultaneous supplementation with cryoprotective agents (such as bovine somatotropin and antioxidants) further improved response to TAI strategies (Aréchiga *et al.*, 1998; Hansen, 2007). Dirandeh (2014) recently reported better outcome in heat stressed cows when ovsynch was initiated 6 days after estrus detected post the 30th day postpartum. The approach enhanced response to first GnRH, an important determinant of both synchronization and fertility on ovsynch TAI.

• Administration of GnRH during early estrus coinciding with endogenous LH surge enhances LH surge and improves synchrony between estrus-LH surge-ovulation-insemination. Timely ovulation, competent oocytes and enhanced luteal progesterone secretion during first 30 days of gestation improves fertilization and embryo survival. Better summer pregnancy rates of 18% to 29 % were reported using this approach (Wolfenson *et al.*, 2000).

• Progesterone supplementation at critical stages of embryonic development was another alternative for improving summer pregnancy rates. Induction of accessory corpora lutea after breeding (by ovulatory doses of hCG or GnRH) and long term application of progesterone supplements by controlled intravaginal drug releasing (CIDR) device to inseminated animals represent the main strategies evaluated. Despite their theoretical soundness, these strategies have thus far failed to unequivocally prove beneficial for improving summer pregnancy rates (Wolfenson *et al.*, 2000).

Conclusion

SI hinders profitable milk production and the problem is escalating with raising global temperatures. Mechanisms underlying SI involve disturbances in development and viability of follicular, luteal, germ, conceptus, endometrial and placental cells. These disturbances are driven by endocrine and energy deficits, physical, oxidative and apoptotic cell injuries and reduced protein synthesis and function. Developments on hormonal interventions assist to alleviate or circumvent certain aspects of SI. Further molecular insights on mechanisms underlying SI can lead to more novel management approaches. Lasting solution to SI requires creating more adaptable dairy herds and/or improving the production environment.

References

Alamer, M. 2011. The role of Prolactin in thermoregulation and water balance during heat stress in domestic animals. Asian J. Anim. Vet. Adv. (12), 1153-1169.

Aréchiga, C.F., Staples, C.R., McDowell, L.R. and Hansen, P.J. 1998. Effects of timed insemination and supplemental betacarotene on reproduction and milk yield of dairy cows under heat stress. J. Dairy Sci. 81(2), 390-402.

Badinga, L., Thatcher, W.W., Diaz, T., Drost, M. and Wolfenson, D. 1993. Effect of environmental heat stress on follicular development and steroidogenesis in lactating Holstein cows, Theriogenology 39, 797-810.

Basiricò, L., Morera, P., Primi, V., Lacetera, N., Nardone, A. and Bernabucci, U. 2011. Cellular thermotolerance is associated with heat shock protein 70.1 genetic polymorphisms in Holstein lactating cows. Cell Stress Chaperon 16, 441-448.

Bilby, T.R., Baumgard, L.H., Collier, R.J., Zimbelman, R.B. and Rhoads, M.L. 2008. Heat stress effects on fertility: Consequences and possible solutions. In the Proceedings of the 2008 South Western Nutritional Conference.

Cavestany, D., El-Whishy, A.B. and Foot, R.H. 1985. Effect of season and high environmental temperature on fertility of Holstein cattle. J. Dairy Sci. 68(6), 1471-1478.

Dirandeh, E. 2014. Starting Ovsynch protocol on day 6 of first postpartum estrous cycle increased fertility in dairy cows by affecting ovarian response during heat stress. Anim. Reprod. Sci. 149(3-4), 135-140.

Ealy, A.D., Drost, M. and Hansen, P.J. 1993. Developmental changes in embryonic resistance to adverse effects of maternal heat stress in cows. J. Dairy Sci. 76, 2899-2905.

Edwards, J.L. and Hansen, P.J. 1996. Elevated temperature increases heat shock protein 70 synthesis in bovine two-cell embryos and compromises function of maturing oocytes. Biol. Reprod. 55, 340-346.

Gilad, E., Meidan, R., Berman, A., Graber, Y. and Wolfenson, D. 1993. Effect of heat stress on tonic and GnRH-induced gonadotrophin secretion in relation to concentration of oestradiol in plasma of cyclic cows. J. Reprod. Fertil. 99, 315-321.

Hansen, P.J. 2012. Solutions to Infertility Caused by Heat Stress. eXtension: http://www.extension.org/pages/64288/solutions-to-infertility-caused-by-heat-stress

Hansen, P.J. 2009. Effects of heat stress on mammalian reproduction. Phil. Trans. R. Soc. B. 364, 3341-3350.

Hansen, P.J. 2007. Exploitation of genetic and physiological determinants of embryonic resistance to elevated temperature to improve embryonic survival in dairy cattle during heat stress. Theriogenology 1(68), Suppl. 1, 242-249.

Hansen, P.J. 2004. Physiological and cellular adaptations of zebu cattle to thermal stress. Anim. Reprod. Sci. 82-83, 349-360.

Hansen, P.J. 2002. Embryonic mortality in cattle from the embryo's perspective. J. Anim. Sci. 80, 33-44.

Hansen, P.J. and Aréchiga, C.F. 1999. Strategies for managing reproduction in the heat stressed. J. Biol. Sci. 1(1), 1-8.

Ju, J.C. 2005. Cellular responses of oocytes and embryos under thermal stress: hints to molecular signaling. Anim. Reprod. 2(2), 79-90.

Kennedy, B.S. 1999. Thermoregulation and the Effects of Heat Stress on Dairy Cattle. Mississippi State University College of Veterinary Medicine, Production Medicine Graduate Program. (http://gpvec.unl.edu/heatdrought/HSDairyReview.htm)

Khodaei-Motlagh, M.M., Zare Shahneh, A., Masoumi, R. and Fabio, D. 2011. Alterations in reproductive hormones during heat stress in dairy cattle. Afr. J. Biotechnol. 10(29), 5552-5558.

Lucy, M.C. 2002. Reproductive loss in farm animals during heat stress. In the Proceeding of 2002 15th Conference on Biometeorology and Aerobiology and the 16th International Congress of Biometeorology, pp: 50-53.

Mihm, M., Baguisi, A., Boland, M.P. and Roche, J.F. 1994. Association between the duration of dominance of the ovulatory follicle and pregnancy rate in beef heifers. J. Reprod. Fertil.102, 123-130.

Nardone, A., Ronchi, B., Lacetera, N., Ranieri, M.S. and Bernabucci, U. 2010. Effects of climate changes on animal production and sustainability of livestock systems. Livest. Sci. 130, 57-69.

Paula-Lopes, F.F. and Hansen, P.J. 2002 Apoptosis is an adaptive response in bovine preimplantation embryos that facilitates survival after heat shock. Biochem. Bioph. Res. Co. 295, 37-42.

Robert, C., Gagne, D., Bousquet, D., Barnes, F.L. and Sirard, M.A. 2001. Differential display and suppressive subtractive hybridization used to identify granulosa cell messenger RNA associatedwith bovine oocyte developmental competence. Biol. Reprod. 64(6), 1812-1820.

Sakatani, M., Alvarez, N.V., Takahashi, M. and Hansen, P.J. 2012. Consequences of physiological heat shock beginning at the zygote stage on embryonic development and expression of stress response genes in cattle. J. Dairy Sci., 95(6), 3080-3091.

Singh, M., Chaudhari, B.K., Singh, J.K., Singh, A.K. and Maurya, P.K. 2013. Effects of thermal load on buffalo reproductive performance during summer season. J. Biol. Sci. 1(1), 1-8.

Sirard, M.A. 2001. Resumption of meiosis: mechanism involved in meiotic progression and its relation with developmental competence. Theriogenology 55, 1241-1254.

Sunil Kumar, B.V., Kumar, A. and Kataria, M. 2011. Effect of heat stress in tropical livestock and different strategies for its amelioration. J. Stress Physiol. Biochem. 7 (1), 45-54.

Vale, W.G. 2007. Effects of environment on buffalo reproduction. Italian J. Anim. Sci. 6(2), 130-142.

Wolfenson, D., Bartol, F.F., Badinga, L., Barros, C.M., Marple, D.N., Cummings, K., Wolfe, D., Lucy, M.C., Spencer, T.E. and Thatcher, W.W. 1993. Secretion of PGF2a and oxytocin during hyperthermia in cyclic and pregnant heifers. Theriogenology 39, 1129-1141.

Wolfenson, D., Lew, B.J., Thatcher, W.W., Graber, Y. and Meidan, R. 1997. Seasonal and acute heat stress effects on steroid production by dominant follicles in cow. Anim. Reprod. Sci. 47, 9-19.

Wolfenson, D., Roth, Z. and Meidan, R. 2000. Impaired reproduction in heat stressed cattle: basic and applied aspects. Anim. Reprod. Sci. 60-61, 535-547.

Yousef, M.K. 1985. Stress Physiology in Livestock. Vol.1. Boca Raton: CRC Press, pp: 67-73.

Zeron, Y., Ocheretny, A., Kedar, O., Borochov, A., Sklan, D. and Arav, A. 2001. Seasonal changes in bovine fertility: relation to developmental competence of oocytes, membrane properties and fatty acid composition of follicles. Reprod. 121, 447-454.

6

The eye of the Barbary sheep or aoudad (*Ammotragus lervia*): Reference values for selected ophthalmic diagnostic tests, morphologic and biometric observations

G.A. Fornazari[1], F. Montiani-Ferreira[1,*], I.R. de Barros Filho[1], A.T. Somma[1] and B. Moore[2]

[1]*Universidade Federal do Paraná, Programa de Pós-Graduação em Ciências Veterinárias, Rua dos Funcionários 1540, 8035-050, Curitiba, PR. Brazil*

[2]*Veterinary Specialty Hospital of San Diego, 10435 Sorrento Valley Road, San Diego, CA 92121, USA*

Abstract

The purpose of this study was to describe the normal ocular anatomy and establish reference values for ophthalmic tests in the Barbary sheep or aoudad (*Ammotragus lervia*). Aoudad eyes are large and laterally positioned in the head with several specialized anatomic features attributed to evolutionary adaptations for grazing. Normal values for commonly used ophthalmic tests were established, Schirmer tear test (STT) - 27.22 ± 3.6 mm/min; Predominant ocular surface bacterial microbiota - *Staphylococcus* sp.; Corneal esthesiometry- 1.3 ± 0.4 cm; Intraocular pressure by rebound tonometry- 19.47 ± 3.9 mmHg; Corneal thickness- 630.07 ± 20.67 μm, B-mode ultrasonography of the globe- axial eye globe length 29.94 ± 0.96 mm, anterior chamber depth 5.03 ± 0.17 mm, lens thickness 9.4 ± 0.33 mm, vitreous chamber depth 14.1 ± 0.53 mm; Corneal diameter- horizontal corneal diameter 25.05 ± 2.18 mm, vertical corneal diameter 17.95 ± 1.68 mm; Horizontal palpebral fissure length- 34.8 ± 3.12 mm. Knowledge of these normal anatomic variations, biometric findings and normal parameters for ocular diagnostic tests may assist veterinary ophthalmologists in the diagnosis of ocular diseases in this and other similar species.

Keywords: Barbary sheep, Biometry, Ocular parameters, Wild caprid.

Introduction

The Barbary sheep or aoudad (*Ammotragus lervia*) is a species of wild caprid (goat-antelope), whose natural habitat includes northern Africa in Algeria, Tunisia, northern Chad, Egypt, Libya, northern Mali, Mauritania, Morocco, Niger and Sudan (west of the Nile, and in the Red Sea Hills east of the Nile). It is also known as waddan, arui, and arruis (Cassinello, 1998; Wacher *et al.*, 2002; Cassinello *et al.*, 2004). The binomial name *Ammotragus lervia* derives from the Greek ammos "sand", referring to the sand-coloured coat) and tragos ("goat"). The species name *lervia* derives from the wild sheep of northern Africa (Cassinello, 1998; Wacher *et al.*, 2002). In its native distribution in northern Africa the aoudad was classified as a "vulnerable" species by the 2012 Red List of the International Union of Conservation of Nature (IUCN) due to natural habitat loss and poaching (Alados and Shackleton, 1997; Hilton-Taylor, 2000; Cassinello *et al.*, 2008). It has, however, been successfully introduced to North America, Europe and elsewhere primarily for trophy-hunting purposes. These introduced populations contain a large number of individuals and are free-ranging, commonly competing with the native mammals for resources (Cassinello *et al.*, 2008). The aoudad is a stocky, heavily built wild ruminant, with short legs and a rather long skull (Kingdon, 1997;

Stuart and Stuart, 1997). Both sexes have horns that sweep backwards and outwards in an arch; those of the male are much thicker and reach up to 50 cm. Aoudads' weight can vary from 40 to 140 kg. Males also differ from females by their significantly heavier weight, up to twice that of females (Kingdon, 1997), and the notably longer curtain of hair that hangs from the throat, chest and upper part of the forelegs (Kingdon, 1997; Stuart and Stuart, 1997; Cassinello, 1998). The coat is woolly during the winter, but moults to a finer, sleek coat for the hot summer months. It has a sandy-brown color, darkening with age, with a slightly lighter underbelly and a darker line along the back (Kingdon, 1997; Stuart and Stuart, 1997). The eyes of the aoudad are bright and apparently large in relation to its body size, more consistent with a cervid- or antelocaprid-like morphology than a caprid one. Concerning aoudads in the scientific literature, hormonal parameters and studies about applied reproductive techniques have been published (Hamon and Heap, 1990; Crenshaw *et al.*, 2000; Abáigar *et al.*, 2012; Santiago-Moreno *et al.*, 2013). Additionally, genetic studies (McLelland *et al.*, 2005; Manca *et al.*, 2006; Mereu *et al.*, 2008), epidemiologic surveys and reports of specific infectious diseases (Yeruham *et al.*, 2004; Candela *et al.*, 2009; Pirastru *et al.*, 2009; Portas *et al.*, 2009; Münster *et al.*, 2013; Morikawa *et al.*, 2014) and parasites (Pence and

*Corresponding Author: Fabiano Montiani-Ferreira. Universidade Federal do Paraná, Programa de Pós-Graduação em Ciências Veterinárias, Rua dos Funcionários 1540, 8035-050, Curitiba, PR. Brazil. E-mail: montiani@ufpr.br

Gray, 1981; Cho *et al.*, 2006; Mayo *et al.*, 2013) were investigated. An additional case report of pemphigus foliaceus has been published in this species (Brenner *et al.*, 2009). However, no ophthalmic investigations or even reports of ocular diseases on this species were available, possibly because baseline values for diagnostic tests have not yet been established for aoudads. Knowledge of baseline values is essential for both making appropriate diagnoses and properly treating ocular diseases in zoo and exotic animals. Important parameters to be established in wild animals include tear production (Schirmer tear test, STT) and intraocular pressure (IOP), echobiometric findings as well as normal conjunctival bacterial microbiota (Prado *et al.*, 2005; Kudirkiene *et al.*, 2006; Montiani-Ferreira *et al.*, 2006, 2008b; Martins *et al.*, 2007; Wang *et al.*, 2008; Ribeiro *et al.*, 2009; Lima *et al.*, 2010; Ghaffari *et al.*, 2012). These normal ophthalmic parameters in domestic, exotic and zoo animals become important references for the veterinary clinician and other researchers once published. The purpose of this study was to describe normal ophthalmic parameters in aoudads, including morphological features, biometry of anatomical structures, corneal ultrasonic pachymetry, globe echobiometry, tear production (Schirmer's tear test, STT), intraocular pressure (IOP), corneal sensitivity, bacterial conjunctival microbiota, and fundus photography.

Materials and Methods

All ophthalmic procedures using live aoudads were conducted in accordance with UFPR's Animal Use Committee and with the ARVO Statement for the Use of Animals in Ophthalmic and Vision Research. Eighteen adult captive aoudads (11 males and 7 females) of different ages (varying from 1.5 to 7 years of age, mean 4 ± 2.0 years) belonging to Curitiba's Zoo (Zoológico de Curitiba), Curitiba-PR, Brazil (25°25′S and 49°16′W) were captured for clinical evaluation as part of a health survey by the park authority (Fig. 1) during the winter of 2014 on three different occasions. A detailed ophthalmic evaluation including all the tests cited here was performed in this survey. Physical examinations, including a complete blood count panel, were performed before ocular examinations to exclude animals with indications of systemic disease. Aoudads with evidence of ocular or systemic diseases were excluded. Procedures and tests necessary to produce this work were split between the investigators. However, to avoid discrepancies related to inter-observer repeatability, the same person always performed the same ocular test on each occasion.

Ophthalmic tests

Clinical tests were performed while the aoudads were physically restrained by two experienced handlers using ropes, taking care to keep the animal comfortable. When the head was manually stabilized

for taking measurements special attention was given to avoid applying pressure to the neck region with hands or ropes, to prevent iatrogenic alterations in IOP. The sequence of procedures performed in this study was, (i) ocular inspection (including photography), (ii) Schirmer tear test (STT), (iii) collection of material for bacterial culture analysis, (iv) corneal esthesiometry, (v) tonometry, (vi) central corneal thickness (CCT) measurement with an ultrasonic pachymeter, (vii) B-mode ultrasonography of the globe, (viii) fundoscopy and lastly (ix) corneal and palpebral fissure measurements (Fig. 2).

Ocular inspection

A total of 36 eyes, from 18 healthy adult aoudads were selected and used in this investigation. The anterior ocular structures were evaluated using a Finoff transilluminator (3.5 V halogen fiber optic, Welch Allyn, Skaneateles Falls, NY, USA) and a slit lamp biomicroscope (Hawk Eye; Dioptrix, L'Union, France). The funduses were evaluated using an indirect ophthalmoscope (Heine Omega 180 Headworn Binocular Indirect Ophthalmoscope, Dover, NH) and photographed with a 7.2 megapixel reflex digital camera with a Carl Zeiss™ lens and 12x of optical zoom (DSC-H5; Sony™, Minato, Tokyo, Japan) (Fig. 3a).

Schirmer tear test

Sterile standardized STT strips (Schering Plough Animal Health, Union, NJ, USA) were used to perform the Schirmer type I test (Fig. 2a), which measures the basal plus a portion of the reflex tear production.

Microbiological analysis

For the microbiological analysis, samples were obtained by carefully touching the conjunctival sac and ocular surface (cornea and bulbar conjunctiva) with a sterile cotton swab (Fig. 2e). No topical anesthetic was

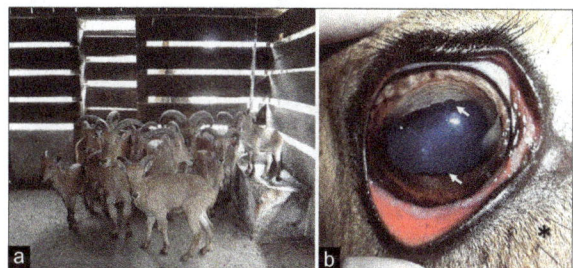

Fig. 1. (a) Part of the group of aoudads (*Ammotragus lervia*) from Curitiba's Zoo investigated in this study. The picture shows a mixed-aged group but only the adult animals were investigated. (b) A representative example of the general external appearance of the eye of the aoudad. True cilia (longer and thicker at the upper eyelid) are visible. Below the lower eyelid margin are two rows of sparsely distributed longer hairs (asterisk). Note in the anterior uvea the extensive iris collarette and the presence of an upper and a lower (more discrete) corpora nigra (arrows). The pupillary aperture shape was oval with the long axis horizontal. The limbus is relatively large and heavily pigmented.

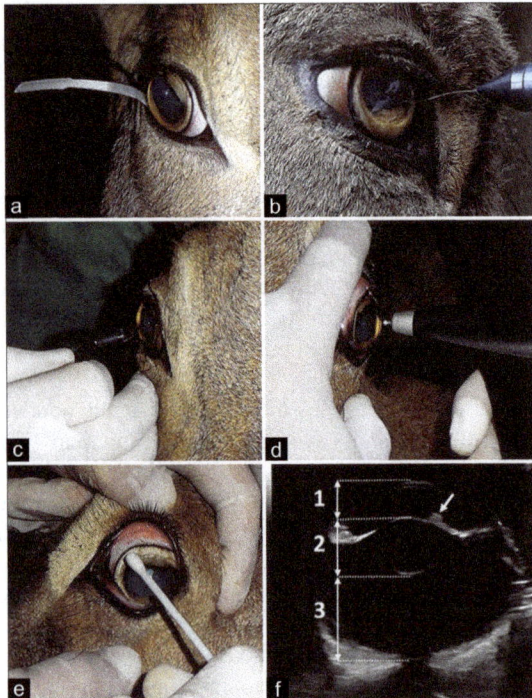

Fig. 2. Photographs of selected ocular tests performed in aoudads. (a) Schirmer tear test; (b) Esthesiometric analysis of central cornea; (c) Corneal pachymetry; (d) Rebound tonometry; (e) Swabbing the conjunctiva and eyelid margins; and (f) B-mode ocular echobiometry. Besides the globe axial length, the following echobiometric measurements were taken, 1- Anterior chamber depth (axial anterior chamber length); 2- Lens thickness (axial lens length); 3- Vitreous chamber depth (axial vitreous chamber length). Note the superior *corpora nigra* (arrow).

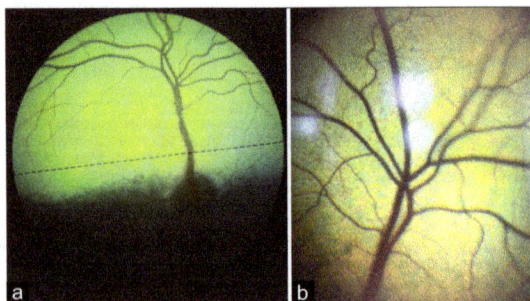

Fig. 3. Aoudad's fundoscopic appearance captured using TEFIT (a) and an indirect lens coupled with a slit lamp biomicroscope (Hawk Eye; Dioptrix, L'union, France). Note the extensive *tapetum lucidum* (a) the holangiotic retinal vascular pattern - (a) and (b). The *tapetum* has a granular or speckled appearance where *stelullae* of Winslow are present (b). The optic disc is grayish in color, oval in shape and located just inferior to the inferior border of the *tapetum lucidum* (a). The major blood vessels of the aoudad's retina radiate from the center of the optic nerve. (a) Blood vessels arising from the dorsal and ventral quadrants taper toward a region just above the inferior border of the *tapetum lucidum*. At this region no blood vessels are present and an imaginary line can be traced creating a streak where thin retinal blood vessels are rare or absent (a).

used prior to sample collection as this may interfere with the growth of organisms (Mullin and Rubinfeld, 1997). Aerobic bacterial culture of the microorganisms was performed in BHI broth (brain–heart infusion), and on 5% sheep blood agar and MacConkey plates, which were incubated at 37°C in an aerobic environment for 24–48 h. The same bacterial growth media used in this research was also used elsewhere to establish normal conjunctival microbiota of the opossum, raccoon, ferret and chinchilla in other investigations (Pinard *et al.*, 2002; Manca *et al.*, 2006; Montiani-Ferreira *et al.*, 2006, 2008b). Bacterial colonies were identified by Gram's stain and standard procedures.

Corneal esthesiometry

For the normal corneal sensitivity analysis, all aoudads were manually restrained, and a Cochet-Bonnet esthesiometer (Luneau Ophtalmologie, Chartres Cedex, France) was used (Fig. 2b). This instrument contains an adjustable nylon filament with a defined diameter, length and surface (0.12 mm diameter, 60 mm length, and 0.0113 mm^2 surface), which was applied at different lengths to the center of the cornea. A stimulus produced by the instrument's nylon monofilament that reaches the corneal touch threshold induces a corneal reflex, consisting of prompt eyelid closure, and discrete retraction of the globe. In this study only the center of the cornea was analyzed for corneal touch threshold, which was repeated five times using the same length of the nylon filament. The length of the nylon filament was then decreased at 5-mm increments until each aoudad responded with a corneal blink reflex. The corneal touch threshold was then quantified in millimeters length of the filament necessary to cause a blink reflex. The length of the filament, indicating a corresponding pressure at which the corneal blink reflex was positive, was deemed the central corneal sensitivity or central corneal touch threshold.

Intraocular pressure

Intraocular pressure (IOP) was measured in 36 eyes, using a veterinary rebound tonometer (Tonovet, Veterinary Division of S&V Technologies AG, Henningsdorf, Germany) (Fig. 2d) with the P setting, which was a preset for other animals except dogs and horses. Six measurements were taken and averaged by the tonometer's internal software.

Central corneal thickness

Central corneal thickness (CCT) measurements were taken after the instillation of sterile topical anesthetic (proparacaine hydrochloride 0.5% ophthalmic solution USP; Alcon Laboratories, Forth Worth, TX, USA). CCT was measured using an ultrasonic pachymeter (Model 200P+; Micropach, Sonomed, Lake Success,NY, USA), with the speed of sound in the cornea preset at 1640 m/s (Fig. 2c).

B-mode ultrasonographic biometry

B-mode scan ultrasonography was performed using

a Sonix SP High Performance B-mode System (Ultrasonix, Richmond, BC, Canada). A drop of topical local anesthetic (0.5% proxymetacaine chlorohydrate, Anestalcon®, Alcon Laboratórios do Brasil, São Paulo, SP, Brazil) was instilled on each eye before ultrasonography. The B-scan 14-MHz probe was gently placed on the corneal surface perpendicular to the center of the cornea using ultrasonic transmission gel (Aquasonic-100; Parker Laboratories Inc., Fairfield, NJ, USA). Care was taken during probe placement to avoid corneal indentation. Reflected ultrasonic waves were captured. Optimal positioning was confirmed when the posterior wall of the eye globe could be clearly visualized on the B-scan ultrasonogram and the image appeared symmetrical and the reflections from the four principal landmarks (cornea, anterior lens surface, posterior lens surface and retinal surface) along the optic axis were perpendicular. The optimal image was frozen on the screen and then all echobiometric measurements were taken (Fig. 2f).

Fundoscopy

After B-mode ultrasonographic biometry the aoudads' eyes were gently rinsed twice with 0.9% saline solution in order to remove the ultrasonic transmission gel. Subsequently the aoudad's funduses were examined using an indirect ophthalmoscope (Heine Omega 180 Headworn Binocular Indirect Ophthalmoscope, Dover, NH) and photographed using the topical endoscopy fundus imaging technique (TEFIT) (Fig. 3a) or a slit lamp containing a built-in indirect ophthalmoscopy lens (Digital 1.0x Imaging Lens, Hawk Eye, Dioptrix, L'Union, France) (Fig. 3b). For the TEFIT procedure a rigid, 8-mm-diameter laparoscope with a 0 degree angle and a crescent-shape illumination tip (WeckTM, Pilling Weck, Markham, ON, Canada) was used. Both the rigid arthroscopy probe and the rigid laparoscope were connected to an adapter of a 7.2 megapixel

reflex digital camera with a Carl ZeissTM lens and 12x of optical zoom (the same previously cited). The light source was a 175W xenon lamp (Karl StorzTM, Tuttlingen, Germany) linked to the arthroscopy probe and the rigid laparoscope by a flexible fiber optic cable. Pupillary dilation for fundoscopy and fundus photography was performed following instillation of the following eyedrops, tropicamide 1% and phenylephrine 10% (Frumtost, São Paulo, SP, Brazil) one drop of each in each eye, with approximate 3-min intervals, every 10 min three times.

Corneal and palpebral fissure biometry

Palpebral fissure length, vertical and horizontal corneal diameters were measured using a stainless steel caliper ruler with an LCD display and an accuracy of ±0.02 mm (Neiko Tools, Klamath Falls, OR, USA).

Statistical analyses

The obtained data were submitted to a Kolmogorov-Smirnov Goodness-of-Fit Test. Unpaired t-tests were used for data comparison between, right and left eyes and males and females. P-values < 0.05 were deemed significant. JMP (SAS Institute, Inc., Cary, NC, USA) software was used to perform both descriptive and inferential statistical analyses. Measurements are reported as mean ± standard deviation (SD).

Results

All continuous numeric data obtained for all ophthalmic tests in the population used in this investigation were normally distributed according to the Kolmogorov-Smirnov Goodness-of-Fit Test. Table 1 contains the condensed results of the descriptive statistical analyses.

Morphological features of the normal aoudad eye

Ophthalmic examinations revealed that the normal anterior ocular structures in the aoudad include dorsal and ventral puncta. Additionally, aoudads possess true cilia (eyelashes) at the upper (Fig. 1b) and lower eyelid margins; with the lower cilia being thinner

Table 1. Results obtained for selected ophthalmic diagnostic tests and echobiometric findings for the aoudad (*Ammotragus lervia*) eye.

Ophtalmic Test or Parameter	Unit	Mean	Standard Deviation	95% Confidence Interval
Schirmer tear test	mm/min	27.22	3.6	26.04-28.4
Esthesiometry	cm	1.3	0.4	1.18-1.43
Intraocular pressure	mmHg	19.47	3.9	18.2-20.74
Central corneal thickness	μm	630.07	20.67	623.32-636.82
Axial globe length	mm	28.43	0.88	26.65-28.43
Anterior chamber depth	mm	5.03	0.17	4.7-5.4
Lens thickness	mm	9.4	0.33	8.73-10.06
Vitreous chamber depth	mm	14.1	0.53	12.93-15.06
Palpebral fissure length	mm	34.8	3.12	33.77-35.82
Corneal horizontal length	mm	25.05	2.18	24.34-25.77
Corneal vertical length	mm	17.95	1.68	17.40-18.50

and more sparsely distributed. Aoudads have a third eyelid (nictitating membrane) which moves across the surface of the cornea from the nasal canthus to the temporal canthus. The leading edge of the third eyelid is pigmented. Above the upper eyelid margin and below the lower eyelid margins, two rows of modified-sparsely distributed longer hairs, resembling vibrissae, also called "tactile hair", were found in all individuals (Fig. 1b). There were approximately 16 to 18 pairs located above and 6 to 8 pairs below the eye. The iris colors of individual animals varied from a yellowish-brown to a grayish-brown. The iris collarette showed no crypts of Fuchs visible, being somewhat flat (Fig. 1b). *Corpora nigra* were present at the ciliary margin (the peripheral border of the iris). The lower *corpora nigra* were considerably more discrete (Fig. 1b). The pupillary aperture shape was oval with the long axis being horizontal. The presence of corpora nigra makes the pupil gain a rectangular appearance when observed from a distance.

Schirmer tear test (STT)

No significant STT differences were determined between right and left eyes or between sexes. Mean STT results for both eyes was 27.22 ± 3.6 mm/min.

Microbiological analysis

Bacteria were isolated in microbiological samples from 33 out of 36 eyes. Five different genera of gram-positive bacteria species were identified. The genera of the isolates were, *Corynebacterium*, *Micrococcus*, *Bacillus*, *Streptococcus* and *Staphylococcus* sp. Four different genera of gram-negative bacteria were isolated. The genera of the isolates were, *Escherichia*, *Acinetobacter*, *Enterobacter* and *Citrobacter* sp. A single genus of bacteria was isolated from 11 eyes. Two genera of bacteria were isolated from 20 eyes. Three genera of bacteria were isolated from two eyes. *Staphylococcus* sp. were the most common bacteria isolated, being present in 13 eyes (prevalence of 36.1%). *Micrococcus* sp. and *Bacillus* sp. were the second most common bacteria isolated, being present in 9 eyes each (prevalence of 25%). Lastly, *Corynebacterium* sp. was present in 5 eyes (prevalence of 13.88%).

Corneal esthesiometry

There were no significant differences between males and females or between left and right eyes. The mean central corneal sensitivity was 1.3 ± 0.4 cm.

Intraocular pressure (IOP)

The mean value for IOP was 19.47 ± 3.9 mmHg. There was no significant difference in IOP between males and females and no significant differences between left and right eyes.

Central corneal thickness (CCT)

The mean CCT was 630.07 ± 20.67 μm. There was no significant difference in CCT between males and females and no significant differences between left and right eyes.

B-mode ultrasonographic biometry

No significant biometric differences were determined between right and left eyes or between sexes. The mean axial globe length was 29.94 ± 0.96 mm. Mean anterior chamber depth (axial anterior chamber length) was 5.03 ± 0.17 mm. Mean lens thickness (axial length) was 9.4 ± 0.33 mm. Mean vitreous chamber depth (axial chamber length) was 14.1 ± 0.53 mm.

Fundus examination and fundus photography

As viewed by the ophthalmoscope, it was possible to observe that the aoudad retina possess an extensive *tapetum lucidum* usually of a greenish-yellow to a yellowish-green color with a typical holangiotic retinal vascular pattern (Fig. 3). The *tapetum* has a granular or speckled appearance (Fig. 3). The optic disc was oval in shape and located just inferior to the inferior border of the *tapetum lucidum*. The major blood vessels of the retina radiate from the center of the optic nerve (Fig. 3). Blood vessels arising from the dorsal and ventral quadrants taper toward a region just above the inferior border of the *tapetum lucidum*. At this region no blood vessels are present and an imaginary line can be traced creating a streak where retinal blood vessels are rare or absent (Fig. 3a).

Corneal and palpebral biometry

The transition between cornea and the sclera (limbus) is relatively large and heavily pigmented and appears as a dense thick band (Fig. 1b). Mean horizontal corneal diameter (or width) of both eyes was 25.05 ± 2.18 mm and the mean vertical corneal diameter of both eyes was 17.95 ± 1.68 mm. The mean horizontal palpebral fissure length of both eyes was 34.8 ± 3.12 mm.

Discussion

This study established normal values and ranges of several ophthalmic tests and biometric measurements of the eyes of a group of clinically normal aoudads (*Ammotragus lervia*), which was previously unavailable in the scientific literature.

The eyes of the aoudad are relatively large for the size of its head and body, and are therefore prominent. For instance, Barbary sheep eyes are bigger than the ones of the normal goat or sheep and other wild same size animals belonging to the Order Artiodactyla. The eyelashes and eyelid vibrissae are long and add to the distinctive appearance. In other species already investigated, vibrissae are considered to be true sensory organs located in anatomical areas where protective reflexes are important such as around the eye, or where environmental light is limited (McGreevy, 2004). Aoudads have a fairly elongated head and their eyes are placed laterally and posteriorly. These features together are similar to the horse head morphology (McGreevy, 2004) and are probably evolutionary adaptations to prevent tall grass from obstructing the view when grazing in both species. The presence of an elongated horizontally oval pupil observed here in the aoudad but also in other ungulates such as horses (Murphy and Arkins, 2007), cows, sheep and goats (Walls, 1943) allows for wide lateral vision (Murphy and Arkins, 2007). This type of pupil alternatively called "rectangular" (Prince, 1956) is also present in the deer, camel and hyrax. Optical analyses show that this horizontal pupillary elongation expands the field of view horizontally allowing terrestrial prey animals to see objects near the ground both in front of and behind them (Sprague et al., 2013).

Another evolutionary adaptation found in the eye of the aoudad is the corpora nigra, which are pigmented projections found on the upper and lower margins of the pupillary aperture. This anatomic structure already described in ungulates (Walls, 1943) is known to have many functions including contribution to pupillary constriction, prevention of actinic damage during grazing and possibly functions as an anti-glare device (Davidson, 1991). In the eye of the aoudad the upper corpora nigra is considerably larger than the lower ones. The authors believe that this feature accentuates information from the inferior visual field (Davidson, 1991).

The horizontal palpebral fissure length of the aoudad (34.8 mm) is only a bit smaller than that of the cow (44.4 mm) and that of the horse (39.5 mm) (Wieser et al., 2013), which are both larger and heavier animals. It is however, considerably bigger than that reported for animals with similar sizes and weight such as the sheep (27.0 mm), goat (28.8 mm) (Wieser et al., 2013), dwarf goat (21.6 mm) (Olopade and Onwuka, 2004) and the Red Sokoto goat (25.0 mm) (Olopade and Onwuka, 2003). The cornea also follows this same trend and can be considered absolutely and relatively large. Its curvature was not evaluated but its external appearance is very prominent. Like in other ungulates the horizontal (transverse) corneal width is invariably considerably larger than the height (Henderson, 1950; Grinninger et al., 2010). The width and height were similar to the ones reported for the miniature horse, which were 25.8 mm and 19.4 mm respectively (Plummer et al., 2003).

The greenish tapetum lucidum observed is similar to the typical fibrosum type found in cow, sheep, goat and horse (Ollivier et al., 2004). The dark specks visible in the tapetal fundus of all aoudads investigates are identical to previously describe structures called "Stars of Winslow" (stelullae of Winslow) in other ungulates such as sheep, goats and horses. These structures represent deep choroidal vessel communications with other blood vessels from the choriocapillaris layer and the specks are the sites of tapetal penetration (Galán et al., 2006). The presence of this normal anatomic feature was not previously described in aoudads.

The linear avascular region in the aoudad fundus presumably represents a retinal specialization called a 'visual streak', which is similar to the macula in humans and the area centralis in dogs and cats, where an increased density of retinal neurons affords higher visual acuity. Early ophthalmoscopic observations of visual streaks reported a band-like thickening across the retina (Chievitz, 1889, 1891; Slonaker, 1897), which has since been shown by microscopic examination to be a high density of retinal ganglion cells. Although further histologic characterization is required to be able to define a visual streak in the aoudad, it is likely that the fundic morphology described in the aoudad fundus represents a visual streak considering the presence of a streak in other previously studied ungulates: cattle (Hebel, 1976), sheep (Hebel, 1976; Shinozaki et al., 2010), goats (Hughes and Whitteridge, 1973; Gonzalez-Soriano et al., 1997), giraffes (Coimbra et al., 2013), black rhinoceros (Pettigrew and Manger, 2008). The visual streak is not unique to ungulates. It has been found in other taxa including reptiles e.g. American garter snake (Wong, 1989), several species of birds e.g. Canada goose (Fernández-Juricic et al., 2011), ostrich (Boire et al., 2001), manx shearwater (Hayes et al., 1991), over 30 species of fish, and many other non-ungulate mammals including carnivores (spotted hyena Crocuta crocuta (Calderone et al., 2003)), aquatic mammals (common dolphin (Dral, 1983)), and marsupials (scrub wallaby (Tancred, 1981)). The visual streak determines visual acuity in a particular part of the visual field and its presence may have ecological correlations with habitat-type, anti-predator behaviors, and orientation behaviors (Johnson, 1901; Pumphrey, 1948; Luck, 1965; Hughes, 1977; Fernández-Juricic et al., 2011). The visual streak has been described to provide panoramic vision (Johnson, 1901; Vincent, 1912; Collin, 1999), and in combination with laterally placed eyes reduces the size of the blind area and offers a wide field of visual coverage (Hughes, 1977; Fernández-Juricic et al., 2011) thus reducing the need to sample visually by moving the eyes or head (Collin, 1999). Combined with the oval-shaped pupillary aperture, a visual streak in the aoudad would likely greatly enhance vision in the horizontal plane.

The STT is considered the gold standard test used to diagnose keratoconjunctivitis sicca (KCS) in domestic and wild animals. It is therefore important to perform a STT in all aoudads with ocular disease to rule out KCS as a cause of chronic eye disease such as corneal ulcers, conjunctivitis, keratitis and ocular discharge (Brooks, 2010; Trbolova et al., 2012). Although there has been no report of KCS in aoudads to date, it likely occurs in the species as it is a common ocular disease in most animals and human beings. It may be that the disease is underreported in aoudads due to the lack of knowledge of normal values for this test. When comparing STT values found in available studies of other species of ruminants, STT results in aoudads are quite high, similar but even higher to those reported for sheep (26.40 ± 17.70 mm/min) (Wieser *et al.*, 2013), llamas (17.3 ± 1.1 mm/min) (Trbolova *et al.*, 2012), goats (14.50 ± 3.78 mm/min) (Wieser *et al.*, 2013), and pigmy goats (15.8 ± 5.7 mm/min) (Broadwater *et al.*, 2007). Normal STT results obtained for the Barbary sheep (27.22 ± 3.6) are quite high comparing to other caprids (subfamily Caprinae) and other species of Artiodactyla. It is significantly higher than the one from llamas (P=0.0001), goats (P=0.0001) and pigmy goats (P=0.001). The observed STT mean value in Barbery sheep is higher than the one from sheep, however, due to the large variation reported for the sheep STT (SD = 17.70) (Wieser *et al.*, 2013), the analysis showed that the difference is not statistically significantly.

Normal conjunctival bacterial microbiota has been studied in several wild mammals such as the opossum (Pinard *et al.*, 2002), bison (Davidson *et al.*, 1999), deer (Dubay *et al.*, 2000), and elephant (Tuntivanich *et al.*, 2002). In the vast majority of these reports, gram-positive bacteria were the most common isolates and the present report is no exception. Both pathogenic and nonpathogenic bacteria were found in this investigation. *Escherichia coli*, *Enterobacter* sp and *Citrobacter* sp were isolated from the eyes of aoudads in this study. The presence of these gram-negative bacteria suggests possible eye contamination with fecal material and/or may represent a transient agent of the conjunctiva. Nonetheless, *Escherichia coli* was also isolated from normal conjunctival microbiota of dogs (Prado *et al.*, 2005; Wang *et al.*, 2008) and horses (Pisani *et al.*, 1997; Andrew *et al.*, 2003). *Enterobacter* sp and *Citrobacter* sp were isolated from the conjunctiva of clinically normal eyes of horses and human beings working as health professionals in a hospital environment (Pisani *et al.*, 1997; Trindade *et al.*, 2000). Additional studies are still necessary to try to determine whether or not some of these gram-negative bacteria are normal inhabitants of the aoudad's ocular microbiota. The label pathogenic versus non-pathogenic is misleading because it is known that in some cases of bacterial conjunctivitis, a formerly nonpathogenic conjunctival bacterium can overgrow and cause an imbalance of the ocular surface microbiota population, becoming pathogenic (Samuelson, 1999).

The Cochet–Bonnet esthesiometer estimates the degree of sensitivity of the cornea by evaluating the corneal touch threshold (Chan-Ling, 1989; Barrett *et al.*, 1991). The mean corneal touch threshold obtained in this investigation was similar to that of the foal (1.4 cm) (Brooks *et al.*, 2000), chinchilla (1.24 cm) (Lima *et al.*, 2010), Guinea pig (1.35 cm) (Wieser *et al.*, 2013) and rabbit (1.47 cm) (Wieser *et al.*, 2013), demonstrating that aoudads possess a less sensitive cornea compared to other species such as the adult horse, cat and cow (Wieser *et al.*, 2013). These results should be interpreted with caution because of the well-known low precision of the Cochet–Bonnet esthesiometer in the 0.5- to 2.0-cm filament length range (Wieser *et al.*, 2013). The aoudad's corneal sensitivity encountered in this investigation was exactly within that range. The pressure applied to the surface of the cornea by the examiner also can vary. It is known that these parameters affect this test results significantly (Boberg-Ans, 1956). In the present study, the temperature and humidity were not assessed in order to be able to correct the corneal sensitivity measurements with the nylon filament. Unfortunately, no formula or correction table exists at this time for the nylon filament currently used and the temperature or humidity conditions, which imposes a challenge for extrapolating corneal sensitivity data obtained with the Cochet-Bonnet esthesiometer. In light of all these possible variables and interferences produced by the examiner, some authors claim that a new esthesiometer, which can display the pressure applied to the surface of the cornea, should be created in order to make the measurement of the CTT more sensitive and comparisons between investigations more precise. Additionally, it might be worth considering a non-contact esthesiometer, since comparing to the Cochet-Bonnet esthesiometer the former allows for superior stimulus reproducibility and better control over stimulus characteristics, in addition to the ability for exploration of the response of all different types of neuro-receptors on the ocular surface (Golebiowski *et al.*, 2011).

Tonometry is a fundamental part of a complete ophthalmic evaluation in any animal species. The main value of tonometry lies in the ability to detect pressure increases as an important clinical sign of glaucoma. However, a normal range of values for each species needs to be established. IOP measurements in the aoudads using the rebound tonometer resulted in means and ranges that were slightly higher than those reported for most other wild and domestic ungulates (Ofri *et al.*, 2000, 2001; Willis *et al.*, 2000). For instance, normal reported mean IOP for sheep was 16.36 ± 2.19 mmHg (Pigatto *et al.*, 2011), which was significantly lower (P=0.0018) than that found in the aoudad (19.47 ± 3.9 mmHg). The aoudad's IOP seems to be similar to other ungulates with higher IOP such as the zebra (Ofri *et al.*, 1998) and dairy cattle (Gum *et al.*, 1998). However, comparison is difficult since most of the normal ranges for IOP previously reported in ungulates were obtained with applanation tonometers, and some even with indentation tonometry (Ofri *et al.*, 1998). Before comparing and extrapolating IOP data from one study to others, researchers need to make sure the tonometry method was the same. It was shown that the Tonovet rebound tonometer may significantly overestimate the IOP values compared to the applanation tonometer, at least in one study using normal Eurasian eagle owls (Jeong *et al.*, 2007). Another study conversely showed that results for the TonoVet-D calibration are similar to those obtained for dogs (Knollinger *et al.*, 2005). Even though the rebound tonometer is tolerated well by most animal species because of its rapid and minimal stress-inducing method, another factor to be considered when establishing IOP in wild and exotic species is stress. It is known that IOP values increase if the animal is firmly restrained, particularly in wild animal species (Jeong *et al.*, 2007). All animals examined in this study were physically restrained and thus it is possible that stress could have influenced our results, though care was taken to avoid neck pressure.

Ultrasonic corneal pachymetry is an accurate and reliable *in vivo* method to measure corneal thickness in animals and human beings (Korah *et al.*, 2000). It was shown that ultrasonic pachymetry set at a standard velocity of 1636 m/s overestimates CCT as compared to optical coherence tomography (Alario and Pirie, 2014). However, correlation between the two mentioned modalities is excellent. Mean central corneal thickness (CCT) acquired with an ultrasonic pachymeter has been the subject of a number of reports investigating the cornea of human beings (Korah *et al.*, 2000), several domestic (Stapleton and Peiffer, 1979; Gilger *et al.*, 1991, 1998), exotic and wild animals (Montiani-Ferreira *et al.*, 2006, 2008a, 2008b; Lima *et al.*, 2010). In our investigation, mean CCT of the aoudad was not significantly different between males and females. The aoudad CCT is slightly thicker than adult dogs (598.54 µm) (Alario and Pirie, 2014) and slightly thinner than the horse (785.60 µm) (Plummer *et al.*, 2003). It is similar to that of adult Saanen goats using a high-resolution 20-MHz A- and B-mode ultrasonography transducer (Ribeiro *et al.*, 2009).

Echobiometric data of the globe obtained using A- and B-mode ultrasonography were reported in children (Kurtz *et al.*, 2004) several domestic (Schiffer *et al.*, 1982; Rogers *et al.*, 1986; Cottrill *et al.*, 1989; Gilger *et al.*, 1998; Tuntivanich *et al.*, 2002; Plummer *et al.*, 2003; Ribeiro *et al.*, 2009), exotic and wild mammal species (Fernandes *et al.*, 2003; Hernández-Guerra *et al.*, 2007; Montiani-Ferreira *et al.*, 2008a; Lima *et al.*, 2010; Ruiz *et al.*, 2015). The aoudad´s axial globe length, lens thickness, and chamber depths were not significantly different according to the eye (left or right) studied or gender. This lack of difference was also observed in dog eyes and eyes of most other wild and exotic animals studied using B-mode ultrasonography. The eye of the aoudad is large in both ways, absolutely and relative to its body size. The axial globe length found for adult aoudads is larger than that obtained in other large mammals including cadaveric eyes of Ramboullet sheep (El-maghrabmy *et al.*, 1995), Ile de France Sheep (Brandão *et al.*, 2004) and Saneen goats (Ribeiro *et al.*, 2009). The dimension of the internal structures such as anterior chamber depth,

lens thickness and vitreous chamber depth follow the same pattern, being all comparable but larger than the sheep (Brandão *et al.*, 2004) and goat (Ribeiro *et al.*, 2009). Only the bovine (Potter *et al.*, 2008), buffalo (*Bos bubalis*) (Kassab, 2012; Assadnassab and Fartashvan, 2013) and the dromedary eye (Osuobeni and Hamidzada, 1999; Kassab, 2012) demonstrated similar echobiometric dimensions, with equivalent lens thickness and vitreous chamber depth even though these are considerable larger ungulates in terms of body size.

In conclusion, this study provides novel data for normal values and reference ranges for several ophthalmic tests and ocular biometric parameters in healthy aoudads. The eyes are large and laterally placed in the head with several anatomic features that are likely evolutionary adaptations for grazing, which was also previously observed in other prey species of ungulates, such as horses, sheep and cattle.

Often a complete ocular examination of zoo animals is not routinely performed (Townsend, 2010) due to limitations such as lack of appropriate instruments (ophthalmoscopes, tonometers), disposable diagnostic test material (such as STT strips, fluorescein strips and eyedrops) and proper facilities (safe, large dark rooms). Nevertheless, the results of this study may assist veterinarians and veterinary ophthalmologists in the diagnosis of ocular diseases in aoudads.

Acknowledgements

The authors wish to thank Gillian Shaw for her help in the preparation of this manuscript.

Conflict of interest

The authors declare that there is no conflict of interest.

References

Abáigar, T., Domené, M.A. and Cassinello, J. 2012. Characterization of the estrous cycle and reproductive traits of the aoudad (*Ammotragus lervia*) in captivity. Theriogenology 77, 1759-1766.

Alados, C. and Shackleton, D.M. 1997. Regional Summary. In, Shackleton, D.M. Wild Sheep and Goats and Their Relatives, Status Survey and Conservation Action Plan for Caprinae. Gland, Switzerland, IUCN, pp: 47-48.

Alario, A.F. and Pirie, C.G. 2014. Central corneal thickness measurements in normal dogs, a comparison between ultrasound pachymetry and optical coherence tomography. Vet. Ophthalmol. 17, 207-211.

Andrew, S.E., Nguyen, A., Jones, G.L. and Brooks, D.E. 2003. Seasonal effects on the aerobic bacterial and fungal conjunctival flora of normal thoroughbred brood mares in Florida. Vet. Ophthalmol. 6, 45-50.

Assadnassab, G. and Fartashvan, M. 2013. Ultrasonographic evaluation of buffalo eyes. Turk. J. Vet. Anim. Sci. 37, 395-39.

Barrett, P.M., Scagliotti, R.H., Merideth, R.E., Jackson, P.A. and Alarcon, F. 1991. Absolute corneal sensitivity and corneal trigeminal nerve anatomy in normal dogs. Vet. Comp. Ophthalmol. 1, 245-254.

Boberg-Ans, J. 1956. On the corneal sensitivity. Acta Ophthalmol. 34, 149-162.

Boire, D., Dufour, J.S., Theoret, H. and Ptito, M. 2001. Quantatative analysis of the retinal ganglion cell layer in the ostrich, Struthio Camelus. Brain Behav. Evol. 58, 343-355.

Brandão, C.V.S., Chiurciu, J.L.V., Ranzani, J.J.T., Mamprim, M.J., Zanini, M., Rodrigues, G.N., Cremonini, D.N., Lima, L.S.A., Peixoto, T.P., Marinho, L.F.L.P. and Teixeira, C.R. 2004. Comparação entre ultra-sonografia modo-A, modo-B e medidas diretas em olhos de ovinos. Braz. J. Vet. Res. Anim. Sci. 41, 68-69.

Brenner, D.J., Stokking, L., Donovan, T.A. and Lamberski, N. 2009. Pemphigus foliaceus in a barbary sheep (*Ammotragus lervia*). Vet. Rec. 165, 509-510.

Broadwater, J.J., Schorling, J.J., Herring, I.P. and Pickett, J.P. 2007. Ophthalmic examination findings in adult pygmy goats (*Capra hicus*). Vet. Ophthalmol. 10, 269-273.

Brooks, D.E., Clark, C.K. and Lester, G.D. 2000. Cochet-Bonnet aesthesiometer-determined corneal sensitivity in neonatal foals and adult horses. Vet. Ophthalmol. 3, 133-137.

Brooks, D.E. 2010. Ocular diseases, In, Taylor F.G.R., Brazil T., Hillyer M.H. (Ed.), Diagnostic Techniques in Equine Medicine. 2nd ed. Elsevier Limited, Amsterdam, pp: 305-322.

Calderone, J.B., Reese, B.E. and Jacobs, G.H. 2003. Topography of photoreceptors and retinal ganglion cells in the spotted hyena (*Crocuta crocuta*). Brain Behav. Evol. 62, 182-192.

Candela, M.G., Serrano, E., Martinez-Carrasco, C., Martín-Atance, P., Cubero, M.J., Alonso, F. and Leon, L. 2009. Coinfection is an important factor in epidemiological studies, the first serosurvey of the aoudad (*Ammotragus lervia*). Eur. J. Clin. Microbiol. Infect. Dis. 28,481-489.

Cassinello, J., Cuzin, F., Jdeidi, T., Masseti, M., Nader, I. and de Smet, K. 2008. *Ammotragus lervia*. The IUCN Red List of Threatened Species. Version 2014.3. <www.iucnredlist.org>. Downloaded on 12 January 2015.

Cassinello, J., Serrano, E., Calabuig, G. and Pérez, J.M. 2004. Range expansion of an exotic ungulate (*Ammotragus lervia*) in southern Spain, Ecological and conservation concerns. Biodivers. Conserv. 13, 851-866.

Cassinello, J. 1998. *Ammotragus lervia*, a review on systematics, biology, ecology and distribution. Ann. Zool. Fenn. 35, 149-162.

Chan-Ling, T. 1989. Sensitivity and neural organization of the cat cornea. Vet. Comp. Ophthalmol. 30, 1075-1082.

Chievitz, J.H. 1889. Untersuchungen über die Area centralis retinae. Arch Anat Physiol Anat Abt Suppl. 139-194.

Chievitz, J.H. 1891. Ueber das Vorkommen der area centralis retinae in den höheren Wirbetierklassen. R. Anat. Entwichlingsgesch. Suppl. 139, 311-334.

Cho, H.S., Shin, S.S. and Park, N.Y. 2006. Balantidiasis in the gastric lymph nodes of Barbary sheep (*Ammotragus lervia*), an incidental finding. J. Vet. Sci. 7, 207-209.

Coimbra, J.P., Hart, N.S., Collin, S.P. and Manger, P.R. 2013. Scene from above, retinal topography and spatial resolving power in the giraffe (*Giraffa camelopardalis*). J. Comp. Neurol. 521, 2042-2057.

Collin, S.P. 1999. Behavioural ecology and retinal cell topography. In Adaptive Mechanisms in the Ecology of Vision. Eds., Archer, S., Djamgoz, M.B., Loew, E. Partridge, J.C. and Vallerga, S. Kluwer Academic Publishers, Dordrecht, pp: 509-535.

Cottrill, N.B., Banks, W.J. and Pechman, R.D. 1989. Ultrasonographic and biometric evaluation of the eye and orbit of dogs. Am. J. Vet. Res. 50, 898-903.

Crenshaw, C.C., Martin, L.M., Mains C.R., Wright, R.D., Dart, M.G., Perkins, R.M., Purdy, P.H. and Ericsson, S.A. 2000. The use of buck and ram extenders and two packaging systems to cryopreserve aoudad (*Ammotragus lervia*) spermatozoa. Theriogenology 54, 69-74.

Davidson, H.J., Vestweber, J.G., Brightman, A.H., Van Slyke, T.H., Cox, L.K. and Chengappa, M.M. 1999. Ophthalmic examination and conjunctival bacteriologic culture results from a herd of North American bison. J. Am. Vet. Med. Assoc. 215, 1142-1144.

Davidson, M.G. 1991. Equine ophthalmology. In, Gelatt, K.N. (Ed.), Veterinary Ophthalmology. 2nd ed. Lea & Febiger, Philadelphia, pp: 576-610.

Dral, A.D.G. 1983. The retinal ganglion cells of *Delphinus delphis* and their distibution. Aquat Mamm. 10, 57-68.

Dubay, S.A., Williams, E.S. and Mills, K. 2000. Bacteria and nematodes in the conjunctiva of mule deer from Wyoming and Utah. J. Wildl. Dis. 36, 783-787.

El-maghrabmy, H.M., Nyland, T.G. and Bellhorn, R.W. 1995. Ultrasonographic and biometric evaluation of sheep and cattle eyes. Vet. Radiol. Ultras. 36, 148-151.

Fernandes, A., Bradley, D.V., Tigges, M., Tigges, J. and Herndon, J.G. 2003. Ocular measurements throughout the adult life span of rhesus monkeys. Invest. Ophthalmol. Vis. Sci. 44, 2373-2380.

Fernández-Juricic, E., Moore, B.A., Doppler, M., Freeman, J., Blackwell, B.F., Lima, S.L. and

DeVault, T.L. 2011. Testing the terrain hypothesis, Canada geese see their world laterally and obliquely. Brain Behav. Evol. 77, 147-158.

Galán, A., Martín-Suárez, E.M. and Molleda, J.M. 2006 Ophthalmoscopic characteristics in sheep and goats, comparative study. J. Vet. Med. A Physiol. Pathol. Clin. Med. 53, 205-208.

Ghaffari, M.S., Hajikhani, R., Sahebjam, F., Akbarein, H. and Golezardy, H. 2012. Intraocular pressure and Schirmer tear test results in clinically normal long-eared hedgehogs (Hemiechinus auritus), reference values. Vet. Ophthalmol. 15, 206-209.

Gilger, B.C., Davidson, M.G. and Howard, P.B. 1998. Keratometry, ultrasonic biometry, and prediction of intraocular lens power in the feline eye. Am. J. Vet. Res. 59, 131-134.

Gilger, B.C., Whitley, R.D. and Mclaughlin, S.A. 1991. Canine corneal thickness measured by ultrasonic pachymetry. Am. J. Vet. Res. 10, 1570-1572.

Golebiowski, B., Papas, E. and Stapleton, F. 2011. Assessing the sensory function of the ocular surface: implications of use of a non-contact air jet aesthesiometer versus the Cochet-Bonnet aesthesiometer. Exp. Eye Res. 92, 408-413.

Gonzalez-Soriano, J., Mayayo-Vicente, S., Martinez-Sainz, P., Contreras-Rodriguez, J. and Rodriguez-Veiga, E. 1997. A quantitative study of ganglion cells in the goat retina. Anat. Histol. Embryol. 26, 39-44.

Grinninger, P., Skalicky, M. and Nell, B. 2010. Evaluation of healthy equine eyes by use of retinoscopy, keratometry, and ultrasonographic biometry. Am. J. Vet. Res. 71, 677-681.

Gum, G.G., Gelatt, K.N., Miller, D.N. and MacKay, E.O. 1998. Intraocular pressure in normal dairy cattle. Vet. Ophthalmol. 1, 159-161.

Hamon, M.H. and Heap, R.B. 1990. Progesterone and oestrogen concentrations in plasma of Barbary sheep (aoudad, Ammotragus lervia) compared with those of domestic sheep and goats during pregnancy. J. Reprod. Fertil. 90, 207-211.

Hayes, B., Martin, G.R. and Brooke, M.D.L. 1991. Novel area serving binocular vision in the retina of procellariiform seabirds. Brain Behav. Evol. 37, 79-84.

Hebel, R. 1976. Distribution of retinal ganglion cells in five mammalian species (pig, sheep, ox, horse, dog). Anat. Embryol. 150, 45-51.

Henderson, T. 1950. Principles of Ophthalmology. Heinemann Medical Books. London, UK.

Hernández-Guerra, A.M., Rodilla, V. and López-Murcia, M.M. 2007. Ocular biometry in the adult anesthetized ferret (Mustela putorius furo). Vet. Ophthalmol. 10, 50-52.

Hilton-Taylor, C. 2000. IUCN Red List of Threatened Species. 1st ed. IUCN, Gland, Switzerland.

Hughes, A. 1977. The topography of vision in mammals of contrasting life style, comparative optics and retinal organization. In, The visual system in vertebrates (Ed. by F. Crescitelli), New York, Springer-Verlag, pp: 615-756.

Hughes, A. and Whitteridge, D. 1973. Receptive Fields And Topographical Organization Of Goat Retinal Ganglion-Cells. Vision Res. 13, 1101-1114.

Jeong, M.B., Kim, Y.J., Yi, N.Y., Park, S.A., Kim, W.T., Kim, S.E., Chae, J.M., Kim, J.T., Lee, H. and Seo, K.M. 2007. Comparison of the rebound tonometer (TonoVet) with the applanation tonometer (TonoPen XL) in normal Eurasian Eagle owls (Bubo bubo). Vet. Ophthalmol. 10, 376-379.

Johnson, G.L. 1901. Contributions to the comparative anatomy of the mammalian eye chiefly based on ophthalmoscopic examination. Philos. T. R. Soc. B 194, 1-82.

Kassab, A. 2012. Ultrasonographic and macroscopic anatomy of the enucleated eyes of the buffalo (Bos bubalis) and the one-humped camel (Camelus dromedarius) of different ages. Anat. Histol. Embryol. 41, 7-11.

Kingdon, J. 1997. The Kingdon Field Guide to African Mammals. 1st ed. Academic Press Ltd, London, pp: 496.

Knollinger, A.M., La Croix, N.C., Barrett, P.M. and Miller, P.E. 2005. Evaluation of a rebound tonometer for measuring intraocular pressure in dogs and horses. J. Am. Vet. Med. Assoc. 227, 244-248.

Korah, S., Thomas, R. and Muliyil, J. 2000. Comparison of optical and ultrasound pachymetry. Indian J. Ophthalmol. 48, 279-283.

Kudirkiene, E., Zilinskas, H. and Siugzdaite, J. 2006. Microbial flora of the dog eyes. Vet. Zootech-Lith 34, 18-21.

Kurtz, D., Manny, R. and Hussein, M. 2004. Variability of the ocular component measurements in children using A-scan ultrasonography. Optometry Vision Sci. 81, 35-43.

Lima, L., Montiani-Ferreira, F., Tramontin, M., Leigue dos Santos, L., Machado, M., Lange, R.R. and Russ, H. 2010. The chinchilla eye, morphologic observations, echobiometric findings and reference values for selected ophthalmic diagnostic tests. Vet. Ophthalmol. 13 Suppl. 14-25.

Luck, C.P. 1965. The comparative morphology of the eyes of certain African suiformes. Vision Res. 5, 283-297.

Manca, L., Pirastru, M., Mereu, P., Multineddu, C., Olianas, A., el Sherbini, el S., Franceschi, P., Pellegrini, M. and Masala, B. 2006. Barbary sheep (Ammotragus lervia), the structure of the adult beta-globin gene and the functional properties of its hemoglobin. Comp. Biochem. Physiol. B Biochem. Mol. Biol. 145, 214-219.

Martins, B.C., Oriá, A.P., Souza, A.L., Campos, C.F., Almeida,D.E.,Duarte,R.A.,Soares,C.P.,Zuanon,J.A., Neto, C.B., Duarte, J.M., Schocken-Iturrino, R.P. and Laus, J.L. 2007. Ophthalmic patterns of captive brown brocket deer (*Mazama gouazoubira*). J. Zoo Wildl. Med. 38, 526-532.

Mayo, E., Ortiz, J., Martínez-Carrasco, C., Garijo, M.M., Espeso, G., Hervías, S. and Ruiz de Ybáñez, M.R. 2013. First description of gastrointestinal nematodes of Barbary sheep (*Ammotragus lervia),* the case of *Camelostrongylus mentulatus* as a paradigm of phylogenic and specific relationship between the parasite and its ancient host. Vet. Res. Commun. 37, 209-215.

McGreevy, P. 2004. Equine Behavior, A Guide for Veterinarians and Equine Scientists. 1st ed. Saunders, Philadelphia.

McLelland, D.J., Kirkland, P.D., Rose, K.A., Dixon, R.J. and Smith, N. 2005. Serologic responses of Barbary sheep (*Ammotragus lervia*), Indian antelope (*Antilope cervicapra*), wallaroos (*Macropus robustus*), and chimpanzees (*Pan troglodytes*) to an inactivated encephalomyocarditis virus vaccine. J. Zoo Wildl. Med. 36, 69-73.

Mereu, P., Palici, di Suni M., Manca, L. and Masala, B. 2008. Complete nucleotide mtDNA sequence of Barbary sheep (*Ammotragus lervia*). DNA Seq. 19, 241-245.

Montiani-Ferreira, F., Mattos, B.C. and Russ, H.H. 2006. Reference values for selected ophthalmic diagnostic tests of the ferret (*Mustela putorius furo*). Vet. Ophthalmol. 9, 209-213.

Montiani-Ferreira, F., Shaw, G., Mattos, B.C., Russ, H.H. and Vilani, R.G. 2008a. Reference values for selected ophthalmic diagnostic tests of the capuchin monkey (*Cebus apella*). Vet. Ophthalmol. 3, 197-201.

Montiani-Ferreira, F., Truppel, J., Tramontin, M.H., Vilani, R.G. and Lange, R.R. 2008b. The capybara eye, clinical tests, anatomic and biometric features. Vet. Ophthalmol. 11, 386-394.

Morikawa, V.M., Zimpel, C.K., Paploski, I.A., Lara, Mdo, C., Villalobos, E.M., Romaldini, A.H., Okuda, L.H., Biondo, A.W. and Barros Filho, I.R. 2014. Occurrences of anti-*Toxoplasma gondii* and anti-*Neospora caninum* antibodies in Barbary sheep at Curitiba zoo, southern Brazil. Rev. Bras. Parasitol. Vet. 23, 255-259.

Mullin, G.S. and Rubinfeld, R.S. 1997. The antibacterial activity of topical anesthetics. Cornea 16, 662-665.

Münster, P., Fechner, K., Völkel, I., von Buchholz, A. and Czerny, C.P. 2013. Distribution of *Mycobacterium avium* ssp. paratuberculosis in a German zoological garden determined by IS900 semi-nested and quantitative real-time PCR. Vet. Microbiol. 163, 116-123.

Murphy, J. and Arkins, S. 2007. Equine learning behaviour. Behav. Processes 76, 1-13.

Ofri, R., Horowitz, I.H. and Kass, P.H. 1998. Tonometry in three herbivorous wildlife species. Vet. Ophthalmol. 1, 21-24.

Ofri, R., Horowitz, I.H. and Kass, P.H. 2000. How low can we get? Tonometry in the Thomson gazelle (*Gazella thomsoni*). J. Glaucoma 9, 187-189.

Ofri, R., Horowitz, I.H., Levison, M. and Kass, P.H. 2001. Intraocular pressure and tear production in captive eland and fallow deer. J. Zoo Wildl. Med. 37, 387-390.

Ollivier, F.J., Samuelson, D.A., Brooks, D.E., Lewis, P.A., Kallberg, M.E. and Komáromy, A.M. 2004. Comparative morphology of the tapetum lucidum (among selected species). Vet. Ophthalmol. 7, 11-22.

Olopade, J.O. and Onwuka, S.K. 2003. A preliminary investigation into some aspects of the craniofacial indices of the Red Sokoto (Maradi) goat in Nigeria. Folia Vet. 47, 57-59.

Olopade, J.O. and Onwuka, S.K. 2004. Morphometric studies of the cranio-facial region of the west african dwarf goat in Nigeria. Int. J. Morphol. 22, 145-148.

Osuobeni, E.P. and Hamidzada, W.A. 1999. Ultrasonographic determination of the dimensions of ocular components in enucleated eyes of the one-humped camel (*Camelus dromedarius*). Res. Vet. Sci. 67, 125-129.

Pence, D.B. and Gray, G.G. 1981. Elaeophorosis in Barbary sheep and mule deer from the Texas Panhandle. J. Wildl. Dis. 17, 49-56.

Pettigrew, J.D. and Manger, P.R. 2008. Retinal ganglion cell density of the black rhinoceros (*Diceros bicornis*), Calculating visual resolution. Visual Neurosci. 25, 215-220.

Pigatto, J.A.T.P., Pereira, F.Q., Albuquerque, L., Corrêa, L.F.D., Bercht, B.S., Hünning, P.S., Silva, A.A.R. and De Freitas, L.V.R.P. 2011. Intraocular pressure measurement in sheep using an applanation tonometer. Rev. Ceres 58, 685-689.

Pinard, C.L., Brightman, A.H., Yeary, T.J., Everson, T.D., Cox, L.K., Chengappa, M.M. and Davidson, H.J. 2002. Normal conjunctival flora in the North American opossum (*Didelphis virginiana*) and raccoon (*Procyon lotor*). J. Wildl. Dis. 38, 851-855.

Pirastru, M., Multineddu, C., Mereu, P., Sannai, M., El Sherbini, el S., Hadjisterkotis, E., Nàhlik, A., Franceschi, P., Manca, L. and Masala, B. 2009. The sequence and phylogenesis of the globin genes of Barbary sheep (*Ammotragus lervia*), goat (*Capra hircus*), European mouflon (*Ovis aries musimon*) and Cyprus mouflon (*Ovis aries ophion*). Comp. Biochem. Physiol. 4, 168-173.

Pisani, E.H.R., Barros, P.S.M. and Avila, F.A. 1997. Microbiota conjuntival normal de eqüinos. Braz. J.

Vet. Res. Anim. Sci. 34, 261-265.

Plummer, C.E, Ramsey, D.T. and Hauptman, J.G. 2003. Assessment of corneal thickness, intraocular pressure, optical corneal diameter, and axial globe dimensions in Miniature horses. Am. J. Vet. Res. 64, 661-665.

Portas, T.J., Bryant, B.R., Jones, S.L., Humphreys, K., Gilpin, C.M. and Rose, K.A. 2009. Investigation and diagnosis of nontuberculous mycobacteriosis in a captive herd of aoudad (*Ammotragus lervia*). J. Zoo Wildl. Med. 40, 306-315.

Potter, T.J., Hallowell, G.D. and Bowen, I.M. 2008. Ultrasonographic anatomy of the bovine eye. Vet. Radiol. Ultras. 49, 172-175.

Prado, M.R., Rocha, M.F., Brito, E.H., Girão, M.D., Monteiro, A.J., Teixeira, M.F. and Sidrim, J.J. 2005. Survey of bacterial microorganisms in the conjuntival sac of clinically normal dogs and dogs with ulcerative keratitis in Fortaleza, Ceará, Brazil. Vet. Ophthalmol. 8, 33-37.

Prince, J.H. 1956. Comparative Anatomy of the Eye. Charles C Thomas, Springfield.

Pumphrey, R.J. 1948. The theory of the fovea. J. Exp. Biol. 25, 299-312.

Ribeiro, A.P., Silva, M.L., Rosa, J.P., Souza, S.F., Teixeira, I.A. and Laus, J.L. 2009. Ultrasonographic and echobiometric findings in the eyes of Saanen goats of different ages. Vet. Ophthalmol. 12, 313-317.

Rogers, M., Cartee, R.E., Miller, W. and Ibrahim, A.K. 1986. Evaluation of the extirpated equine eye using B-mode ultrasonography. Vet. Radiol. 27, 24-29.

Ruiz, T., Campos, W.N., Peres, T.P., Gonçalves, G.F., Ferraz, R.H., Néspoli, P.E., Sousa, V.R. and Ribeiro, A.P. 2015. Intraocular pressure, ultrasonographic and echobiometric findings of juvenile Yacare caiman (*Caiman yacare*) eye. Vet. Ophthalmol. 1, 40-45.

Samuelson, D.A. 1999. Ophthalmic anatomy. In, Gelatt, K. N. (Ed.), Veterinary Ophthalmology. 3rd ed. Lippincott Williams and Wilkins, Philadelphia, pp: 31-50.

Santiago-Moreno, J., Castaño, C., Toledano-Díaz, A., Esteso, M.C., López-Sebastián, A., Guerra, R., Ruiz, M.J., Mendoza, N., Luna, C., Cebrián-Pérez, J.A. and Hildebrandt, T.B. 2013. Cryopreservation of aoudad (*Ammotragus lervia sahariensis*) sperm obtained by transrectal ultrasound-guided massage of the accessory sex glands and electroejaculation. Theriogenology 79, 383-391.

Shinozaki, A., Hosaka, Y., Imagawa, T. and Uehara, M. 2010. Topography of ganglion cells and photoreceptors in the sheep retina. J. Comp. Neurol. 518, 2305-2315.

Slonaker, J.R. 1897. A comparative study of the area of acute vision in vertebrates. J. Morphol. 13, 445-494.

Sprague, W., Helft, Z., Parnell, J., Schmoll, J., Love, G. and Banks, M. 2013. Pupil shape is adaptive for many species. J. Vision. 13, 607.

Stapleton, S. and Peiffer, R. 1979. Specular microscopic observations of the clinically normal canine corneal endothelium. Am. J. Vet. Res. 40, 1803-1804.

Stuart, C. and Stuart, T. 1997. Field Guide to the Larger Mammals of Africa. 3rd ed. Struik Publishers, Cape Town.

Tancred, E. 1981. The distribution and sizes of ganglion cells in the retinas of five Australian marsupials. J. Comp. Neurol. 196, 585-603.

Townsend, W.M. 2010. Examination techniques and therapeutic regimens for the ruminant and camelid eye. Vet. Clin. North Am. Food. Anim. 26, 437-458.

Trbolova, A., Gionfriddo, J.R. and Ghaffari, M.S. 2012. Results of Schirmer tear test in clinically normal llamas (*Lama glama*). Vet. Ophthalmol. 15, 383-385.

Trindade, R.C., Bonfim, A.C.R. and Resende, M.A. 2000. Conjunctival Microbial Flora of Clinically Normal Persons Who Work in a Hospital Environment. Braz. J. Microbiol. 31, 12-16.

Tuntivanich, P., Soontornvipart, K., Tuntivanich, N., Wongaumnuaykul, S. and Briksawan, P. 2002. Conjunctival microflora in clinically normal Asian elephants in Thailand. Vet. Res. Commun. 26, 251-254.

Vincent, S.B. 1912. The mammalian eye. J. Anim. Behav. 2, 249-255.

Wacher, T., Baha El Din, S., Mikhail, G. and Baha El Din, M. 2002. New observations of the "extinct" Aoudad *Ammotragus lervia ornata* in Egypt. Oryx 36, 301-304.

Walls, G.L. 1943. The vertebrate eye and its adaptive radiation. Michigan, The Cranbrook Press.

Wang, L., Pan, Q., Zhang, L., Xue, Q., Cui, J. and Qi, C. 2008. Investigation of bacterial microorganisms in the conjunctival sac of clinically normal dogs and dogs with ulcerative keratitis in Beijing, China. Vet. Ophthalmol. 11, 145-149.

Wieser, B., Tichy, A. and Nell, B. 2013. Correlation between corneal sensitivity and quantity of reflex tearing in cows, horses, goats, sheep, dogs, cats, rabbits, and guinea pigs. Vet. Ophthalmol. 16, 251-262.

Willis, A.M., Anderson, D.E., Gemensky, A.J., Wilkie, D.A. and Silveira, F. 2000. Evaluation of intraocular pressure in eyes of clinically normal llamas and alpacas. Am. J. Vet. Res. 61, 1542-1544.

Wong, R.O.L. 1989. Morphology and distribution of neurons in the retina of the American garter snake Thamnophis sirtalis. J. Comp. Neurol. 283, 587-601.

Yeruham, I., David, D., Brenner, J., Goshen, T. and Perl, S. 2004. Malignant catarrhal fever in a Barbary sheep (*Ammotragus lervia*). Vet. Rec. 155, 463-465.

7

Foreign body-induced changes in the reticular contraction pattern of sheep observed with M-mode ultrasonography

A.A. Morgado[1,*], M.C.A. Sucupira[1], G.R. Nunes[1] and S.C.F. Hagen[2]

[1]*Department of Clinical Science, Faculdade de Medicina Veterinária e Zootecnia da Universidade de São Paulo, 05508 270, Sao Paulo, SP, Brazil,*

[2]*Department of Surgery, Faculdade de Medicina Veterinária e Zootecnia da Universidade de São Paulo, 05508 270, Sao Paulo, SP, Brazil*

Abstract

In the pre-experimental period of a clinical trial, an apparently clinically healthy sheep fitted with ruminal and abomasal cannulas showed changes in the reticular contraction pattern visualized in M-mode ultrasonogram. Radiographic examination revealed a blunt metal screw in its reticulum. By the time change in the reticular motility through the ultrasound examination was detected, the animal had still not expressed any behavioral changes. A description of the clinical case, follow-up of the findings and laboratory data, like white blood cell count, serum pepsinogen and fibrinogen concentrations, were presented. The foreign body was removed through the ruminal cannula and reticular contraction tended to normal. An association of the contraction pattern with measured clinical data was possible, leading to the conclusion that use of M-mode ultrasonography has a potential application in similar clinical situations.

Keywords: Blunt object, M-mode curve, Reticulum, Ruminant.

Introduction

Ultrasonography has been considered an excellent diagnostic tool to investigate disorders of the pre-stomachs, abomasum and intestines of ruminants. Indeed, this technique is non-invasive, has no known side effect, provides images in real time and does not require sedation (Braun, 2009).

This technique has been used successfully to evaluate the rumen, reticulum, omasum, abomasum and some portions of intestines, providing important information to clinicians, avoiding the need of invasive diagnostic procedures (Streeter and Step, 2007; Braun *et al.*, 2011; Braun *et al.*, 2013a,b).

Despite its potential and possibilities, there is limited literature available and the references found used only B-mode (Streeter and Step, 2007; Braun *et al.*, 2011; Braun *et al.*, 2013a,b). No records on utilization of pre-stomachs ultrasound in adult sheep were found (SCOPUS, PUBMED, GOOGLE SCHOLAR, researched on March of 2015). In Brazil, there is scant reference to ruminant gastrointestinal ultrasound and no specific publication on ultrasound of pre-stomach was identified. One of the authors, in his 25 years of activity in local market, registered only sporadic use of gastrointestinal ultrasound in ruminants, most of which in academic environment.

A detailed analysis of the movement of the reticulum is necessary to obtain significant information, and B-mode ultrasound can be used to observe the frequency and amplitude of the reticular phase contraction as well as its speed and the duration of the organ relaxation (Streeter and Step, 2007; Braun, 2009). In M-mode, the behavior of a reading line during a certain period is represented, and temporal changes can be observed in the generated graph. In our experience, the biphasic curve obtained in M-mode representing the reticular contraction facilitates its evaluation; standardization is easier and the measured points of dynamic aspects of reticular contraction are precisely shown.

Case Details

The technique using M-mode ultrasonography was standardized in an effort to design a study in which the reticular motility of sheep that received ranitidine intravenously would be evaluated (Morgado *et al.*, 2014). For this experiment all sheep had ruminal and abomasal cannulas. The animals were examined while standing, held by a halter with no additional mechanical or chemical restraint. Hair was clipped at a small area (2×3 cm), caudal and adjacent to the sternum. Scanning was performed with 3.5-5.0 MHz probe, adjusted to 15 cm of depth. Scan head was positioned caudal and adjacent to the xiphoid cartilage in the medial plane and scan beam directed cranially (max 30°) (Fig. 1), applying slight pressure until capturing a representative image. The images obtained were printed on thermal paper through a Sony UP701 video printer.

During the standardization of the technique, a constant pattern of reticular contraction curves was observed. The reticular contraction waves viewed by M-mode ultrasonography of the animal in question were particularly well defined and had the standard biphasic pattern (Fig. 2) (Akester and Titchen, 1969;

*Corresponding Author: Aline A. Morgado. Department of Clinical Science, Faculdade de Medicina Veterinária e Zootecnia da Universidade de São Paulo, 05508 270, Sao Paulo, SP, Brazil. E-mail: *aline.morgado@usp.br*

Streeter and Step, 2007; Braun, 2009; Kandeel *et al.*, 2009) and triphasic pattern (Braun and Rauch, 2008) during rumination. Suddenly, lower amplitude in both contraction phases and longer return time to the starting position were observed in comparison with their previous examinations (Fig. 3).

The B-mode ultrasonogram showed minor signs of a little quantity of fibrin and low amount of totally anechoic content around the reticulum, which were interpreted as signs of non-specific inflammation. Clinically, only bruxism and mild dehydration were noted.

The initial suspicion was abomasal problems resulting from the cannula surgery that occurred one month prior to the change in M-mode pattern, so the animal was forwarded to the diagnostic imaging section and was examined by contrasted radiographic exam with the administration of 50 ml of barium sulfate through the abomasal cannula (day 0). The images were obtained

with the animal in standing position, with the current technique (KV 60, MAS 3.2) and right-left lateral projection.

The radiographic examination revealed the presence of a blunt screw in the animal's reticulum (Fig. 4). No sign of reticular commitment was identified. Because the animal was fitted with a ruminal cannula, it was possible to remove the gastric contents and to retrieve the blunt screw in the reticulum by direct palpation. During the process, no adherence to the mucosa was noted. As the ruminal content had an acid smell, healthy contents were replaced via the ruminal cannula. After these procedures, the animal was more active and showed appetite.

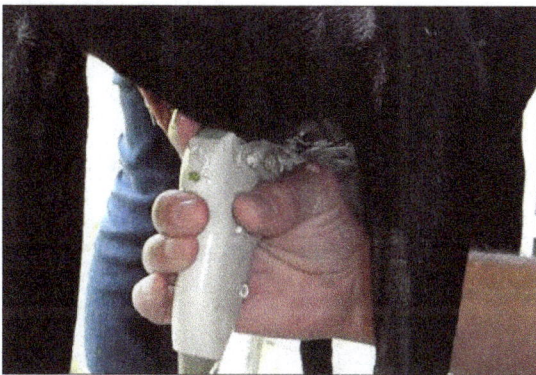

Fig. 1. Scanning was performed with the probe positioned caudal and adjacent to the xiphoid cartilage in the medial plane and directed cranially (max 30º).

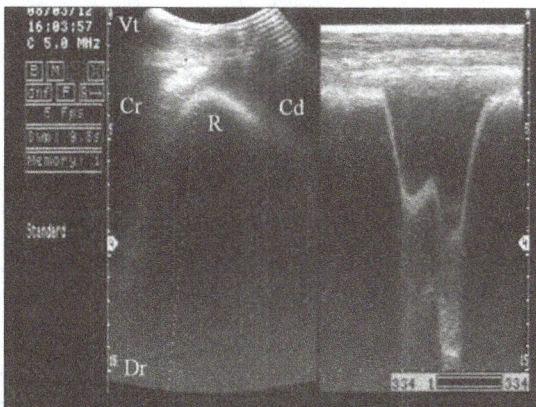

Fig. 3. B-mode (left) and M-mode (right) ultrasonographic images of an abnormal biphasic pattern of reticular contraction of the same animal shown in Fig. 2. (Cr = Cranial; Cd = Caudal; Vt = Ventral abdominal wall; Dr = Dorsal abdominal wall; R = Reticulum).

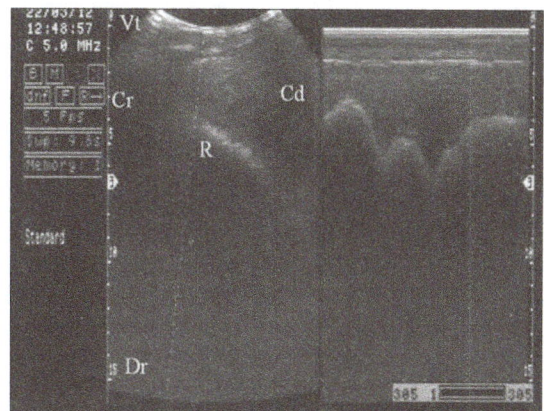

Fig. 2. B-mode (left) and M-mode (right) ultrasonographic images of the normal biphasic pattern of reticular contraction in a cannulated sheep before swallowing a foreign body. (Cr = Cranial; Cd = Caudal; Vt = Ventral abdominal wall; Dr = Dorsal abdominal wall; R = Reticulum).

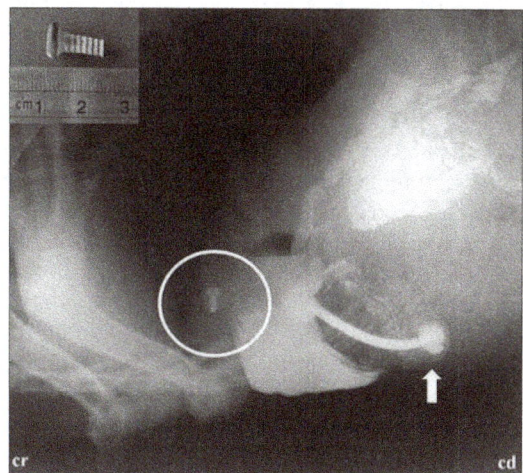

Fig. 4. Radiographic image revealing the presence of blunt screw in the reticulum of a sheep (circle). The left small image shows the size of the screw removed from the animal. Animal was standing, right-left lateral projection. The circle shows the screw in the reticulum; the white arrow points the abomasal cannula. (Cr = Cranial; Cd = Caudal).

A non-steroidal anti-inflammatory drug (2.2 mg/kg of flunixin meglumine) was administered intravenously for three consecutive days, and preventive antibiotic therapy with penicillin (40,000 IU of benzathine penicillin/kg of body weight) was administered intramuscularly for five days (day 0 to 6).

Daily blood samples were collected before, during and after treatment to determine the blood count (automatic hematological counter, ABC Vet, ABX, Gurnee, Illinois, USA), differential leukocyte count (evaluation of a blood smear by microscopy), and serum fibrinogen(Schalm *et al.*, 1981) and pepsinogen (Paynter, 1992) concentrations.

On day 1, the animal showed leukocytosis $(14.9 \times 10^9$ leukocytes/L) with neutrophilia $(12.5 \times 10^9$ neutrophils/L) (Fig. 5). These findings in addition to the B-mode ultrasonography images confirmed a mild inflammatory process. The serum total protein was 88 g/L, and the cell volume was normal.

On subsequent days, the leukocyte count returned to the normal range for sheep, with a neutrophil: lymphocyte rate close to ideal for small ruminants(Byers and Kramer, 2010). Serum pepsinogen (Fig. 6) has increasedon day 0 (8.89 IU/L), reflecting changes in the gastrointestinal tract, and returned to normal values on day 1 (Mesarič, 2005). The fibrinogen concentration has increased on day 2 (Byers and Kramer, 2010) (Fig. 6).

After the removal of the screw, the animal showed occasional kyphosis but all other clinical parameters were normal; it presented an appetite and the rumen was filled. Although the animal had mild dehydration, the PCV was within normal range and the total protein values were close to normal.

From day 1 to the last ultrasonographic examination (day 4), M-mode sonography revealed a biphasic pattern of reticular contraction, with a longer return time in comparison with their previous examinations (Fig. 7).

Discussion

Radiography is the gold standard for identifying metallic foreign bodies in the forestomach of small ruminants. The gas content in the gastric compartments is a physical barrier for the use of ultrasound and an obstacle for the detection of foreign bodies by ultrasonography. M-mode ultrasonography, however, identified the effects of the presence of a foreign body on reticular motility by representing a contraction curve, thereby enabling measurement. In this sheep, changes in the pattern of reticulum contraction were observed even before clinical manifestations were noted, showing the potential of ultrasonography. M-mode ultrassonography can be an important tool to monitor reticular contraction, including the possibility of diagnostic support in foreign body ingestion.

Conflict of interest

The authors declare that there is no conflict of interest.

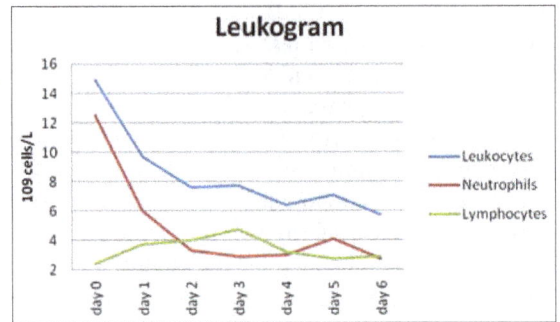

Fig. 5. Leukogram changes of the sheep from the day of diagnosis of a foreign body up to the six subsequent days.

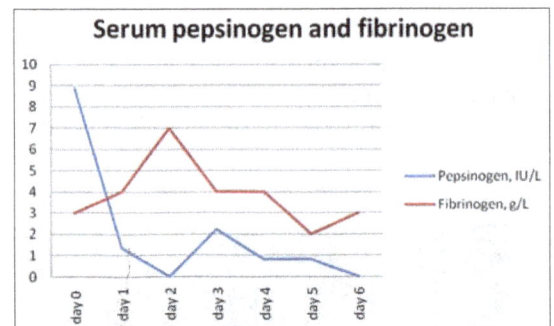

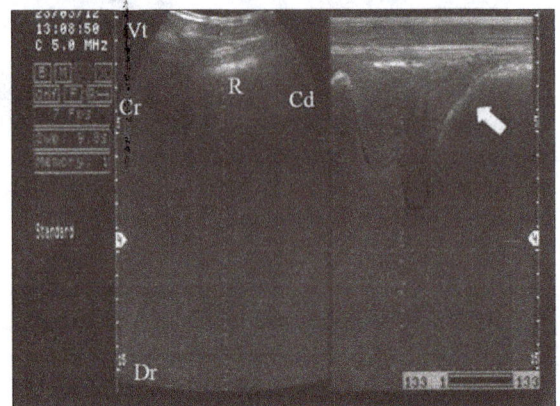

Fig. 6. Serum pepsinogen and fibrinogen changes of the sheep from the day of diagnosis of a foreign body up to the six subsequent days.

Fig. 7. B-mode (left) and M-mode (right) ultrasonographic images of the biphasic curve of reticular contraction in a cannulated sheep four days after foreign body removal showing a longer return time to the starting position (arrow). (Cr = Cranial; Cd = Caudal; Vt = Ventral abdominal wall; Dr = Dorsal abdominal wall; R = Reticulum).

References

Akester, A.R. and Titchen, D.A. 1969. Radiographic studies of the reticulo-rumen in the sheep. J. Anat. 104(1), 137-152.

Braun, U. 2009. Ultrasonography of the gastrointestinal tract in cattle. Vet. Clin. North Am. Food Anim. Pract. 25(3), 567-590.

Braun, U., Jacquat, D. and Hässig, M. 2011. Ultrasonography of the rumen in 30 Saanen goats. Schweiz Arch. Tierheilkd. 153(9), 393-399.

Braun, U., Jacquat, D. and Steininger, K. 2013a. Ultrasonographic examination of the abdomen of the goat. I. Reticulum, rumen, omasum, abomasum and intestines. Schweiz Arch. Tierheilkd. 155(3), 173-184.

Braun, U. and Rauch, S. 2008. Ultrassonographic evaluation of reticular motility during rest, eating, rumination and stress in 30 healthy cows. Vet. Rec. 163, 571-574.

Braun, U., Schweizer, A. and Trösch, L. 2013b. Ultrassonography of the rumen of dairy cows. BMC Vet. Res. 44(9), 1-6.

Byers, S.R. and Kramer, J.W. 2010. Normal hematology of sheep and goats. In Schalm's Veterinary Hematology, Eds., Weiss DJ, Wardrop KJ. Ames, IO: Wiley-Blackwell. pp: 837.

Kandeel, A.E., Omar, M.S.A., Mekkawy, N.H.M., El-Seddawy, F.D. and Gomaa, M. 2009. Anatomical and ultrasonographic study of the stomach and liver in sheep and goats. Iraqi J. Vet. Sci. 23 Suppl. 2, S181-191.

Mesarič, M. 2005. Role of serum pepsinogen in detecting cows with abomasal ulcer. Vet. Arhiv. 75, 111-118.

Morgado, A.A., Nunes, G.R., Martins, A.S., Hagen, S.C.F., Rodrigues, P.H.M. and Sucupira, M.C.A. 2014. Metabolic profile and ruminal and abomasal pH in sheep subjected to intravenous ranitidine. Pesq. Vet. Bras. 34, Suppl. 1, S17-22.

Paynter, D.I. 1992. Pepsinogen activity: determination in serum and plasma. In: Corner LA, Bagust TJ, editors. Australian standard diagnostic techniques for animal diseases. East Melbourne: CSIRO.

Schalm, W., Jain, N.C. and Carroll, E.J. 1981. Hematologia Veterinaria. 1st Ed. Español. Editorial Hemisferio Sur. S.A. Buenos Aires. Argentina. pp: 89-228.

Streeter, R.N. and Step, D.L. 2007. Diagnostic ultrasonography in ruminants. Vet. Clin. North Am. Food Anim. Pract. 23, 541-574.

8

Clinical management of dietary induced urolithiasis associated with balanoposthitis in a Boer goat

Y. Abba[1], F.F.J. Abdullah[2,3], N.H. Bin Abu Daud[4], R. Bin Shaari[4]*, A. Tijjani[1], M.A. Sadiq[2], K. Mohammed[2], L. Adamu[2] and A.M.L. Mohd[1]

[1]Department of Veterinary Pathology and Microbiology, Faculty of Veterinary Medicine, Universiti Putra Malaysia, 43400 UPM Serdang, Selangor, Malaysia

[2]Department of Veterinary Clinical Studies, Faculty of Veterinary Medicine, Universiti Putra Malaysia, 43400 UPM Serdang, Selangor, Malaysia

[3]Research Centre for Ruminant Disease, Faculty of Veterinary Medicine, Universiti Putra Malaysia, 43400 UPM Serdang, Selangor, Malaysia

[4]Faculty of Veterinary Medicine, Universiti Malaysia Kelantan, Locked Bag 36, Pengkalan Chepa, 16100 Kota Bharu, Kelantan, Malaysia

Abstract

A Boer-Kajang cross male goat was presented to the Veterinary Hospital, University Malaysia Kelantan with a history of dysuria, hematuria and restlessness. The goat was intensively managed (confined to the pen) and fed with only palm kernel cake for the last three months. Physical examination revealed that the goat was dull, depressed, having an inflamed penis and prepuce with blood stained urine dripping from the penis. The differential diagnoses were obstructive urolithiasis, urinary tract infection and balanoposthitis. Based on the history, clinical signs, physical examination, urinalysis, ultrasonagraphy and feed analysis, the goat was diagnosed with obstructive urolithiasis and balanoposthitis. Treatment was instituted by amputation of the urethral process and retrograde urohydropulsion to relieve the blockade. Sulfadiazine-trimethoprim (Norodine®24) 15mg/kg, I.M; flunixin meglumine 2.2mg/kg, I.M; vitamin B complex 1ml/10kg, I.M and ammonium chloride 300mg/kg orally were administered. The goat responded well to treatment and was recovering well during a follow up visit.

Keywords: Balanoposthitis, Boer goat, Obstructive urolithiasis, Palm kernel cake

Introduction

Urolithiasis is a condition associated with the formation of urinary calculi in the urinary system. Thus, obstructive urolithiasis is usually associated with the obstruction of the urethra by one or more uroliths which results in blockage of urine outflow (Radostits et al., 2007; Ewoldt et al., 2008). Nutritional disease is considered the primary factor for ruminant urolithiasis, while sex and hormonal changes are also considered as predisposing factors (Kahn et al., 2005). Animals affected with obstructive urolithiasis usually show signs of abdominal pain, restlessness, groaning and grunting while straining to urinate but passing only a few drops of blood stained urine. However, these conditions usually go unnoticed in many food animals. Balanoposthitis which is an inflammation of the penis and prepuce can be found in male animals with urethral obstruction (Radostits et al., 2007). This can be due to self-inflicted trauma or caused by Corynebacterium renale which is capable of hydrolyzing urea. Animals affected will show signs of swelling around the prepuce (Kahn et al., 2005). Balanoposthitis can be a secondary lesion due to obstructive urolithiasis.

Dietary imbalances resulting from disproportionate calcium-phosphorus ratios (Ca:P ratios) have been incriminated in formation of uroliths and crystals in the urine (Makhdoomi and Ghazi, 2013). Palm kernel cake (PKC) is an important oil palm by-product used as animal feed (Kum and Zahari, 2011). However, PKC contains an imbalance of calcium-phosphorus ratio and excess quantities in the feed may lead to the formation of uroliths (Wan Zahari and Alimon, 2012). The optimum level of PKC to be fed to goats is 30% (MPOB, 2002). This clinical case reports the management of dietary induced obstructive urolithiasis associated with balanophosthitis in a Boer goat.

Case History

A 2 year-old Kajang cross male goat weighing about 30kg with a body condition score of 3/5 was presented to the Veterinary Hospital, University Malaysia Kelantan with a history of dysuria, hematuria and restlessness lasting for five days. Vaccination and deworming statuses were not up to date. The goat was intensively managed and fed with a commercially bought palm kernel cake for the past three months.

Clinical examination

On clinical evaluation, the goat was found to be dull, depressed and recumbent. There was pyrexia and

*Corresponding author: Rumaizi Bin Shaari. Faculty of Veterinary Medicine, Universiti Malaysia Kelantan, Locked Bag 36, PengkalanChepa, 16100 Kota Bharu, Kelantan, Malaysia. E-mail: rumaizi@umk.edu.my

tachypnoea. The mucous membrane was pale pink with capillary refill time and skin recoil of 3 seconds. The prepuce and penis were inflamed, hemorrhagic and necrotic (Fig. 1). Upon abdominal palpation, the urinary bladder was turgid and enlarged. Palpation of the inguinal region revealed pain at the point of sigmoid flexure.

Diagnostic Work-up and results

Urinalysis, radiography, ultrasonography and feed mineral analysis were done for the diagnostic work-ups. The urinalysis results showed the presence of leucocytes (+1), nitrite, proteins (+3), and red blood cells (+4). Urinary sediments were also observed under the microscope where calcium phosphate crystals (Fig. 2) and struvite crystals (Fig. 3) were seen.

Radiography of the right lateral view showed an absence of the urinary bladder line and a ground glass appearance of the abdomen, which was interpreted as ruminal distention. The glans penis and the prepuce were observed to be radiopaque (Fig. 4).

Ultrasonographic examination showed collection of hyperechoic sediments at the dorsal part of the enlarged

and turgid bladder which measured approximately 10cm in diameter (Fig. 5).

Feed analysis of the palm kernel cake showed that calcium and phosphorus level in feed were 0.25% and 0.59%, respectively.

Based on the history, clinical signs, physical examination and urinalysis, the definitive diagnosis for this case were obstructive urolithiasis associated with balanoposthitis.

Management

Management of obstructive urolithiasis generally involves establishing a patent urethra (Ewoldt et al., 2008). Thus, urethral process amputation and retrograde urohydropulsion were indicated in this case. The penis was grossly inflamed with presence of multifocal necrotic patches on the preputial surface. The goat was placed in a squatting position and the hair around the prepucial area was shaved and disinfected

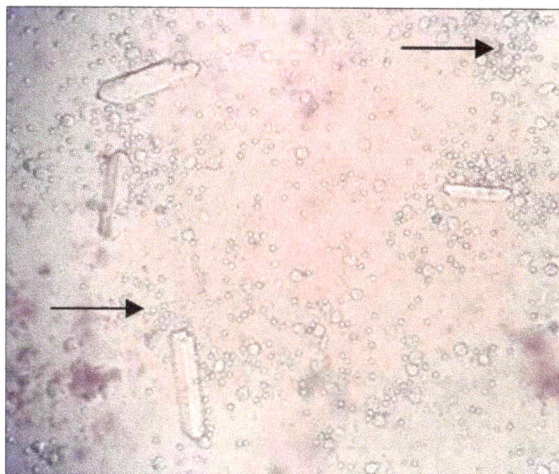

Fig. 3. Struvite crystals; colorless, 3-dimensional, prism-like crystals from urine smear (arrows).

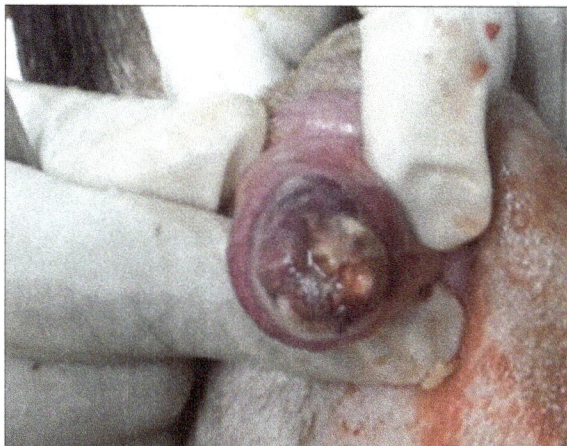

Fig. 1. Inflamed and necrotic penis and prepuce.

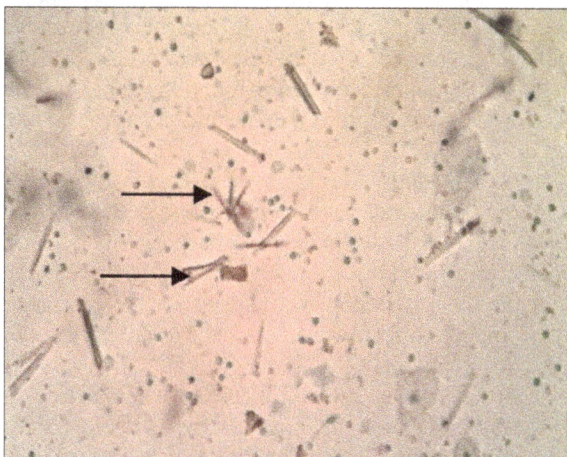

Fig. 2. Calcium phosphate crystals from urine smear (arrows).

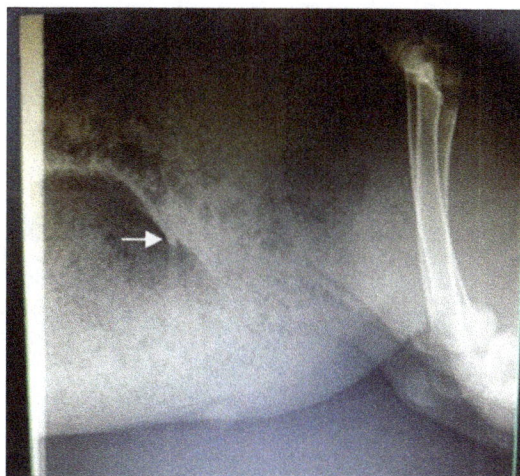

Fig. 4. Radiograph showing right lateral view of the abdomen. Note opaque distended urethra due to obstruction (arrow).

using chlorhexidine, alcohol and povidone-iodine. The glans penis and urethral process were extruded out by pushing back the prepuce (Fig. 6). A 2 % lidocaine hydrocholoride injection (3ml) was injected into the glands penis and the urethral process was transected with a scissors, while the surrounding necrotic penile tissue was debrided. The incised urethral process was examined for presence of uroliths and crystals. In order to initiate retrograde urohydropulsion, a urethral catheter was inserted into the urethra up to the level of the sigmoid flexure and the urinary bladder was manually expressed to evacuate the urine until the bladder was empty.

Sulfadiazine-trimethoprim (Norodine® 24) 15mg/kg, I.M, SID, for 10 days as broad spectrum antibiotic, Flunixine meglumine 2.2mg/kg, I.M, SID, for 10 days as analgesic and anti-inflammatory, ammonium

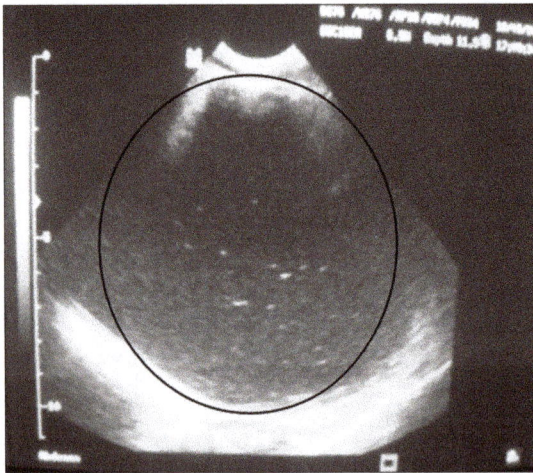

Fig. 5. Ultrasonograph of the distended bladder (10cm) showing opaque bodies. Note the uniformly distributed echoes resulting from cystitis. Transducer was placed on the ventral abdomen in the standing position.

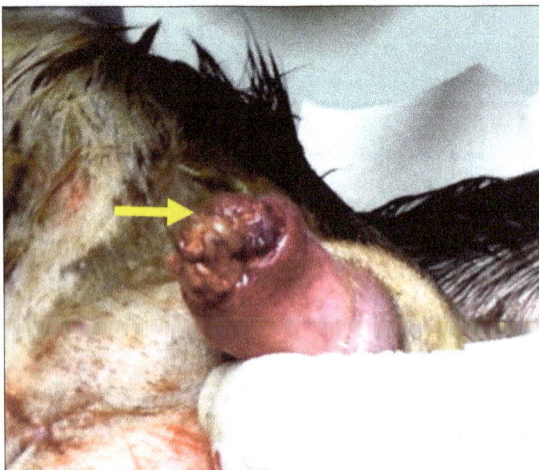

Fig. 6. Urethral process amputation (arrow).

chloride 300mg/kg, P.O, SID, for 1 month as urine acidifier and Vitamin B complex 1ml/10 kg, SID, I.M for 3 days were administered.

Discussion

The prevalence of urolithiasis is high in ruminants fed with high grain diet. These animals are at increased risk of developing struvite uroliths due to the high phosphorus level in the feed (Kahn *et al.*, 2005). The formation of calculi and the development of urolithiais occurs in phases; from the formation of nidus, concentration of urine and lastly precipitation of various minerals such as phosphorus from which struvite crystals are formed (Makhdoomi and Ghazi, 2013). The distal aspect of sigmoid flexure and urethral process of sheep and goats are the most common sites for formation of uroliths due to the narrow lumen (Parrah *et al.*, 2010). The goat in this case was fed solely with PKC for a few months, which predisposed it to struvite uroliths formation resulting from the imbalance of calcium-phosphorus ratio in the feed. Another predisposition is the sex of the goat, thus making the uroliths to be easily lodged at the sigmoid flexure and the urethral process. On the other hand, the presence of inflammation around the penis and prepuce, which was presumed to be secondary to the urolith formation, might have contributed to obstruction of the urethral process. Complete obstruction around the urethral process will usually lead to perforation and inflammation around the prepuce and glans penis (Kahn *et al.*, 2005).

According to Kahn *et al.* (2005), the Ca: P ratio in the diet should be 2:1. Thus, any feeding program incorporating concentrate feeding must include appropriate calcium supplements in the diet. Ammonium chloride supplementation at 2.25% has been shown to maintain urinary pH of goats at 6.5 for up to 24 hrs (Mavangira *et al.*, 2010). Since maintenance of urinary pH at 5.5-6.5 is paramount in preventing the formation of uroliths, incorporation of ammonium chloride in goat feed is essential. A high P:Ca ratio has been shown to predispose to osteopenia and fibrous osteodystrophy in confined goats fed with high phosphate diet (Bandarra *et al.*, 2011). High dietary phosphate and magnesium has also been shown to increase urinary excretion of phosphate and predisposes to the formation of struvite crystals and phosphate calculi (Makhdoomi and Ghazi, 2013). In an experimental study using cotton seed feed and magnesium oxide for induction of urolithiasis in goats, Wang et al. (2008) and Sun *et al.* (2010) reported that the most important component for the formation of a urolith was magnesium, which contributed to the development of struvite calculi. The authors also observed that crystals formed were made up of magnesium ammonium phosphate (MAP) before stone formation and potassium magnesium phosphate (MKP) after stone formation. In Malaysia, most concentrates are oil palm based, where PKC is used as animal feed. The Ca:P ratio in PKC is 1:2; hence the phosphorus level is two times higher than calcium level (MPOB, 2002). As a result, feeding high quantities of PKC predisposes the animals to uroliths and crystal formation in the urine just as we observed in this report.

Surgical intervention through tube cystotomy and chemical dissolution is the most widely practiced management procedure, especially when the stones are located proximal to the sigmoid flexure and urethral catheter insertion fails (Dubey *et al.*, 2006). In our case, insertion of a urethral catheter coupled with normograde retro-hydropulsion was able to restore urine flow to normal because the urolith was small and the obstruction was distal to the sigmoid flexure. On the other hand, large uroliths that are proximal and which are impossible to dislodge through this procedure will require a perineal urethrostomy and cystotomy as previously described by other researchers (Ewoldt *et al.*, 2008). Although currently the most effective approach is tube cystototmy, future approach is aimed at using laser lithotripsy to break down stones within the bladder. Since dietary cation differences have been identified as the most important factor in its development, preventive measures such as controlled salt level in diet, use of urine acidifiers and reduced concentrate coupled with increased roughage intake is recommended to reduce incidence of this condition in farm animals (Jones *et al.*, 2009; Makhdoomi *et al.*, 2013).

Conclusion

It is important to limit feeding of concentrate to goats and other livestock due to imbalance in the Ca:P ratio. The best feeding regime is 70% roughage and 30% concentrate feed based on dry matter. It is also crucial to educate farmers on the clinical signs associated with obstructive urolithiasis in order to ensure institution of early treatment for better prognosis.

Acknowledgement

The authors wish to acknowledge the staff of Veterinary Hospital, Faculty of Veterinary Medicine, University Malaysia Kelantan for their technical help and support.

References

Bandarra, P.M., Pavarini, S.P., Santos, A.S., Antoniassi, N.A.B., Cruz, C.E. and Driemeier, D. 2011. Nutritional fibrous osteodystrophy in goats. Pesquisa Vet. Brasil. 31(10), 875-878.

Dubey, A., Pratap, K., Amarpal, Aithal, H.P., Kinjavdekar, P., Singh, T.I. and Sharma, M.C. 2006. Tube cystotomy and chemical dissolution of urethral calculi in goats. Indian J. Vet. Surg. 27(2), 98-103.

Ewoldt, J.M., Jones, M.L. and Miesner, M.D. 2008. Surgery of obstructive urolithiasis in ruminants. Vet. Clin. North Am. Food Anim. Pract. 24(3), 455-465.

Jones, M.L., Streeter, R.N. and Goad, C.L. 2009. Use of dietary cation difference for control of urolithiasis risk factors in goats. Am. J. Vet. Res. 70, 147-155.

Kahn, C.M. and Line, S. 2005. The Merck Veterinary Manual 9th Edition. USA: Merial.

Kum, W.H. and Zahari, M.W. 2011. Utilisation of oil palm by-product as ruminant feed in Malaysia. J. Oil Palm Res. 23, 1029-1035.

Makhdoomi, D.M. and Ghazi, M.A. 2013. Obstructive urolithiasis in ruminants- A review. Vet. World 6(4), 233-238.

Malaysia Palm Oil Board, MPOB. 2002. Palm kernel cake as animal feed.

Mavangira, V., Cornish, J.M. and Angelos, J.A. 2010. Effect of ammonium chloride supplementation on urine pH and urinary fractional excretion of electrolytes in goats. J. Am. Vet. Med. Assoc. 237(11), 1299-1304.

Parrah, J.D., Hussain, S.S., Moulvi, B.A., Singh, M. and Athar, H. 2010. Bovine uroliths analysis: A review of 30 cases. Isr. J. Vet. Med. 65(3), 103-107.

Radostits, O.M., Gay, C.C., Hinchcliff, K.W. and Constable, P.D. 2007. A textbook of the diseases of cattle, horses, sheep, pigs and goats. Veterinary Medicine, 10th ed. London: Saunders. pp:1548-1551.

Sun, W.D., Wang, J.Y., Zhang, K.C. and Wang, X.L. 2010. Study on precipitation of struvite and struvite-K crystal in goats during onset of urolithiasis. Res. Vet. Sci. 88(3), 461-466.

Wang, J.Y., Sun, W.D. and Wang, X.L. 2009. Comparison of effect of high intake of magnesium with high intake of phosphorus and potassium on urolithiasis in goats fed with cottonseed meal diet. Res. Vet. Sci. 87(1), 79-84.

Wan Zahari, M. and Alimon, A.R. 2012. Recent advances in the utilization of oil palm by-products as animal feed. In: International Conference on Livestock Production and Veterinary Technology (ICARD), Ciawi, Bogor, Indonesia.

9

Comparison of several methods of sires evaluation for total milk yield in a herd of Holstein cows in Yemen

F.R. Al-Samarai[1,*], Y.K. Abdulrahman[1], F.A. Mohammed[2], F.H. Al-Zaidi[2] and N.N. Al-Anbari[3]

[1]Department of Veterinary Public Health/College of Veterinary Medicine, University of Baghdad, Iraq
[2]Department of Animal Resources, Directorate of Baghdad Agriculture, Ministry of Agriculture, Iraq
[3]Department of Animal Resources, College of Agriculture, University of Baghdad, Iraq

Abstract

A total of 956 lactation records of Holstein cows kept at Kaa Albon station, Imuran Governorate, Yemen during the period from 1991 to 2003 were used to investigate the effect of some genetic and non-genetic factors (Sire, parity, season of calving, year of calving and age at first calving as covariate) on the Total Milk Yield (TMY), Lactation Length (LL), and Dry Period (DP). Components of variance for the random effects (mixed model) were estimated by Restricted Maximum Likelihood (REML) methodology. Sires were evaluated for the TMY by three methods, Best Linear Unbiased Prediction (BLUP) using Harvey program, Transmitting Ability (TA) according to the Least Square Means of sire progeny (TALSM) and according to Means (TAM). Results showed that TMY and DP were affected significantly (P < 0.01) by all factors except season of calving and age at first calving, while LL was affected significantly (P< 0.01) only by year of calving and parity. The averages of the TMY, LL, and DP were 3919.66 kg, 298.28 days, and 114.13 days respectively. The corresponding estimates of heritability (h²) were 0.35, 0.06, and 0.14 respectively. The highest and lowest BLUP values of sires for the TMY were – 542.44 kg and 402.14 kg, while the corresponding estimates for TALSM and TAM were – 470.38, 380.88 kg and – 370.12, 388.50 kg respectively. The Spearman rank correlation coefficients among BLUP, TALSM and TAM ranged from 0.81 to 0.67. These results provide evidence that the selection of sires will improve the TMY in this herd because of the wide differences in genetic poetical among sires, and a moderate estimation of heritability.

Keywords: BLUP, Genetic evaluation, Heritability, Holstein cows.

Introduction

Milk yield is an important economic trait in livestock species. It represents a major source of income in most dairy enterprises. Economic traits are generally controlled by genetic factors but environmental influences like, year, calving season, age at first calving and parity have significant effects on milk yield (Pirzada, 2011). These environmental factors may suppress the animal's true genetic ability and create a bias in the selection of animals. Therefore these environmental effects have to be taken into account to estimate the genetic factor in milk yield (Djemali and Berger, 1992).

The aim of the animal breeding is not only to produce superior individual animals but also to cause a general improvement in a herd by selecting genetically superior sires and dams as parents for future generations (Bourdon, 1997). Quantitative genetics has a large applicability in animal husbandry. The main goal in animal breeding is to select those cows, which can produce offspring with improved phenotypes. In order to establish effective breeding programs it is necessary to know the genetic inheritance of a certain character (Bugeac et al., 2013). The potential for genetic improvement of a trait largely depends upon genetic variation existing in the population of interest. The genetic variability for a particular trait in a herd or population is measured by heritability estimate of a trait under given environmental conditions (Goshu et al., 2014).

Thus, the estimation of heritability and evaluation of sires could be one of the best methods to accomplish this aim. The use of an appropriate method for genetic evaluation of sires is an important aspect of dairy cattle improvement, so various methods have been proposed for use in the genetic evaluation of dairy cattle (Kheirabadi et al., 2013).

Heritability is required to calculate genetic evaluations, to predict response to selection, and to help producers decide if it is more efficient to improve traits through management or through selection. In view of these facts, several researchers estimated the heritability of total milk yield in Holstein cows. Estimation ranged from 0.06 to 0.39 (Klopcic et al., 1997; Ojango and Pollott 2001; Hermiz et al., 2005; Cilek and Sahin 2009; Ayied et al., 2011; Usman et al., 2012; Nawaz et al., 2013; Hamrouni et al., 2014), while heritability of LL ranged from 0.02 to 0.49 (Hermiz et al., 2005; Ayied et al., 2011; Usman et al., 2012; Nawaz et al., 2013).

*Corresponding Author: Firas R. Al-Samarai. Department of Veterinary Public Health, College of Veterinary Medicine, University of Baghdad, Iraq. Email: firas_rashad@yahoo.com

Estimation of heritability of DP ranged from 0.07 to 0.78 (Funk *et al.*, 1987; Hermiz *et al.*, 2005; Kuhn *et al.*, 2005; Ayied *et al.*, 2011; Usman *et al.*, 2012). The purpose of this research was to investigate the effect of some genetic and non-genetic factors on the productive traits of Holstein cows in Yemen and to estimate the phenotypic trend and heritability of studied traits in addition to utilizing the genetic evaluation of sire for TMY using several methods.

Materials and Methods

Data

The data that included lactation records of 956 belong to 281 cows and 81sires for the period extending from 1991 to 2006. Pedigree information and the data used in this study were obtained from the Kaa Alboon Station, Imuran Governorate, Yemen. Prior to analyses, abnormal records for the lactation length (less than 200 and greater than 400 days) were excluded from the data set (Ayied *et al.*, 2011). As a result of the low number of records for the last three years, -with no specific reason- these records were included into the year of 2003. The calving months were grouped into four seasons: December to February (winter), March to May (spring), June to August (summer), and September to November (autumn). Parity greater than 6 considered as 6.

Statistical analysis

Two models were used to analyze the data: the first was fixed model which included both of genetic and non-genetic effects (sire, parity, season and year of calving and age at first calving as covariate), and the second model was mixed model (considered sire as a random) which included the same effects mentioned in the first model except of season of calving and age at first calving as they are non-significant. This model was used to estimate BLUP of sires for TMY (Harvey, 1990) and heritability. The σ^2s and σ^2e were estimated by the Restricted Maximum Likelihood (REML) methodology. Minimum and Maximum No. of daughter per sire were 2 and 8 respectively (with average of 3.47 daughter per sire). Phenotypic trends were estimated from regression for each trait on year of calving.

A formula (Bourdon, 1997) was used for calculating Transmitting Ability (TA) for Least Square Means (LSM) as these means were adjusted for all factors in the employed model and Means (M) of sires (raw means not adjusted) were as follow:

$$TA = b*(P_i - P) \dots\dots (1)$$

where $b = (n*h^2) / ((n-1)*h^2 + 4)$

TA : Transmitting ability of sire

b: Regression coefficient

P_i: Average result of the sire's offspring

P: Average result of the comparison group

h^2: Heritability for the trait

n: Number of offspring.

The formula (1) mentioned above was used to estimate the TA of sires according to its progeny Mean (TAM) and according to progeny Least Square Means (TALSM). Best Linear Unbiased Prediction (BLUP) for each sire was estimated using Harvey program (Harvey, 1990). Accuracy was estimated for BLUP using the following equation (Bourdon, 1997):

$$\text{Accuracy} = \text{sqr } [(n*h^2) / ((n-1)*h^2 + 4)] \dots\dots (2)$$

Results

Total milk yield:

The overall mean of the TMY in the current study was 3919.66 ±42.99 kg (Table 1).

Table 1. Means±SE of some productive traits in Holstein cows.

Trait	No. of records	Max	Min	Mean	SE
Total milk yield	956	5890	1720	3919.66	42.99
Lactation length	956	340	200	298.28	5.48
Dry period	956	165	45	114.13	1.95

The effect of sire, parity and year of calving was significant (P< 0.01) (Table 2), while the effect of season of calving and age at first calving was non-significant.

Table 2. Analysis of variance of factors affecting TMY in Holstein cows.

Sources of variation	DF	Mean square	F value	Pr > F
Sire	80	2112741.2	2.24	<.0001
Parity	5	3804790.0	4.03	0.0013
Season of calving	3	363472.1	0.38	0.7639
Year of calving	13	4028171.1	4.27	<.0001
Age at first calving	1	1783882.1	1.89	0.1696
Error	854	944184		
Corrected Total	956			

Parity 4th had the highest average TMY of 4132.84 kg as compared with other parities. Mean of the TMY fluctuated across years with significant (P < 0.01) reduction in phenotypic trend along with advance years (- 196.92 kg/year). Heritability estimate for the TMY was 0.35 (Table 3). BLUP values of sires were between – 471.88 and 443.80 kg, while the corresponding estimates for TALSM and TAM were between – 470.38 and 380.88 kg and between –370.12 and 338.50 kg respectively (Table 4). The spearman rank correlation coefficients among BLUP, TALSM and TAM were between 0.81and 0.67 (Table 5). The accuracy of the three methods of sire evaluation was between low (0.40) to moderate (0.65) (Table 4).

Table 3. Phenotypic trends and heritability of TMY, LL, and DP in Holstein cows.

Trait	Phenotypic trend	Heritability (h²)±SE
TMY	-196.92 kg/year**	0.35±0.12
LL	0.35 days/year*	0.06±0.04
DP	-0.26 days/year**	0.14±0.07

TMY= Total milk yield; LL= Lactation length; DP= Dry period.
* (P < 0.05) **(P < 0.01)

Table 4. Estimates of BLUP, TALSM and TAM of total milk yield for Holstein sires.

BLUP	TALSM	TAM	ACC
-471.88	-470.38	-370.12	0.28 – 0.61
443.80	380.88	388.50	
915.68	851.26	758.62	

BLUP = Beast Linear Unbiased Prediction; TALSM = Transmitting ability according least square means; TAM = Transmitting ability according means; ACC = Accuracy of BLUP.

Table 5. Spearman rank correlation coefficients of BLUP, TALSM and TAM for Holstein sires.

	TALSM	TAM
BLUP	0.81**	0.67**
TALSM		0.72**

** P < 0.01

Lactation length:

The result of the present study revealed that the mean of LL was 298.28±5.48 days (Table 1). Parity and year of calving had a significant (P < 0.01) effect on LL, while the effect of sire, season of calving and age at first calving was non-significant (Table 6).

Table 6. Analysis of variance of factors affecting LL in Holstein cows.

Sources of variation	DF	Mean square	F value	Pr > F
Sire	80	197.55751	1.01	0.4540
Parity	5	696.55303	3.57	0.0034
Season of calving	3	449.01616	2.30	0.0760
Year of calving	13	598.66926	3.07	0.0003
Age at first calving	1	19.14333	0.10	0.7543
Error	854	195.2886		
Corrected Total	956			

The highest average of LL was found in 4th parity (303.07 days) and lowest was found in 5th parity (293.34 days). The average LL increased significantly (P < 0.05) along with advance years with positive phenotypic trend (0.35 days/year) and heritability estimate for LL was 0.06 (Table 3).

Dry period:

The mean DP of Holstein cows was 114.13±1.95 days (Table 1). Sire, parity, and year of calving had a significant (P < 0.01) effect on DP while the effect of season of calving and age at first calving was non-significant (Table 7).

Table 7. Analysis of variance of factors affecting DP in Holstein cows.

Sources of variation	DF	Mean square	F value	Pr > F
Sire	80	9349.4355	1.68	0.0003
Parity	5	30670.5986	5.52	<.0001
Season of calving	3	6756.3321	1.22	0.3031
Year of calving	13	41867.0695	7.53	<.0001
Age at first calving	1	500.3670	0.09	0.7607
Error	830	5559.633		
Corrected Total	932			

Cows had the lowest DP at 5th parity (106.76 days) and the highest DP at 4th parity (126.58 days). Results showed that there was a significant (P < 0.01) decreasing of – 0.26 days/year in phenotypic trend of DP across years. Heritability estimate of DP was 0.14 (Table 3).

Discussion

Total milk yield:

It was reported that the range of the average TMY of Holstein cows in tropical regions was from 2772.76 kg to 3986 kg (Abdullah, 2005; Hermiz et al., 2005; Sattar et al., 2005; Tadesse et al., 2010). TMY in the present study was in line with the above mentioned studies. The significant (P < 0.01) effect of sire on TMY was consistent with Ayied et al. (2011) and Nawaz et al. (2013). The significant (P < 0.01) effect of parity on TMY was confirmed in previous studies obtained by Lateef et al. (2008), Tadesse et al. (2010) and Al-Masri et al. (2012). Nevertheless, the result differed from that of Habib et al. (2003) who found non-significant (P>0.05) effect of parity on milk yield. In the present study, the highest TMY was found in parity 4. Similar finding were reported by Abdel-Gader et al. (2007) and Al-Masri et al. (2012).

On the other hand the present results disagreed with Lateef et al. (2008) who reported that the highest TMY was in 3rd parity. These differences could be attributed to differences between age at first calving and calving intervals. Al-Samarai (1988) stated that "increasing of age at first calving and calving interval will lead the cow to reach high milk yield synchronized with lower parity". Significant (P < 0.01) effect of year of calving on TMY revealed that the management and environment were unstable during these years.

According to Fontaneli et al. (2005) differences in performance between years reflected the effects of environmental variations, which had marked effects on the quantity and quality of herbage available. The effect of year of calving on milk yield was confirmed by Abou-Bakr (2009) who concluded that the variation in milk yield from one year to another could be attributed to the changes in age of the animals, attacks of different diseases and management practices level followed from year to another, e.g. fluctuations in feed availability, and quality and prices. However Tavirimirwa et al. (2012) attributed that to the differences in rainfall, which will lead to mark differences between years in quality and quantity of forage available. The non-significant effect of season of calving was in agreement with the results obtained by Abou-Bakr (2009) and Al-Masri et al. (2012).

The phenotypic trend of TMY indicated that milk yield decreased significantly (P < 0.01) by – 196.92 kg/year. This reduction could be caused by several reasons such as involuntary culling of high milking cows, no improvement program was applied and reduction in the level of management. Thus it was very imperative to conduct some studies to investigate reasons of such reduction in TMY. Similarly, Abou-Bakr (2009) detected a significant (P< 0.02) negative phenotypic trend in milk yield with an overall rate of - 91.6 ± 35.16 kg per year for the same breed in Egypt.

The heritability of the TMY ranged widely from 0.06 to 0.39 (Klopcic et al., 1997; Ojango and Pollott, 2001; Hermiz et al., 2005; Cilek and Sahin, 2009; Ayied et al., 2011; Usman et al., 2012; Nawaz et al., 2013; Hamrouni et al., 2014). Differences in heritability estimates among various studies for the same trait of the same breed could be due to differences in the records number used, the correction for different non-genetic factors, the model used and the methodology for estimating heritability of the trait (Abou-Bakr, 2009) in addition to herd size, level of production and region in the same country (Hamrouni et al., 2014).

Moderate heritability (0.35) estimated in this study refers to a considerable genetic variation among sires. Our estimate was close to the estimate of 0.32 reported by Nawaz et al. (2013). The estimate of heritability decreased from 0.35 to 0.31 when LL was included as a covariate in the model. Ojango and Pollott (2001) reported that the heritability estimate for milk yield, considering lactation length as a covariate, was moderate (0.25 ± 0.04) and less than the estimate for total milk yield ignoring lactation length (0.30 ± 0.04). Madalena (1988) noted that using lactation length as a covariate in analyses of milk yield tended to reduce differences between animals, making low-producing animals seem to produce more milk.

Although the animal model was more accurate than sire model for genetic evaluation, we used sire model because the required relationship information was not available. The BLUP values of sires for the TMY ranged from -471.88 to 443.80 with marginal

difference of 915.68 kg between lower and higher value.

The corresponding values of TALSM and TAM were – 470.38 to 380.88 kg and 851.26 kg, respectively. Similarly, Abubakar et al., (1986) with 15512 lactation records of daughters of 138 sires found that BLUP of 305 milk yield ranged from – 400 to 400 kg. Abdel-Glil (1991) with 1653 lactation records of daughters of 163 sires found that BLUP values ranged from – 466 to 681 kg. Also, Atil and Khattab (1999) with 1931 lactation records of daughters of 76 sires found that the BLUP values ranged from – 506 to 675 kg with marginal difference of 1181 kg and TALSM values ranged from – 964 to 895 kg with marginal difference of 1859 kg. Although the accuracy for three methods was not high and this could be attributed to low No. of daughter per sire (3.51), the present study detected the existence of a considerable genetic variation which could be used to improve TMY.

The spearman rank correlation coefficient between BLUP and TALSM (0.81) was higher than 0.71 obtained by Glil and Parmar (1988) and lower than 0.88 and 0.98 reported by Vij and Tiwana (1988) and Atil and Khattab (1999) respectively. Low correlation was found between BLUP and TAM. The differences among estimates of Spearman rank correlation indicated that the three methods were not equal for the evaluation of the sires. The accuracy of the three methods of sire evaluation is between low (0.28) to moderate (0.61) (Table 4). The low estimations of accuracy could be attributed to low number of progeny per sire. Hence it is very imperative to increase the number of progeny per sire to get high estimations of accuracy.

Lactation length:

The range of LL was reported to be from 291.86 to 362 days (Tadesse and Dessie 2003; Hermiz et al., 2005; Sattar et al., 2005; Nawaz et al., 2013). Although, the average LL in the study was within the range, it was lower than the ideal value (305 days). Non-significant effect of sire on LL indicated the importance of non-genetic factors in the variation of this trait.

The significant (P < 0.01) effect of parity on LL was reported by several workers (Lakshmi et al., 2009; Topaloğlu and Güneş, 2010). It was found that year of calving had a significant effect (P <0.01) on LL. A similar finding was obtained by Nyamushamba et al. (2013) who reported that differences between years were a normal phenomenon which was caused by unforeseen fluctuations in environmental conditions that are difficult to control; particularly this trait had low heritability. Results showed that heritability of LL was low (0.06). The present estimate was parallel to 0.06 that was reported by Lakshmi et al. (2009) and close to 0.04 that was recorded by Ayied et al. (2011).

The low estimate of heritability indicated that larger proportion of phenotypic variance was due to environment and improvement through direct selection would be slow.

Ojango and Pollott (2001) found that the heritability of LL was 0.09 for the same breed in Kenya. They concluded that low estimation of heritability implied that the variation in lactation length was more a result of variation in management and feeding in the given environment of lactation rather than the genetic factors. On the other hand the effect of season of calving and age at first calving was non-significant. Although, phenotypic trend of LL (0.35 days/year) was positive and significant ($P < 0.05$), more efforts are needed to extend LL as its average was lower than optimum length.

Dry period:

Mean DP of 114.13 days in this study was within the range of 100.26 to 281.33 days obtained by several researches (Abdullah, 2005; Hermiz et al., 2005; Sattar et al., 2005; Suhail et al., 2010; Hossein-Zadeh and Mohit, 2013). Dairy cows are usually dried-off for two months prior to the next calving. This rest period is necessary to maximize milk production in subsequent lactation. It was reported that the dry period was required for the renewal of udder glandular tissue (Capuco et al., 1997; Annen et al., 2004). Two studies that were carried out in Poland by Borkowska et al. (2006) and Winnicki et al. (2008) indicated that in practice the extended or excessively shortened dry period, caused a reduction in milk production as compared to the recommended optimum.

Hossein-Zadeh and Mohit (2013) divided cows according to DP into 14 classes from < 10 days through > 130 days. They found that cows with group of DP between 51 -60 and 61 - 70 days had the highest milk yield.

Long DP found in this study will decrease the average annual production of the cow by extending the calving interval beyond the normal 13-14 month interval and causing a decrease in the lifetime production of the dairy cow.

DP was affected significantly ($P < 0.01$) by sire. This result was in agreement with Hermiz et al. (2005), Ayied et al. (2011) and Usman et al. (2012). On the contrary some workers (Kuhn et al., 2005; Suhail et al., 2010) observed that sire had a non-significant effect on the DP. Results revealed that DP was affected significantly ($P < 0.01$) by parity. A similar finding was reported by Hossein-Zadeh and Mohit (2013). The differences could be attributed to the differential culling which may account for part of the differences between parities (Kuhn et al., 2005). It was found that DP of 4th parity was the highest while the lowest was at 5th parity. This estimation was parallel to the corresponding estimation of LL. Kuhn

et al., (2005) who reported that the longer lactations were associated with longer dry periods. Year of calving had a significant ($P < 0.01$) effect on DP. Our results confirmed results that were obtained by Hossein-Zadeh and Mohit (2013).

Heritability of DP (0.14) in this study was higher than 0.07 reported by Funk et al. (1987) and Kuhn et al. (2005) and lower than 0.22 that reported by Hermiz et al. (2005). The low estimate of heritability indicated that the large phenotypic variation in DP was due to the environmental factors.

The significance ($P < 0.05$) of each of positive phenotypic trend of DP, positive trend of LL and negative phenotypic trend of TMY, all together was referred to the absence of applying suitable improvement program in this herd. In conclusion, many efforts are required to enhance the productive performance of the herd. The poor production of this herd could be attributed to the sub optimal performance of cows as a result of unplanned breeding and inadequate feeding, management and disease control measures.

Thus, improving environmental conditions and management practices, coupled with improved genetic potential of dairy animals would be more effective approaches for high milk production. Although, the results showed that the values of spearman correlation coefficients for the three methods were moderate, the accuracy of the sire evaluation was low to moderate ($0.28 - 0.61$). Hence, we recommend to adopt the BLUP for selection of sires.

References

Abdel-Gader, A., Mohamed-Khair, A.A., Musa, L.M.-A. and Peters, K.J. 2007. Milk yield and reproductive performance of Friesian cows under Sudan tropical conditions. Arch. Tierz. Dum. 50, 155-164.

Abdel-Glil, M.F. 1991. Sire differences for milk production traits in Friesian cattle. Ph.D. Thesis Faculty of Agric. Zarazig Univ. Egypt.

Abdullah. 2005. Factors effecting productive and reproductive traits, genetic and phenotypic correlation of various parameters of black and white Danish Friesian cattle at government dairy farm Quetta. M.Sc. Thesis, Khyber Pakhtunkhwa Agricultural University Peshawar, Pakistan. pp: 29-80.

Abou-Bakr, S. 2009. Genetic and phenotypic trends of 305-day milk yield of Holstein cows raised at commercial farm in Egypt. Egyptian J. Anim. Prod. 46, 85-92.

Abubakar, B.Y., McDowell, R.E., Wellington, K.E. and Van Vleck, L.D. 1986. Estimating genetic values for milk production in the tropics. J. Dairy Sci. 69, 1087-1092.

Al-Masri, O.A., Salhab, S.A. and Mousa, S.K. 2012. Factors affecting the total milk yield in Holstein Friesian cattle at Kharabo dairy station. J. Damascus Univ. 28, 259-272.

Al-Samarai, F.R. 1988. Genetic evaluation of some productive and reproductive performance of Friesian cows in two farms 7th of April and Abu-Gharib. A Thesis. College of Agriculture, Univ. of Baghdad. Iraq. (*In Arabic*).

Annen, E.L., Collier, R.J., Mcguire, M.A. and Vicini, J.L. 2004. Effect of dry period length on milk yield and mammary epithelial cells. J. Diary Sci. 87, Suppl., E66-E76.

Atil, H. and Khattab, A.S. 1999. Seasonal age correction factors for 305 day milk yield in Holstein cattle. Pakistan J. Bio. Sci. 2, 296-300.

Ayied, S.A., Jadoa, A.J. and Abdulrada, A.J. 2011. Heritabilties and breeding values of production and reproduction traits of Holstein cattle In Iraq. J. Basrah Res. (Sciences) 37, 66-70.

Borkowska, D., Januś, E. and Malinowska, K. 2006. Zależność pomiędzy długością okresu zasuszenia krów a ich produkcyjnością w następnej laktacji (Relation between the dry period length and productivity of cows in subsequent lactation). Roczniki Naukowe PTZ. 2, 27-32.

Bourdon, R.M. 1997. Understanding Animal Breeding. Prentice-Hall, Inc. USA.

Bugeac, T., Maciuc, V. and Creangă, Ş.T. 2013. Genetic parameters of milk yield and quality traits in Holstein-Friesian cows. Bulletin UASVM Anim. Sci. Bio. 70, 150-154.

Capuco, A.V., Awers, R.M. and Smith, J.J. 1997. Mammary growth in Holstein cows during the dry period: qualification of nucleic acids and histology. J. Dairy Sci. 80, 477-487.

Cilek, S. and Sahin, E. 2009. Estimation of some genetic parameters (heritability and repeatability) for milk yield in the Anatolian population of Holstein cows. Arch. Zoo. 12, 57-64.

Djemali, M. and Berger, P.G. 1992. Yield and reproduction characteristics of Friesian cattle under North African conditions. J. Dairy Sci. 75, 3568-3575.

Fontaneli, R.S., Sollenberger, L.E., Littell, R.C. and Staples, C.R. 2005. Performance of lactating dairy cows managed on pasture–based or in freestall barn–feeding systems. J. Dairy Sci. 88, 1264-1276.

Funk, D.A., Freeman, A.E. and Berger, P.J. 1987. Effects of previous days open, previous days dry, and present days open on lactation yield. J. Dairy Sci. 70, 2366-2373.

Glil, G.S. and Parmar, O.S. 1988. Genetic merits of Red Dane bulls used in a crossbreeding projeet. Indian J. Anim. Sci. 58, 811-813.

Goshu, G., Singh, H., Petersson, K.J. and Lundeheim, N. 2014. Heritability and correlation among first lactation traits in Holstein Friesian cows at Holeta Bull Dam Station, Ethiopia. Int. J. Livest. Prod. 5, 47-53.

Habib, M.A., Bhuiyan, A.K.F.H., Bhuiyan, M.S.A. and Khan, A.A. 2003. Performance of Red Chittagong Cattle in Bangladesh Agricultural University Dairy Farm. Bangladesh J. Anim. Sci. 32, 101-108.

Hamrouni, A., Djemali, M. and Bedhiaf, S. 2014. Interaction between genotype and geographic region for milk production traits in Tunisian Holstein cattle. Int. J. Farm. Alli. Sci. 3, 623-628.

Harvey, W.R. 1990. Users guide for LSMLMW and MIXMDL PC-2 version. Ohio State University. pp: 90.

Hermiz, H.N., Juma, K.H., Khalaf, S.S. and Aldoori, T.Sh. 2005. Genetic parameters of production, reproduction and growth traits of Holstein cows. Dirasat Agri. Sci. 32, 157-162.

Kheirabadi, K., Alijani, S., Zavadilová, L., Rafat, S.A. and Moghaddam, G. 2013. Estimation of genetic parameters for daily milk yields of primiparous Iranian Holstein cows. Archiv. Tierzucht. 56, 44, 455-466.

Kuhn, M.T., Hutchison, J.L. and Norman, H.D. 2005. Characterization of days dry for United States Holsteins. J. Dairy Sci. 88, 1147-1155.

Hossein-Zadeh, N.G. and Mohit, A. 2013. Effect of dry period length on the subsequent production and reproduction in Holstein cows. Spanish J. Agri. Res. 11, 100-108.

Klopcic, M., Moning, E.S. and Pagacar, J. 1997. Environmental effects and heritability estimation for milk traits at test days in the Slovenian Brown, Simmental and Black and White cattle population. Stocarstvo 51, 421-426.

Lakshmi, B.S., Gupta, B.R., Sudhakar, K., Prakash, M.G. and Sharma, S. 2009. Genetic analysis of production performance of 642 Holstein Friesian × Sahiwal cows. Tamilnadu J. Vet. Anim. Sci. 5(4), 143-148.

Lateef, M., Ateef, K.Z., Gondal, M., Younas, M., Sarwar, M.I., Mustafa, M.I. and Bashir, M.K. 2008. Milk production potential of pure bred Holstein Friesian and Jersey cows in subtropical environment of Pakistan. Pakistan Vet. J. 28, 9-12.

Madalena, F.E. 1988. A note on the effect of variation of lactation length on the efficiency of tropical cattle selection for milk yield. Theor. Appl. Genet. 76, 830-834.

Nawaz, A., Nizamani, A.H., Marghazani, I.B., Nasrullah and Fatih, A. 2013. Influence of genetic and environmental factors on lactation performance of Holstein Friesian cattle in Balochistan. J. Anim. Plant Sci. 23, 17-19.

Nyamushamba, G.B., Tavirimirwa, B. and Banana, N.Y.D. 2013. Non-genetic factors affecting milk yield and composition of Holstein-Friesian cows nested within natural ecological regions of Zimbabwe. Sci. J. Anim. Sci. 2, 102-108.

Ojango, J.M. and Pollott, G.E. 2001. Genetics of milk yield and fertility traits in Holstein-Friesian cattle on large-scale Kenyan farms. J. Anim. Sci. 79, 1742-1750.

Pirzada, R. 2011. Estimation of Genetic Parameters and Variance Components of Milk Traits in Holstein-Friesian and British-Holstein Dairy Cows. Kafkas Univ. Vet. Fak. Derg. 17, 463-467.

Sattar, A., Mirza, R.H., Niazi, A.A.K. and Latif, M. 2005. Productive and Reproductive performance of Holstein- Friesian cows in Pakistan. Pakistan Vet. J. 25, 75-81.

Suhail, S.M., Ahmed, I., Hafeez, A., Ahmed, S., Jan, D., Khan, S. and Rehman, A. 2010. Genetic study of some reproductive traits of Jersey cattle under subtropical conditions. Sarhad J. Agric. 26, 87-91.

Tadesse, M. and Dessie, T. 2003. Milk performance of Zebu, Holstein Friesian and their crosses in Ethiopia. Liv. Res. Rur. Dev. 3, 765-772.

Tadesse, M.J., Thiengtham, J., Pinyopummin, A. and Prasanpanich, S. 2010. Productive and reproductive performance of Holstein Friesian dairy cows in Ethiopia. Livestock Research for Rural Development, 22 (2): cited in http://www.lrrd.org/lrrd22/2/tade22034.htm

Tavirimirwa, B., Manzungu, E. and Ncube, S. 2012. The evaluation of dry season nutritive value of dominant and improved grasses in fallows in Chivi district, Zimbabwe. Online J. Anim. Feed Res. 2(6), 470-474.

Topaloğlu, N. and Güneş, H. 2010. Effects of Some Factors on Milk Yield and Components of Holstein-Friesian Cattle in England. J. Fac. Vet. Med. İstanbul Üniv. 36, 65-74.

Usman, T., Guo, G., Suhail, S.M., Ahmed, S., Qiaoxiang, M.S., Qureshi, M.S. and Wang, Y. 2012. Performance traits study of Holstein cattle under subtropical conditions. J. Anim. Plant Sci. 22, 92-95.

Vij, R.K. and Tiwana, M.S. 1988. A note on evaluation of buffaloes sires. Indian J. Dairy Sci. 41, 500-503.

Winnicki, S., Głowicka-Wołoszyn, R., Helak, B., Dolska, M. and Jugowa, J.L. 2008. Wpływ długości okresu zasuszenia krów na wydajność i jakość mleka w następnej laktacji (Effect of a dry period length on milk production and quality in next lactation). Prace i materiały Zootechniczne. 65, 176-172.

10

Contribution to reconstruction of third degree rectovestibular lacerations in mares

A.H. Elkasapy[1,*] and I.M. Ibrahim[2]

[1]*Department of Surgery, Faculty of Veterinary Medicine, Benha University, Egypt*
[2]*Department of Surgery, Anesthesiology and Radiology, Faculty of Veterinary Medicine, Cairo University, Egypt*

Abstract
The study was conducted on ten mares suffering from third degree rectovestibular laceration. Four uterine washes were performed in all cases by using diluted betadine (mixing 5ml of betadine antiseptic solution in 1 liter of sterile saline) to control vaginal and uterine infections before surgery. Surgical repair of third degree rectovestibular laceration was done by one-stage Goetz technique after four to six weeks of initial injury, with the lateral dissection continued extensively until the two flaps were created and brought to the midline without any tension. Primary healing occurred in all cases without significant complications. The obtained results indicate that mares with third degree rectovestibular lacerations are candidates for uterine wash and one-stage Goetz technique with excessive lateral continuation of the flap.
Keywords: Fertility, Mares, Rectovestibular laceration, Surgery.

Introduction

Third degree rectovestibular lacerations result in disruption of the perineal body, anal sphincter, floor of the rectum and ceiling of the vagina leading to a common opening between vestibule and rectum. Laceration had been classified according to their extent as first, second and third degree lacerations (Aanes, 1988; Emberston, 1990; Farag *et al.*, 2000).

Rectovestibular laceration occasionally occur in mares at first parturition than at any time thereafter. Fetal malposition, large fetal size or aggressive assistance during delivery may play a role. Perineal lacerations are much more common in mares compared to cattle and other domesticated species. The prominence of the vestibulo-vaginal sphincter and remnants of the hymen in mares foaling for the first time are presumed to be responsible for most of these injuries (Kazemi *et al.*, 2010). The powerful expulsive efforts and the rotation of the equine fetus from a dorso-venteral to a dorso-sacral position during parturition (Purohit, 2011) renders the foal's leg to exert undue pressure on the lateral and dorsal walls of the birth canal: thus increasing the chances of laceration (Woodie, 2006).

Surgical interference for acute injury repair should be considered only if it can be performed within a few hours, and if local tissue damage seems compatible with success (Saini *et al.*, 2013). Local debridement of acute injuries may be necessary in some cases and tetanus prophylaxis and temporary antibacterial and anti-inflammatory treatment is recommended. Definitive repair is usually delayed for 4-6 weeks until complete wound contraction and epithelization occurs (Farag *et al.*, 2000; Ghamsari *et al.*, 2008).

Numerous techniques and modifications of techniques have been described. With the basic tenet of all being reconstruction of a shelf between the rectum and vestibule and restoration of the functional perineal body (Aanes, 1988). The principles that need to be observed and fulfilled include appropriate suture material, broad tissue apposition with minimal tension on the suture line. The common methods used are the two-stage repair (Saleh *et al.*, 1988) and the single stage repair using a modifications of the original Goetz-method (Woodie, 2006).

This report aimed to provide details regarding the presurgical considerations and surgical procedures recommended for mares that suffer from third degree perineal lacerations and intended for breeding purpose.

Materials and Methods

This study was performed on ten mares of different ages (3-8 years), and those that suffered from third degree perineal laceration. The cases were eight primiparous and two pluriparous. These cases were referred to the surgery clinic of the Faculty of Veterinary Medicine Cairo and Benha Universities and private practices. The owners of these cases were advised to remain on the same feed regimen for the entire period before and after the operation.

Vaginal and uterine infections were controlled before surgical intervention by making four uterine washes (2 per week) using diluted betadine (mixing of 5 ml of betadine antiseptic solution in 1 liter of sterile saline) (Brinsko *et al.*, 2011). The last wash was performed on the same day of the operation. The surgical repair was performed in the standing position with restrain of the animal in stanchion and under effect of combination of

Corresponding Author: Abdelhaleem Elkasapy. Department of Surgery, Faculty of Veterinary Medicine, Benha University, Egypt. Email: *abdelhaleem_elkasapy@yahoo.com*

sedation of 0.5 mg/kg body weight xylazine HCl (Xylaject, ADWIA, Cairo, Egypt), and posterior epidural analgesia at a dose 8-10 ml lidocaine HCl (Debocaine, Aldebiky, Egypt) (Hall *et al.*, 2001). The tail was bandaged and tied up. The rectum was evacuated from feces as cranial as possible and closed by large tampon. One stay suture or allis tissue forceps was applied on each side of the anal sphincter to provide adequate exposure (Fig. 1A and 1B).

An incision was made along the scar tissue line marking the junction between vestibule/vagina and rectum (Fig. 2A and 2B). Dissection of the rectovestibular shelf was started cranially in a frontal plane and laterally into the submucosal tissues as well as caudally to the level of the perineal skin. Lateral dissection was continued until the two flaps were created and brought to the midline without any tension. Closure suture was made according to the modified Goetz technique (six-bite vertical mattress suture pattern) (Fig. 3). The suture material used to oppose the flaps was a coated multifilament No.2 polyglactin 910 (vicryl, Ethicon Inc.) with a half circle needle.

Prophylactic doses of antitetanic serum, nonsteroidal anti-inflammatory drugs (phenylbutaone) with a dose of 2.2 mg/kg body weight once daily intravenous route (phenyloject, ADWIA, Cairo, Egypt), and broad spectrum antibiotics (Procaine Penicillin 200 mg and Dihydrostreptomycine Sulphate 250 mg) (Pen & Strep, Norbrook labrotories) were injected for five successive days.

Mares were observed frequently after surgery for any evidence of defecation or staining, especially for the first 5 days following surgery. If constipation was found, manual evacuation of the rectum was performed by back racking. Wound healing, recovery and complications were recorded.

Results
Third degree rectovestibular lacerations were recorded in ten mares admitted to the clinic one day after parturition. The tissues was edematous and contaminated with feces and some tissues were not be viable. The repair was delayed 4-6 weeks to allow complete healing of the injured tissues (Fig.1A & 1B).

In eight cases the surgical repair of third degree rectovestibular lacerations healed successfully without any complications. The remaining two cases developed partial wound dehiscence at the anal sphincter that eventually recovered after surgery. The uterine wash using diluted betadine (mixing of 5 ml of betadine antiseptic solution in 1 liter of sterile saline) gave good results on the control of infection. The operated mares were naturally inseminated four months following surgery. Eight pregnant mares delivered normally without complications and two cases showed rectovaginal fistula. Rectovaginal fistula was repaired according to Aanes (1964).

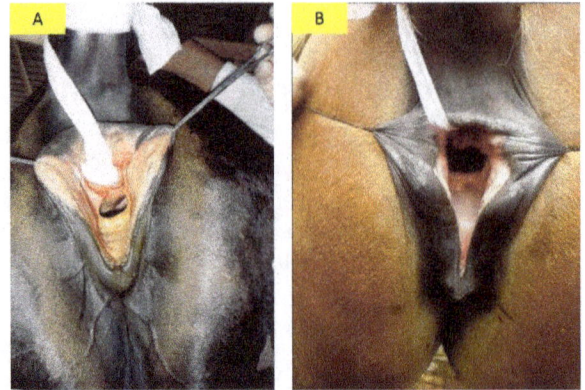

Fig. 1. Third degree rectovestibular lacerations in mares. (A): 45 day post injury, showing absence of vulvar oedema and a band of scar tissue formation. (B): 30day post injury, showing absence of vulvar oedema and a band of scar tissue formation. One stay suture was applied on each side of the anal sphincter to provide adequate exposure.

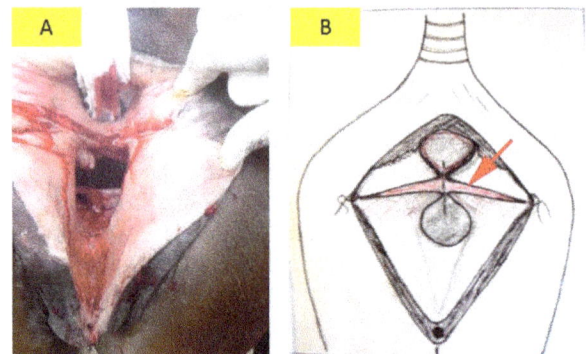

Fig. 2. (A): Dissection along the scar tissue band that separate the rectum from the vestibule. (B): Schematic drawing showing the same (arrow).

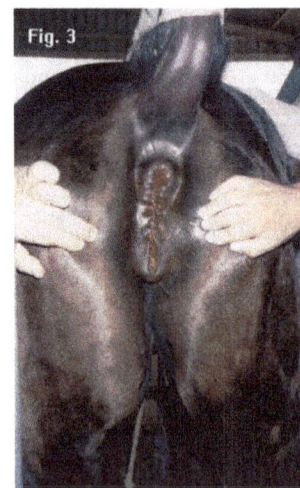

Fig. 3. Suture of the perineal skin with No.2 vicryl.

Discussion
In the present study, all cases occurred at parturition following a dystocia. Out of the ten animals, eight were primiparous. This could be attributed to a

prominent annular fold at the vaginovestibular junction, which could be caught by the foal front foot or nose (McKinnon *et al.*, 1991; Mair *et al.*, 1998; Woodie, 2006; Dabas and Sharma, 2011).

To avoid straining on the suture line after surgery many surgeons prefer keeping the animal fasted for up to 5 days before and 9 days after operation (Aanes, 1988; Hospes and Bleul, 2007). In the present study the owners were advised to keep the animals on the same feed without any change, as the change on the feed lead to hard fecal matter which lead to severe straining and rupture of the suture line.

Because immediate repair of third-degree rectovestibular lacerations is not recommended, the single-stage operation in the cases of this study was delayed for 4-6 weeks, to give chance for the rectal and vestibular walls to heal together and for inflammation to resolve. This findings agree with Flower (1960), Aanes (1964), Vaughan (1974), Farag *et al.* (2000) and Saini *et al.* (2013). On the other hand Woodie (2006) reported that acute repair of third-degree injures should be considered only if it can be performed within a few hours, and if local tissue damage seems compatible with success.

Reconstruction of rectovestibular lacerations was performed in a standing position under the effect of caudal epidural anesthesia with all structures supported in proper relation. These findings agree with that reported by Farag *et al.* (2000) and Mosbah (2012).

However, some studies (Walker and Vaughan, 1880; Saleh *et al.*, 1988; Saini *et al.*, 2013) used dorsal recumbency under effect of general anesthesia. Adams and Fessler (2000) mentioned that dorsal positioning of the cases completely distorted the anatomical relations, and is thus not recommended.

For the success of this surgery, proper selection of the suture material is fundamental. Vicryl (polyglactin 910) is a strong, delayed absorbable and synthetic suture with excellent tissue compatibility. Various suture materials have been used for repair of third-degree rectovestibular lacerations such as monofilament nylon (Stickle *et al.*, 1979), chromic cat gut (Colbern *et al.*, 1985), polyglycolic acid (Shokry *et al.*, 1986; El-Seddawy, 1993), polydioxanone (Karrouf and Zaghloul, 2003; Mosbah, 2012) and polyglactin 910 (Farag *et al.*, 2000; Mehrjerdi *et al.*, 2010).

The success of the surgical repair of the third-degree rectovestibular laceration depends on whether the dissection was sufficiently deepened into sides of the defect to free a thicker rectal and vestibular flap on each side that could be brought together in the midline without any tension. This finding coincides with that reported by Walker and Vaughan (1980), Karrouf and Zaghloul (2003) and Mosbah (2012). They reported that a commonly encountered error was to make division of the tissue planes too shallow. This resulted in excessive tension on the edge of the tissue when they were brought into apposition by the suture causing either wound dehiscence or fistula formation.

There are multiple complications reported in the literature for the repair of third degree perineal laceration in mares. These include rectovestibular fistula, pneumorectum, complete dehiscence of the repair, constipation, tenesmus or reduced performance (Kazemi *et al.*, 2010; Mosbah, 2012). In the present study two mares showed complication of partial wound dehiscence at the anal sphincter that eventually recovered after surgery. However, Kazemi *et al.* (2010) did not report any complication in the seven mares repaired for third degree perineal laceration using one stage Goetze technique.

We concluded that the successful of the surgical interference in third-degree rectovestibular lacerations depend on the control of vaginal and uterine infection by uterine wash and using of one-stage six-bite suture with excessive continuation of dissection of vaginal shelf and rectal floor.

References

Aanes, W.A. 1964. Surgical repair of third-degree perineal laceration and rectovaginal fistula in the mare. J. Am. Vet. Med. Assoc. 144, 485-491.

Aanes, W.A. 1988. Surgical management of foaling injuries. Vet. Clin. North Am. Equine Pract. 4, 417-438.

Adams, S.B. and Fessler, J.F. 2000. Third-degree perineal laceration repair. In: Atlas of equine surgery, 1st ed. Philadelphia, London, Toronto, Sydney: W. B. Saunders Co. pp: 241-244.

Brinsko, S.P., Blanchard, T.L., Varner, D.D., Schumacher, J. and Love, C.C. 2011. Manual of equine reproduction, 3rd edition. Mosby, Inc., an affiliate of Elsevier Inc. pp: 65.

Colbern, G.T., Aanes, W.A. and Stashak, T.S. 1985. Surgical management of perineal lacerations and rectovestibular fistulae in the mare: a retrospective study of 47 cases. J. Am. Vet. Med. Assoc. 186, 265-269.

Dabas, V.S. and Sharma, V.K. 2011. New spiral suture technique to reconstruct third degree perineal laceration in Mare. Indian Vet. J. 88, 36-37.

El-Seddawy, F.D. 1993. Surgical repair of perineal lacerations in mares and Friesian cows. J. Egypt. Vet. Med. Assoc. 534, 681-691.

Emberston, R.H. 1990. Perineal lacerations. In: White NA, Moore JN, editors. Current practice in equine surgery. Philadelphia, PA: J. B. Lippincott. pp: 669-704.

Farag, K.A., Berbish, E.A. and Ghoneim, I.M. 2000. A one-stage repair of third-degree rectovestibular lacerations in the mare: an experimentaland clinical study. J. Egypt. Vet. Med. Assoc. 60(2), 143-151.

Flower, M.E. 1960. The repair of perineal lacerations in the mare. Proc. Am. Assoc. Equine Pract. 6, 106.

Ghamsari, S.M., Nejad, M.M.M. and Moradi, O. 2008. Evaluation of Modified Surgical Technique in Repair of Third-Grade Perineal Lacerations in Mare. Iranian J. Vet. Surg. 3, 71-76.

Hall, L.W., Clarke, K.W. and Trim, A. 2001. Anaesthesia of the horse. In: Veterinary anesthesia 3rd ed. W.B Saunders, pp: 247- 307.

Hospes, R. and Bleul, U. 2007. The effect of extended preoperative fasting in mares undergoing surgery of the perineal region. J. Equine Vet. Sci. 27, 542-545.

Karrouf, G.I. and Zaghloul, A.E. 2003. Surgical correction of third-degree rectovestibular lacerations in equine. Mansoura Vet. Med. J. VI(2), 95-110.

Kazemi, M.H., Sardari, K. and Emami, M.R. 2010. Surgical repair of third-degree perineal laceration by Goetz technique in the mare: 7 cases (2000-2005). Iranian J. Vet. Res. 11, 184-188.

Mair, T., Love, S., Schumacher, J. and Watson, E. 1998. Equine medicine, surgery and reproduction. Philadelphia, PA:W. B. Saunders Co. pp: 177-179.

McKinnon, A.O., Belden, J.O. and Vasey, J.R. 1991. Selected reproductive surgery of the broodmare. Equine reproduction. A seminar for veterinarians, 174. Sydney: Post Graduate Committee in Veterinary Science. pp: 109-125.

Mehrjerdi, K.H., Sardari, K. and Emami, M.R. 2010. Surgical repair of third-degree perineal laceration by Goetz technique in the mare: 7 cases (2000-2005). Iranian J. Vet. Res. 11, 184-188.

Mosbah, E. 2012. A modified one-stage repair of third-degree rectovestibular lacerations in mares. J.

Equine Vet. Sci. 32, 211-215.

Purohit, G.N. 2011. Intrapartum conditions and their management in the mare: A review. J. Livestock Sci. 2, 20-37.

Saini, N.S., Mohindroo, J., Mahajan, S.K., Raghunath, M., Sangwan, V., Kumar, A., Anand, A., Singh, T. and Singh, N. 2013. Surgical management of third degree perineal laceration in young mares. Indian J. Anim. Sci. 83(5), 525-526.

Saleh, M.S., Gohar, H.M., El-Keiey, M.T., Ibrahim, I.M. and Abdel-Hamid, M.A. 1988. Reconstruction of a third-degree rectovestibular laceration in an Arabian mare. J. Egypt. Vet. Med. Assoc. 48(4), 629-635.

Shokry, M., Ibrahim, I.M., Ahmed, A.S. and Abdel-Hamid, M.A. 1986. Preferred suture material in repair of rectovestibular lacerations in mares. Modern Vet. Pract. 67, 546.

Stickle, R.L., Fessler, J.F. and Adams, S.B. 1979. A single-stage technique for repair of rectovestibular lacerations in the mare. Vet. Surg. 8, 25-27.

Vaughan, J.T. 1974. Reconstructive surgery of the perineum, rectum and vagina. In textbook of large animal surgery. Williams and Wilkins, Baltimore; pp: 498-505.

Walker, D.F. and Vaughan, J.T. 1980. Repair of third-degree perineal lacerations. In: Walker DF, Vaughan JT, editors. Bovine and equine urogenital surgery. Philadelphia, PA: Lea and Febiger. pp: 201-210.

Woodie, B. 2006. The vulva, vestibule, vagina and cervix. In: Auer JA, Stick JA, editors. Equine surgery, 3rd ed. Philadelphia, PA: W.B. Saunders Co. pp: 845-852.

11

Cardiotoxicity of *Senna occidentalis* in sheep (*Ovis aries*)

D.I.S. Lopes[1], M.G. Sousa[2,]*, A.T. Ramos[3] and V.M. Maruo[1]

[1]*Federal University of Tocantins (UFT), College of Veterinary Medicine and Animal Science, Araguaina, TO, Brazil*
[2]*Federal University of Paraná (UFPR), Department of Veterinary Medicine, Curitiba, Paraná, Brazil*
[3]*Federal University of Santa Catarina (UFSC), College of Veterinary Medicine, Curitibanos, Santa Catarina, Brazil*

Abstract

The cardiotoxicity of Coffee senna (*Senna occidentalis*) was investigated in sheep that were fed diets containing its seeds, which are recognized as the most poisonous part of such weed. Dianthrone, the main toxic component of *S. occidentalis*, is known to impair mitochondrial oxidative phosphorylation, leading to myofiber degeneration. In this study, fifteen ewes were fed 0%, 2% or 4% of seeds of *S. occidentalis* for 63 days. Non-specific markers of myocyte injury and electrocardiograms were undertaken at baseline, and at 14, 35, and 63 days after the animals were first fed the diets, while histopathology of heart samples was performed at the very end of the study. Our results showed an increase in serum AST and LDH over time, while CK-MB did not change significantly. Changes that could be ascribed to myocardial damage were not documented in the electrocardiograms. Cardiac histopathology demonstrated only mild-to-moderate vacuolar degeneration, myofiber edema and disarray, structural disorganization, and cellular necrosis. In conclusion, *S. occidentalis* caused myocardial fiber degeneration in a dose-dependent fashion, but the electrocardiogram was not able to identify these lesions non-invasively. Because the markers of myofiber injury used in this study lack specificity, they may not be used to support cardiac impairment objectively, despite some of them did change over time.

Keywords: Coffee senna, Electrocardiogram, Myofiber disarray, Plant toxicity.

Introduction

Senna occidentalis, a weed belonging to the family *Caesalpinoideae*, is recognized as one of the most important poisonous plants in veterinary medicine (Tasaka *et al.*, 2000; Górniak, 2008). This leguminous plant is commonly found in summer crops, therefore having its seeds contaminate the harvest, which will later be consumed together with the feed (Riet-Correa *et al.*, 1998; Haraguchi *et al.*, 2003). Poisoning can occur when all the plant is ingested, but most commonly it occurs indirectly when its seeds are not separated from cereal grains. Therefore, it is a concern even for animals under intensive confinement (Górniak, 2008). Although all parts of *S. occidentalis* are poisonous, the seeds are thought to be more toxic (Haraguchi *et al.*, 1998) because of the elevated concentrations of dianthrone, an anthraquinone that interferes with the function of mitochondria, leading to swelling and impairment of its inner structure (Barbosa-Ferreira *et al.*, 2005; Górniak, 2008). Either natural or experimental ingestion of *S. occidentalis* have been investigated in several species and resulted in an afebrile disease, which is characterized by prostration, muscle twitches, diarrhea, myoglobinuria, motor incoordination, and death (Barbosa-Ferreira *et al.*, 2005). Skeletal muscle degeneration has been reported as a common finding in necropsies of several animal species. Alterations in the liver, central nervous system, and heart muscle have been documented as well (Tokarnia *et al.*, 2002). Also, skeletal muscle histopathology demonstrated myofiber atrophy and interstitial edema, while vacuolar degeneration with structural disarray has been recognized in myocardial samples (Górniak, 2008).

To the best of the authors' knowledge, the cardiotoxicity of *S. occidentalis* has never been investigated in ovines fed a diet containing increasing levels of dianthrone. Also, the potential use of electrocardiography as a non-invasive surrogate for myocardial injury was certainly not studied in animals being fed *S. occidentalis*. In this study, we hypothesized that diets containing more seeds of this weed would result in more severe cardiac lesions. Therefore, the purpose of this investigation was threefold: 1) to investigate how the serum levels of non-specific markers of myofiber injury is affected in sheep fed *S. occidentalis*; 2) to determine whether electrocardiography could potentially identify any cardiac lesion caused by the diet; and finally, 3) to use histopathology to assess the changes in cardiac structure.

Material and Methods

Animals

Fifteen mature mixed-breed ewes were recruited into a prospective experimental study. Inclusion criteria included the animals being completely healthy, as determined by a detailed clinical examination and ancillary laboratory tests (CBC and biochemistry) to rule out any conditions that could preclude their inclusion in this investigation. Exclusion criteria included anemia, leukocytosis, atypical biochemistry, as well as any part of physical examination being considered abnormal, such as altered temperature, enlarged lymph nodes, unusual cardiac and/or respiratory auscultation, and abdominal pain. Once enrolled in the study, the sheep were divided into three equal groups. Over a two-month period, each group was fed diets containing 0%, 2% or 4% of *S. occidentalis* seeds. Consumption of the diets was guaranteed by an individual monitoring of each animal throughout the experiment. The analysis of blood markers and the electrocardiograms were undertaken at baseline, and at 14, 35, and 63 days after the animals were first fed the diets. Histopathology of hearts was performed at the very end of the study, which was entirely conducted in accordance with guidelines outlined in the National Institutes of Health *Guide for the Care and Use of Laboratory Animals*.

Plant

S. occidentalis was obtained from rural properties and roadsides of the region (7°11'34.1"S 48°14'05.3"W) in which the study was undertaken. The plant was authenticated and deposited under register #HTO-10035 at the Federal University of Tocantins' herbarium located within Porto Nacional campus. The seeds used to prepare the feed were maintained in tightly sealed containers until the diets were produced at the university premises. The basic feed included 80% cornmeal and 20% soybean meal. Once it was produced, either 0%, 2% or 4% of *S. occidentalis* seeds were manually added in order to reduce the degradation of its active constituent.

Biomarkers of myofiber injury

Blood samples were drawn in sterile tubes. After centrifugation, serum samples were aliquoted and stored at -20°C until the batch analysis was carried out. Using commercially-available kits, we measured the serum levels of aspartate aminotransferase (AST/GOT Liquiform, reference 109, Labtest, Lagoa Santa, Brazil), creatine kinase MB fraction (CK-MB Liquiform, reference 118, Labtest, Lagoa Santa, Brazil), and lactate dehydrogenase (LDH Liquiform, reference 86, Labtest, Lagoa Santa, Brazil). All manufacturer recommendations were strictly followed for laboratory procedures involved with the measurements.

Electrocardiogram

One-minute computer-based electrocardiograms were recorded with a sweep speed of 50 mm/s and an 1 cm = 1 mV sensitivity. The animals were kept standing over a rubber isolation pad, and neither sedatives nor anesthesia were used throughout the procedure. To record a base-apex lead, the negative electrode was placed cranial to the left scapula at the jugular furrow, while the positive electrode was positioned just behind

the left olecranon on the left chest wall (over the apex beat area of the heart) (Fig. 1). Several ECG parameters were measured, including P wave duration (P_{ms}), P wave amplitude (P_{mV}), duration of PR interval (PR), duration of QRS complex (QRS), R wave amplitude (R), S wave amplitude (S), duration of QT interval (QT), T wave amplitude (T_{mV}), and duration of RR interval (RR). Changes in cardiac rhythm were also recorded.

Histopathology of the heart

A total of five cardiac tissue samples, which included the left ventricle free wall, right ventricle free wall, left atrium, right atrium, and the interventricular septum, were harvested from each animal. Samples were immediately fixed in 10% neutral-buffered formalin for 24 hours, and the fixed material was stored in 70% ethanol prior to processing into paraffin. Later, the samples were embedded in paraffin, sectioned at 5 μm, and stained with hematoxylin and eosin staining. All heart samples were semi-quantitatively scored for injuries on a scale of 0 (absent), 1 (mild, small focal lesions), 2 (moderate, multifocal or focally extensive lesions), and 3 (severe, affecting most areas). A positive result was considered when at least one sample was altered in a given animal.

Statistical analysis

The enzyme and electrocardiographic data was tested for normality using the Shapiro-Wilk test. Either a repeated measures analysis of variance or the Friedman test was used to check for differences in these parameters over 63 days of study. Chi-square test was performed to look for an association between diet and the identification of myocardial lesions on histopathology. The software Prism for Windows v. 5.04 (Graphpad Software, San Diego CA, USA) was used for all statistical analyses, and probability < 0.05 was considered significant.

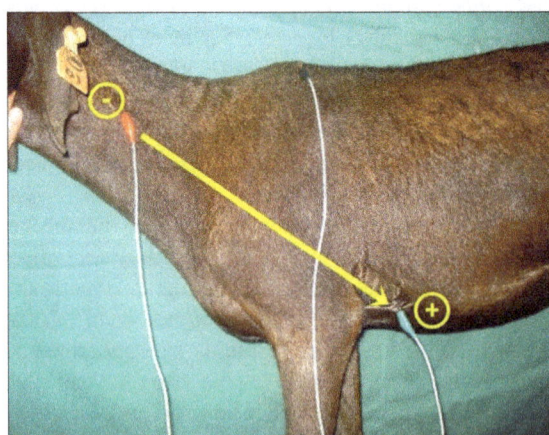

Fig. 1. Electrode placement to record the base apex lead electrocardiogram. The negative electrode (red) is attached to the skin over the jugular furrow, just cranial to the left scapula, while the positive electrode (green) is placed on the apex beat area of the heart, just behind to the left olecranon. The ground electrode (black) is positioned over the thoracic spine. The electrical vector is represented with an arrow.

Results

Table 1 shows the means and standard deviations of the plasma enzymes in all groups. AST and LDH increased significantly over time when diets containing either 2% or 4% of *S. occidentalis* seeds were fed to the animals. No significant alteration was documented for CK-MB data undergoing an analysis of variance. The electrocardiographic data is listed in Table 2, which shows an absence of consistent changes along the experimental period. Only sinus rhythm and sinus arrhythmia were identified throughout the study (Fig. 2). We observed variations in rhythms and sinus arrhythmia became more prevalent over time in ewes being given diets with either 2% or 4% *S. occidentalis* seeds. Nevertheless, an association between diets and rhythms could not be demonstrated by chi-square tests (0% P=0.6444; 2% P=0.1718; 4% P=0.2795).

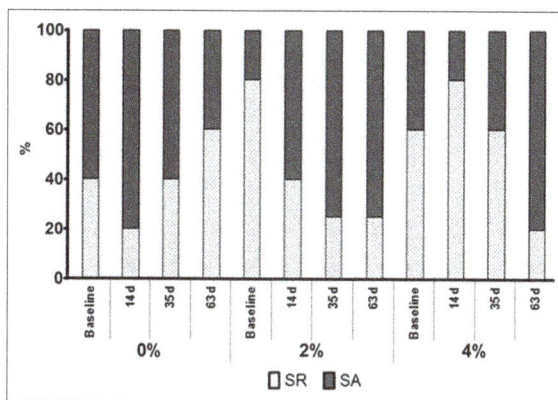

Fig. 2. Distribution of heart rhythms in sheep that were fed diets containing 0%, 2% or 4% of *Senna occidentalis* seeds. Only sinus rhythm (SR) and sinus arrhythmia (SA) were documented over time and no significant association could be demonstrated between diets and heart rhythms.

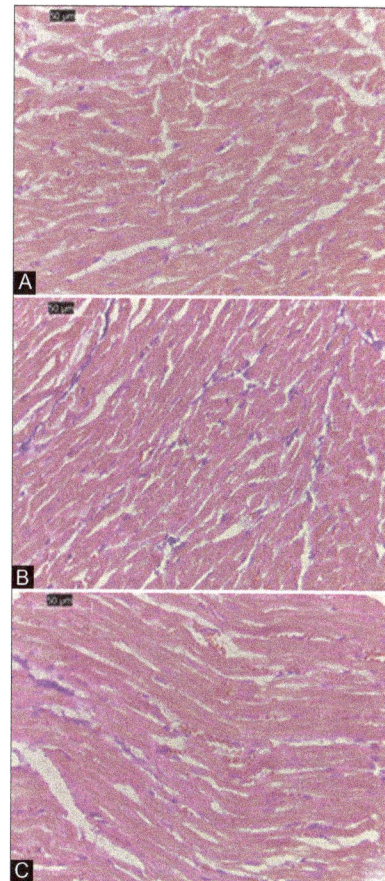

Fig. 3. Representative findings of the histopathological assessment of the left ventricular free wall from ewes fed a diet containing 0% (A), 2% (B) or 4% (C) of *Senna occidentalis* seeds. (A) Normal cardiac myofibers exhibiting a completely normal structural organization; (B) enlarged nuclei are seen within the myofibers; (C) enlarged nuclei and vacuolation of the cytoplasm around the nuclei are shown (H&E, 40x).

Table 1. Serum enzymes [mean (SD)] measured in ewes fed a diet containing 0%, 2% or 4% of *Senna occidentalis* seeds.

Diet (%)	Baseline	14 days	35 days	63 days
AST (U/L)				
0	101.2 (14.9)	105.0 (24.4)	123.0 (9.9)	127.7 (25.5)
2	92.6 (16.6)	98.9 (6.8)	113.1 (4.9)	160.7 (48.4)*
4	77.5 (18.0)	123.0 (25.0)	125.4 (24.3)	149.3 (50.7)*
CK-MB (U/L)				
0	101.7 (96.7)	110.1 (43.9)	135.0 (75.5)	145.0 (45.8)
2	200.0 (44.1)	160.0 (41.0)	258.3 (100.2)	185.8 (75.7)
4	200.0 (67.1)	143.3 (44.5)	188.3 (54.2)	128.8 (45.6)
LDH (U/L)				
0	817.2 (165.4)	666.4 (88.1)	710.4 (140.4)	1023.0 (273.8)
2	276.6 (276.6)	715.2 (220.0)	823.2 (41.5)	1088.7 (506.5)*
4	113.4 (113.4)	815.6 (152.3)*	927.2 (145.6)*	886.6 (240.3)*

*Significantly different (P<0.05) from the baseline measurement at the *post hoc* test. AST: Aspartate aminotransferase, CK-MB: Creatine kinase MB fraction, LDH: Lactate dehydrogenase

Table 2. Results [mean (SD)] of the base-apex electrocardiograms recorded in ewes fed a diet containing 0%, 2% or 4% of *Senna occidentalis* seeds.

Diet (%)	Baseline	14 days	35 days	63 days
P_{ms}				
0	52.60 (4.32)	50.60 (5.75)	60.80 (10.91)	51.40 (3.38)
2	58.80 (8.35)	63.20 (6.43)	62.50 (4.82)	63.20 (8.73)
4	52.80 (3.43)	57.80 (6.68)	59.40 (6.71)	57.20 (6.27)
P_{mV}				
0	0.19 (0.03)	0.12 (0.03)*	0.14 (0.02)	0.16 (0.03)
2	0.15 (0.05)	0.11 (0.03)	0.14 (0.03)	0.17 (0.01)
4	0.15 (0.04)	0.13 (0.02)	0.13 (0.03)	0.17 (0.05)
PR				
0	97.00 (8.00)	95.20 (10.21)	99.40 (16.28)	92.80 (11.30)
2	112.00 (12.93)	118.60 (8.43)	105.25 (11.14)	112.25 (7.19)
4	98.20 (10.54)	107.80 (10.01)	105.80 (21.90)	101.20 (13.48)
QRS				
0	70.60 (9.85)	53.20 (6.71)*	65.20 (9.20)	63.20 (7.81)
2	56.00 (2.68)	56.00 (5.25)	66.75 (15.22)	57.50 (7.63)
4	63.00 (11.02)	57.20 (5.81)	57.20 (8.21)	60.80 (7.14)
R				
0	0.03 (0.01)	0.02 (0.004)	0.03 (0.01)	0.03 (0.01)
2	0.07 (0.06)	0.06 (0.08)	0.05 (0.04)	0.06 (0.04)
4	0.03 (0.01)	0.03 (0.01)	0.02 (0.005)	0.03 (0.01)
S				
0	0.67 (0.26)	0.34 (0.12)	0.44 (0.19)	0.48 (0.06)
2	0.47 (0.17)	0.31 (0.13)	0.40 (0.12)	0.49 (0.16)
4	0.54 (0.19)	0.37 (0.12)	0.43 (0.10)	0.60 (0.25)
QT				
0	279.40 (28.16)	288.80 (20.25)	269.40 (28.09)	280.80 (25.51)
2	279.20 (18.51)	304.60 (38.53)	265.75 (24.77)	256.75 (46.49)
4	294.60 (14.29)	311.80 (36.19)	263.80 (20.57)	284.60 (34.00)
T_{mV}				
0	0.38 (0.15)	0.18 (0.09)	0.25 (0.11)	0.38 (0.21)
2	0.13 (0.10)	0.17 (0.15)	0.19 (0.13)	0.29 (0.05)
4	0.18 (0.06)	0.12 (0.03)	0.18 (0.09)	0.33 (0.14)
RR				
0	527.20 (128.11)	625.60 (86.90)	512.60 (112.14)	524.20 (116.21)
2	646.80 (59.64)	692.80 (140.80)	464.75 (49.06)*	525.75 (85.73)
4	655.60 (99.16)	713.00 (198.93)	502.40 (127.27)	553.40 (59.56)

*Significantly different ($P<0.05$) from the baseline measurement at the *post hoc* test. P_{ms}: P wave duration, P_{mV}: P wave amplitude, PR: Duration of PR interval, QRS: Duration of QRS complex, R: Amplitude of R wave, S: Amplitude of S wave, QT: Duration of QT interval, T_{mV}: Amplitude of T wave, RR: Duration of RR interval

On histopathological examination the microscopic structure of the heart of animals that were fed diets with no *S. occidentalis* appeared normal (Fig. 3A). On the contrary, all animals that were fed diets containing *S. occidentalis* seeds had lesions detected in at least one cardiac sample. When a diet containing 2% of seeds was fed to the ewes, 36% (9/25) of the samples exhibited any abnormality (8/25 mild; 1/25 moderate), which included

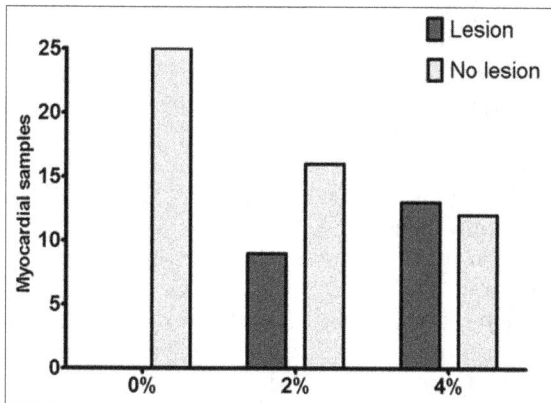

Fig. 4. Identification of myocardial injuries on histopathology in sheep that were fed diets containing 0%, 2% or 4% of *Senna occidentalis* seeds. A significant association ($P=0.0002$) was found to exist between the increasing amount of seeds in diets and the documentation of any cardiac lesions, which included cell vacuolation, myofiber swelling and disarray, pyknotic nuclei, acidophilic cytoplasms, and varying degrees of structural disorganization.

vacuolar degeneration, myofiber edema, and structural disorganization (Fig. 3B). For the animals receiving diets with 4% of seeds, 52% (13/25) of the samples had alterations (9/25 mild; 4/25 moderate), including a complete structural disorganization, with myofiber disarray, small, dark-staining pyknotic nuclei, and acidophilic cytoplasms, which are indicative of cellular necrosis (Fig. 3C). Although Chi-square test found a significant ($P=0.0002$) association to exist between diets and the identification of myocardial lesions on histopathology (Fig. 4), severe lesions affecting most areas were not documented in any animal enrolled in this investigation.

Discussion

In this study we sought to investigate the effects of diets containing increasing concentrations of *Senna occidentalis* seeds, which are recognized as the most poisonous part of that weed. Our main goals were to determine whether diets containing varying concentration of the plant seeds would produce changes, over a two-month period that could be documented by the electrocardiogram, by the serum concentration of some non-specific markers of cardiac injury, and by histopathology of the heart. AST and LDH serum concentrations increased significantly over time (Table 1). However, the non-specific nature of these enzymes, which may be released under a wide array of injuries, including liver damage, preclude its sole use to identify cardiac impairment specifically.

As mentioned before, the ECG disclosed no significant changes when the ewes were fed the diets. The very few changes found on the electrocardiographic data occurred in animals receiving diets with no seed at all (Table 2), except for a reduction in RR interval observed at 35 days in animals fed 2% of seeds. The

RR interval is inversely related to heart rate, therefore indicating an increased heart rate at the same moment. It is worth mentioning, however, that the instantaneous heart rate recorded by the electrocardiogram is heavily influenced by environmental conditions, including those that potentially cause stress to the animals, such as the physical restraint needed for ECG recording (Lago *et al.*, 2009). In a study in which 31 healthy ovines were enrolled, Schultz *et al.* (1972) found the heart rate to range from 60 to 197 bpm, showing its strong variation. Later, another investigation also found an increased mean heart rate of 119 bpm in normal sheep (Tório *et al.*, 1997). In this study, however, the mean heart rates remained within the normal range for ovines at all times. Sinus rhythm was the most prevalent cardiac rhythm at baseline evaluation, which is consistent with prior studies in sheep (Tório *et al.*, 1997; Mir *et al.*, 2000; Lago *et al.*, 2009). However, when diets containing seeds were given to the animals, there was a progressive non-significant change to sinus arrhythmia, which became the most prevalent rhythm at 63 days animals fed either 2% or 4% of *S. occidentalis* seeds. Curiously, sinus arrhythmia is not considered a malignant arrhythmia, since it results from variations in autonomic balance. Therefore, increases in sympathetic tone accelerate the heart rate, while the attenuated sympathetic tone reduces the heart rate. To the authors' knowledge, however, the effects of *S. occidentalis* in the autonomic balance was never investigated, and at this time we might speculate that these findings could be ascribed to the animals being more used to the exam room, therefore having an attenuated sympathetic response along the procedure.

In contrast, the microscopic assessment of heart samples showed varying degrees of structural damage to the myocardial cells, which was more prevalent and severe in animals being given a 4%-seed diet. This condition is likely supportive of the toxicity of *Senna occidentalis* on the heart occurring in a dose-dependent fashion. Interestingly, no changes in QT interval could be observed, suggesting no impairment in ventricular total electrical activity in spite of the structural damage and myofiber disarray. P waves, which represent the atrial electrical activity, were consistently documented in all animals regardless of the diet being fed to them. Prior studies in ovines indicated a positive P wave in the majority of leads (Schultz *et al.*, 1972; Tório *et al.*, 1997), which is similar to our findings. In this study, 100% of the electrocardiograms exhibited positive P wave at lead II. It is likely that myocyte disorientation and myofibrilar disarray were not able to create an electrical milieu and substrate for supraventricular arrhythmias in these animals.

Alterations in cardiac muscle have been documented in several species being given *S. occidentalis*. Necrosis, vacuolar degeneration, structural disorganization, acidophilic cytoplasm, pyknosis, myofiber thinning, swelling and replacement by connective tissue are all reported in many preceding investigations (O'Hara *et al.*, 1969; Martins *et al.*, 1986; Barros *et al.*, 1990; Tasaka *et al.*, 2000). Dianthrone, the main toxic component of *S. occidentalis*, is known to induce the uncoupling of mitochondrial oxidative phosphorylation, which is absolutely necessary to produce energy for the constant pumping action of the heart. Such energy-deprivation impairs the sodium-potassium pump activity and, as a result, water accumulates within the cell leading to myofiber degeneration (Barros *et al.*, 1990). Similarly, feeding diets containing either 2% or 4% *S. occidentalis* seeds to animals in this study for 63 days was enough to produce myocardial lesions that included vacuolation, pyknotic nuclei, acidophilic cytoplasms, and swelling of myofiber bundles, which resulted in varying degrees of structural disarray that are similar to previous reports (Suliman *et al.*, 1982; Suliman and Shommein, 1986; Barros *et al.*, 1999).

Among the several limitations of this investigation are the small number of animals recruited, the relatively short period of time during which the animals were fed the seed-containing diets, the absence of a cardiac-specific biomarkers such as troponin I, and finally, the absence of an echocardiographic assessment of the hearts to evaluate remodeling and function *in vivo*. Also, a more detailed microscopic assessment of the heart samples could reveal information on remodeling of the extracellular matrix, and whether apoptosis also played a role in the degenerative process ascribed to *S. occidentalis*.

Conclusion

In conclusion, diets containing either 2% or 4% of *Senna occidentalis* seeds caused myocardial fiber degeneration in ewes in a dose-dependent fashion. A wide array of lesions was observed, but all animals had at least one lesion documented on cardiac histopathology. Although only mild lesions could be documented, this study found that a few animals that were given diets containing the plant seeds developed lesion within the myocardial tissue. Serum AST and LDH increased over time and might potentially aid in detecting myofiber injury. On the contrary, the electrocardiogram was not able to document any changes that could be related to myocardial damage.

References

Barbosa-Ferreira, M., Dagli, M.L., Maiorka, P.C. and Gorniak, S.L. 2005. Sub-acute intoxications by *Senna occidentalis* seeds in rats. Food Chem. Toxicol. 43, 497-503.

Barros, C.S.L., Ilha, M.R.S., Bezerra Junior, P.S., Langohr, I.M. and Kommers, G.D. 1999. Intoxicação por *Senna occidentalis* (Leg. Caesalpinoidea) em bovinos em pastoreiro. Pesq. Vet. Bras. 19, 68-70.

Barros, C.S.L., Pilati, C., Andujar, M.B., Graça, D.L. Irigoyen, L.F., Lopes, S.T. and Santos, C.F. 1990. Intoxicação por *Cassia occidentalis* (Leg. Caes.) em Bovinos. Pesq. Vet. Bras. 10, 47-58.

Górniak, S.L. 2008. Plantas tóxicas de interesse agropecuário. In: Toxicologia aplicada à Medicina veterinária. Eds., Spinosa, H.S., Górniak, S.L. and Paterno-Neto J. Barueri:Manole, pp: 415-458.

Haraguchi, M., Calore, E.E., Dagli, M.L., Cavaliere, M.J., Calore, N.M.P., Weg, R., Raspantini, P.C. and Górniak, S.L. 1998. Muscle atrophy induced in broiler chicks by parts of *Senna occidentalis* seeds. Vet. Res. Commun. 22, 265-271.

Haraguchi, M., Dagli, M.L.Z., Raspantini, P.C.F. and Górniak, S.L. 2003. The effects of low doses of *Senna occidentalis* seeds on broiler chickens. Vet. Res. Commun. 27, 321-328.

Lago, E.P., Melo, M.M., Araujo, R.B., Nascimento, E.F., Silva, E.F. and Melo, M.B. 2009. Perfis eletrocardiográfico e ecodopplercardiográfico de ovinos após ingestão da suspensão aquosa de *Mascagnia rigida Griseb. (Malpighiaceae)*. Arq. Bras. Med. Vet. Zootec. 61, 853-862.

Martins, E., Martins, V.M.V., Riet-Correa, F., Soncini, R.A. and Paraboni, S.V. 1986. Intoxicação por *Cassia occidentalis* (leguminoseae) em suínos. Pesq. Vet. Bras. 6, 35-38.

Mir, S.A., Naski, A.R. and Raina, R. 2000. Comparative eletrocardiographic studies and differing effects of pentazocine on ECG, heart and respiratory rates in young sheep and goats. Small Rumin. Res. 37, 13-17.

O'hara, P.J., Pierce, K.R. and Kay Read, W. 1969. Degenerative Myopathy Associated with Ingestion of *Cassia occidentalis* L.: Clinical and Pathologic Features of the Experimentally Induced Disease. Am. J. Vet. Res. 30, 2173-2180.

Riet-Correa, F., Soares, M.P. and Mendez Mdel, C. 1998. Poisonings in horses in Brazil. Ciência Rural 28(4), 715-722.

Schultz, R.A., Pretorius, P.J. and Terblanche, M. 1972. An electrocardiographic study of normal sheep using a modified technique. Onderstepoort J. Vet. Res. 39, 97-106.

Suliman, H.B., Wasfi, I.A. and Adam, S.E.I. 1982. The toxicology of *Cassia occidentalis* to goats. Vet. Hum. Toxicol. 24, 326-330.

Suliman, H.B. and Shommein, A.M. 1986. Toxic effect of the roasted and unroasted beans of Cassia occidentalis to goats. Vet. Hum. Toxicol. 28, 6-11.

Tasaka, A.C., Weg, R., Calore, E.E., Sinhorini, I.L., Dagli, M.L.Z., Haraguchi, M. and Górniak, S.L. 2000. Toxicity testing of *Senna occidentalis* seed in rabbits. Vet. Res. Commun. 24, 573-582.

Tokarnia, C.H., Dobereiner, J.D. and Peixoto, P.V. 2002. Poisonous plants affecting livestock in Brazil. Toxicon 40, 1635-1660.

Tório, R., Cano, M., Montes, A., Prieto, F. and Benedito, J.L. 1997. Comparison of two methods for electrocardiographic analysis in Gallega sheep. Small Rumin. Res. 24, 239-246.

12

Isolation of *Staphylococcus sciuri* from horse skin infection

H. Beims[1], A. Overmann[1], M. Fulde[2], M. Steinert[1] and S. Bergmann[1,*]

[1]*Department of Infection Biology, Institute of Microbiology, Technische Universität Braunschweig, Spielmannstr. 7, 38106 Braunschweig, Germany*
[2]*Center for Infection Medicine, Institute of Microbiology and Epizootics, Freie Universität Berlin, Berlin, Germany*

Abstract

Staphylococcus sciuri is known as an opportunistic pathogen colonizing domesticated animals and has also been associated with wound infections in humans. Particularly over the last decade, oxacillin (methicillin) resistant strains had been emerged, which now increase the medical relevance of this species. This report describes the identification of an oxacillin-resistant *S. sciuri* isolate from a wound infection of a horse. We determined the absence of coagulase and hyaluronidase activity and analysed the antibiotic resistance profile.

Keywords: Colonization, Horse, Oxacillin resistance, *Staphylococcus sciuri*.

Introduction

Staphylococcus sciuri is a member of the *S. sciuri*-species group composed of coagulase-negative and novobiocin-resistant bacteria (Nemeghaire *et al.*, 2014a). This group includes *S. sciuri* (with three subspecies), *S. lentus, S. vitulinus, S. fleurettii* and *S. stepanovicii* (Becker *et al.*, 2014a), which are in general considered as commensal animal-associated species (Kloos *et al.*, 1976). *S. sciuri* possesses a certain pathogenic potential and is able to induce infections in both, animals (Frey *et al.*, 2013; Dos Santos *et al.*, 2015) and humans (Stepanovic *et al.*, 2003). Some isolates of the *S. sciuri* group are known to carry different homologues of the methicillin resistance genes *mecA*, B and C and display methicillin/oxacillin resistance (Becker *et al.*, 2014a,b; Harrison *et al.*, 2014).

In the present study, we report the identification of an oxacillin-resistant *S. sciuri* isolate from a purulent skin lesion of a horse, determined activity of coagulase and hyaluronidase and characterized the antibiotic resistance profile.

Case Details

A "Hannoveraner Hengst" at the age of ten presented a purulent skin lesion on the right forehand pastern. The medical prehistory claimed repeated episodes of purulent skin infections, foremost on the bridge of the nose, which poorly healed untreated within a couple of weeks.

One year later, a closed, swollen abscess-like structure was developed on the right forehand pastern. The abscess erupted within two to three days and presented a bloody skin lesion of ~4 cm in length and ~1 cm in width (Fig. 1).

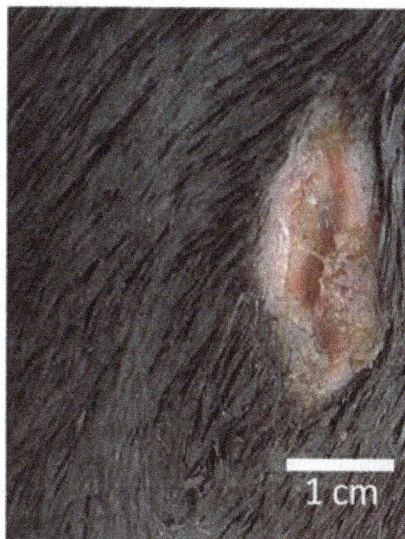

Fig. 1. Erupted abscess-like skin lesion of ~4 cm in length and ~1 cm in width on the right forehand pastern of the horse.

The skin lesion became purulent and was treated with non-antibiotic zinc-containing ointment. No systemic clinical signs were detected.

Culture-based analyses/Identification of S. sciuri

A swab specimen was taken from the purulent skin lesion and cultured onto Columbia blood agar plates (Becton Dickenson) containing 5% sheep blood at 37°C and 5% CO_2. Morphological analyses revealed growth of uniform, non-hemolytic, white opaque colonies after 24 h at 37 °C (Fig. 2A, B). Light microscopy and Gram-stain indicated a pure culture of Gram positive cocci clustered in grape-like aggregates (Fig. 2C).

*Corresponding Author: Simone Bergmann. Department of Infection Biology, Institute of Microbiology, Technische Universität Braunschweig, Spielmannstr. 7, 38106 Braunschweig, Germany. Email: *simone.bergmann@tu-braunschweig.de*

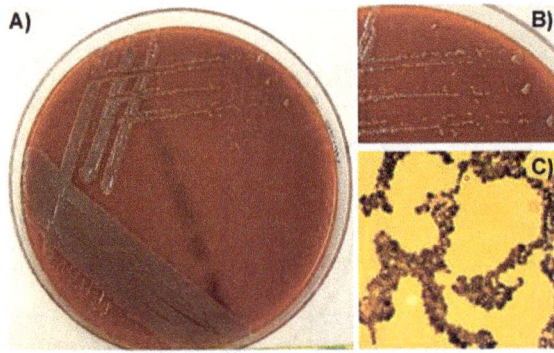

Fig. 2. (A): Morphology of *Staphylococcus sciuri* on Columbia blood agar plates. (B): The zoom in indicates white to light grey staphylococcal colonies without any haemolytic activity. (C): Gram-stain visualized Gram-positive, coccoid bacteria, clustered in grape-like structures.

Strain identification by sequencing of 16S rRNA was conducted from a single colony as described elsewhere (Weisburg, *et al.*, 1991) using the following oligonucleotides: forward primer: 27f 5'-AGA GTT TGA TCM TGG CTC AG-3', reverse primer: 1492 r 5'-CGG TTA CCT TGT TAC GAC TT-3' and was repeated three times using colony material from the same culture plate. After purification of PCR-products using QIA quick PCR Purification Kit (Qiagen) sequencing procedure was performed by GATC-Biotech (Germany).

Blast® search (provided by NCBI, NLM, Bethesda, USA) identified *S. sciuri* in all three independent probes as primary infectious agent. The listed blast results presented in Table 1 confirm the high sequence identity with up to 98% query coverage to *S. sciuri* in all of the tested three independent probes. Results further point to the identification of *carnicatus* or *rodentium* as respective subspecies but the nominal difference to the results given for the third potential subspecies *sciuri* were not significant enough to allow a final determination of the subspecies.

A bacterial colonization analysis from swabs taken from the horse nostrils did not identified *S. sciuri* as constant colonizer of the horse, but identified typical members of horse microflora such as *Aeromonas viridans* and *S. vitulinus* by Maldi Tof.

Verification of strain-identification and MIC-determination

Species identification of the *S. sciuri* isolate was confirmed using the standardized API STAPH V5.0 system and revealed an ID value of 88.4%. The specification of the respective isolate was further confirmed using the bioMérieux VITEK®2 system (Germany) according to the manufacturer recommendations and also independently by the "National Reference Center of Staphylococci and Enterococci" of the Robert Koch Institute (RKI) in Wernigerode, Germany.

Table 1. 16SrRNA-based sequencing results from three independent culture probes as obtained by blast®-sequence alignment (NCBI; NLM).

sample	hit		S. sciuri		
		subsp.	carnicatus	rodentium	sciuri
1	1	Strain	GTC 1227	GTC 844	ATCC 29062
		Query cover	98%	98%	98%
		Ident	85%	85%	85%
		Accession	NR 041327.1	NR 041328.1	AJ421446.1
	2	Strain	GTC 1227	GTC 844	ATCC 29062
		Query cover	98%	98%	40%
		Ident	85%	85%	85%
		Accession	AB233331.1	AB233332.1	AY688097.1
	3	Strain	ATCC 700058	ATCC 70061	
		Query cover	40%	40%	
		Ident	82%	82%	
		Accession	AY688095.1	AY688096.1	
2	1	Strain	GTC 1227	GTC 844	ATCC 29062
		Query cover	96%	96%	95%
		Ident	86%	86%	86%
		Accession			
	2	Strain	GTC 1227	GTC 844	ATCC 29062
		Query cover	96%	96%	35%
		Ident	86%	86%	82%
		Accession	AB233331.1	AB233332.1	AY688097.1
	3	Strain	ATCC 700058	ATCC 70061	
		Query cover	35%	35%	
		Ident	82%	82%	
		Accession	AY688095.1	AY688096.1	
3	1	Strain	GTC 1227	GTC 844	ATCC 29062
		Query cover	95%	95%	95%
		Ident	86%	86%	86%
		Accession	NR 041327.1	NR 041328.1	AJ421446.1
	2	Strain	GTC 1227	GTC 844	ATCC 29062
		Query cover	95%	95%	37%
		Ident	86%	86%	82%
		Accession	AB233331.1	AB233332.1	AY688097.1
	3	Strain	ATCC 700058	ATCC 70061	
		Query cover	37%	37%	
		Ident	82%	82%	
		Accession	AY688095.1	AY688096.1	

Furthermore, automated antimicrobial susceptibility testing was performed at the "National Reference Center for Staphylococci and Enterococci" of the Robert Koch Institute in Wernigerode, Germany via microbouillon-dilution, including the following antibiotics: ß-lactams (benzylpenicillin, oxacillin), macrolides (erythromcycin), lincosamides (clindamycin), oxazolidinone (linezolid), fucidanes (fusidic acid), aminoglycosides (gentamycin), ansamycins (rifampicin), tetracycline (oxytetracyclin), glycopeptides (vancomycin, teicoplanin), gylcylcyclins (tigecyclin), fluoroquinolons (ciprofloxacin, moxifloxacin), cyclic lipopeptides (daptomycin), the epoxid fosfomycin and the folate synthesis inhibitor cotrimoxazol. MIC value determination was evaluated according to the EUCAST standards for human medicine and revealed sensitivity to most of the tested antibiotics (Table 2).

Table 2. Analyses of MIC of different antibiotics by the "National Reference Center of Staphylococci and Enterococci" of the Robert Koch Institute in Wernigerode, Germany, evaluated by EUCAST-based interpretation.

Antibiotics	MIC (µg/ml)	interpretation
Benzylpenicillin	0.125	S
Oxacillin	1.0	R
Fosfomycin	8.0	R
Gentamycin	0.5	S
Linezolide	1.0	S
Erythromycin	0.5	S
Clindamycin	0.25	S
Oxytetracyclin	0.5	S
Tigecyclin	0.125	S
Vancomycin	1.0	S
Teicoplanin	4.0	R
Ciprofloxacin	0.5	S
Moxifloxacin	0.25	S
Daptomycin	1.0	S
Co-trimoxazole	0.5	S
Rifampicin	0.063	S
Fusidic acid	8.0	R

Interestingly, the antibiotic resistance profile covering 17 antibiotics indicated a resistance against fosfomycin, fusidic acid and teicoplanin (Table 2).

Teicoplanin resistance was additionally tested by plating a higher inoculum. In sum, the results point to a heterogenic teicoplanin resistant strain. Moreover, according to the EUCAST standards, the *S. sciuri* strain is resistant against oxacillin. This is remarkable since detection of the common resistance genes *mecA* and

mecC via specific PCR by Reference Center of the RKI (Wernigerode, Germany) was negative.

Additionally, the particular *S. sciuri* was tested negative for coagulase and hyaluronidase activity, respectively. The activities of both virulence factors was analysed by tube test with human and rabbit plasma and by decapsulation test with *S. equi* as described by Essers and Radebold (1980).

Discussion

S. sciuri is mostly recovered from skin and mucous membrane of animals and has long been considered as a non-pathogenic commensal bacterium (Adegoke, 1986). During the last decade of years, it has been associated with several cases of bovine mastitis (Lüthje and Schwarz, 2006; Nam et al., 2010; Frey et al., 2013), as well as from goats suffering from peste des petites ruminants (PPR) (Ugochukwu and Agwu, 1991), from cases of canine dermatitis (Hauschild and Wójcik, 2007; Hauschild et al., 2010), and from several outbreaks of fatal exudative epidermitis in piglets (Chen et al., 2007; Nemeghaire et al., 2014c).

The recurrent manifestation of skin lesions monitored in the present case, initially suggested a permanent colonization of the horse with *S. sciuri*. In contrast to several reports pointing to nasal colonization of horses with *S. sciuri*, so far no data on permanent skin colonization has been reported for horses (Bagcigil et al., 2007; Aslantas et al., 2012; Karakulska et al., 2012). The lack of *S. sciuri* in cultures of nasal swabs in this case may point to the occurrence of a single colonization event or may suggest repeated episodes of temporary colonization.

Interestingly, a transmission in between healthy domestic animals colonized with *S. sciuri* was repeatedly observed (Moodley and Guardabassi, 2009; Aslantas et al., 2012). This transmission may be promoted by insects serving as transmission vectors. In this respect, a report also suggested that the possible source of *S. sciuri* colonization in surgical wounds may be flies perching on open wounds (Kolawole and Shittu, 1997).Thus, it is assumed that frequent contact with healthy domestic and farm animals may also contribute to an at least temporary colonization of the skin, and subsequently the wounds, by *S. sciuri* (Kloos et al., 1976; Nemeghaire et al., 2014b).

Despite the rare occurrence of *S. sciuri* in humans (Marsou et al., 1999; Couto et al., 2000; Nagase et al., 2002), some reports furthermore point to the role of *S. sciuri* as opportunistic pathogens isolated from various clinical specimen and causing serious infections in humans such as endocarditis, peritonitis, septic shock, and wound infections (Hedin and Widerstrom, 1998; Wallet et al., 2000; Horii et al., 2001; Stepanovic et al., 2002, 2003;). Moreover, despite the lack of data regarding *S. sciuri* colonization of the handler, a recurrent transmission from the handler to the horse cannot be excluded. The isolated *S. sciuri* strain was tested negative for coagulase and hyaluronidase activity and the antibiotic profiling confirmed sensitivity against most of the tested antibiotics, which suggested a low general pathogenicity of this strain. Nevertheless, the *S. sciuri* strain revealed resistance against fosfomycin, fusidic acid and teicoplanin (Table 2). According to the information provided by the Reference Center of the RKI in Wernigerode, approximately 80% of the tested *S. sciuri* strains reveal resistance against fusidic acid.

Interestingly, based on the EUCAST definition, the present strain is also resistant against Oxacillin. The *S. sciuri* species cluster group is represented by three *S. siuri* subspecies and also contains the species *S. vitulinus*. This cluster group carries different *mecA* homologues and has been proposed as origin and reservoir of the *S. aureus mecA* gene (Becker *et al.*, 2014a,b; Nemeghaire *et al.*, 2014a). In the genome of the present *S. sciuri* isolate, neither a *mecA* nor a *mecC* gene mediating methicillin/oxacillin resistance could be amplified by specific PCR at the National Reference Center at the RKI in Wernigerode. Thus, it has been reported that phenotypic methicillin (and other β-lactam) -resistance in *Staphylococcaceae* members is conferred not only by *mecA*, but also by different *mecA* allotypes and also by homologous genes such as *mecB* and *mecC* (Becker *et al.*, 2014a,b). Moreover, a hybrid SCC*mec* consisting of a *mecA*-encoding SCC*mec* type VII element and a separate *mecC* region in terms of a ΨSCC*mec* element was published for *S. sciuri* (Harrison *et al.*, 2014; Becker *et al.*, 2014a). These reports might suggest the presence of a further *mec*-homolog or a *mec* gene hybrid within the genome of the isolated *S. sciuri* strain, which could not be amplified by the *mecA* and *mecC*-specific oligonucleotides.

Nevertheless, based on genomic and plasmid encoded genes, multiresistant *S. sciuri* isolates carrying resistance genes against all major classes of antibiotics have already been reported (Li *et al.*, 2016) and support the potential to temporarily serve as a "bacterial shuttle" e.g. by transmitting genetic information between other bacterial species of the horse´s skin microbiome.

In sum, these results suggest the identification of a coagulase-negative *Staphylococcus* exhibiting moderate virulence.

Conflict of interest

The Authors declare that there is no conflict of interest.

References

Adegoke, G.O. 1986. Characteristics of staphylococci isolated from man, poultry and some other animals. J. Appl. Bacteriol. 60, 97-102.

Aslantas, O., Turkyilmaz, S., Yilmaz, M.A., Erdem, Z. and Demir, C. 2012. Isolation and molecular characterization of methicillin-resistant staphylococci from horses, personnel and environmental sites at an equine hospital in Turkey. J. Vet. Med. Sci. 74, 1583-1588.

Bagcigil, F.A., Moodley, A., Baptiste, K.E., Jensen, V.F. and Guardabassi, L. 2007. Occurrence, species distribution, antimicrobial resistance and clonality of methicillin- and erythromycin-resistant staphylococci in the nasal cavity of domestic animals. Vet. Microbiol. 121(3-4), 307-315.

Becker, K., Ballhausen, B., Köck, R. and Kriegeskorte, A. 2014a. Methicillin resistance in *Staphylococcus* isolates: the "mec alphabet" with specific consideration of mecC, a mec homolog associated with zoonotic *S. aureus* lineages. Int. J. Med. Microbiol. 304(7), 794-804.

Becker, K., Heilmann, C. and Peters, G. 2014b. Coagulase-negative staphylococci. Clin. Microbiol. Rev. 27(4), 870-926.

Chen, S., Wang, Y., Chen, F., Yang, H., Gan, M. and Zheng, S.J. 2007. A highly pathogenic strain of *Staphylococcus sciuri* caused fatal exudative epidermitis in piglets. PLoS One 2, e147.

Couto, I., Santos Sanches, I., Sá-Leão, E., and de Lencastre H. 2000. Molecular characterization of *Staphylococcus sciuri* strains isolated from humans. J. Clin. Microbiol. 38, 1136-1143.

Dos Santos, F., Mendoca, L.C., Reis, D.R., Guimaraes, A.S., Lange, C.C., Ribeiro, J.B., Machado, M.A. and Brito, M.A. 2015. Presence of a mecA-positive multidrug-resistant *Staphylococcus epidermidis* in bovine milk samples in Brazil. J. Dairy Sci. 99(2), 1374-1382.

Essers, L. and Radebold, K. 1980. Rapid and Reliable Identification of *Staphylococcus aureus* by a Latex Agglutination Test. J. Clin. Microbiol. 12, 641-643.

Frey, Y., Rodriguez, J.P., Thomann, A., Schwendener, S. and Perreten, V. 2013. Genetic characterization of antimicrobial resistance in coagulase-negative staphylococci from bovine mastitis milk. J. Dairy Sci. 96, 2247-2257.

Harrison, E.M., Paterson, G.K., Holden, M.T., Ba, X., Rolo, J., Morgan, F.J., Pichon, B., Kearns, A., Zadoks, R.N., Peacock, S.J., Parkhill, J. and Holmes, M.A. 2014. A novel hybrid SCC*mec-mecC* region in *Staphylococcus sciuri*. J. Antimicrob. Chemother. 69, 911-918.

Hauschild, T., Slizewski, P. and Masiewicz, P. 2010. Species distribution of staphylococci from small wild mammals. Syst. Appl. Microbiol. 33, 457-460.

Hauschild, T. and Wojcik, A. 2007. Species distribution and properties of staphylococci from canine dermatitis. Res. Vet. Sci. 82, 1-6.

Hedin, G. and M. Widerstrom. 1998. Endocarditis due to *Staphylococcus sciuri*. Eur. J. Clin. Microbiol. Infect. Dis. 17, 673-675.

Horii, T., Suzuki, Y., Kimura, T., Kanno, T., and Maekawa. M. 2001. Intravenous catheter-related septic shock caused by *Staphylococcus sciuri* and *Escherichia vulneris*. Scand. J. Infect. Dis. 33(12), 930-932.

Karakulska, J., Fijałkowski, K., Nawrotek, P., Pobucewicz, A., Poszumski, F. and Czernomysy-Furowicz, D. 2012. Identification and methicillin resistance of coagulase-negative staphylococci isolated from nasal cavity of healthy horses. J. Microbiol. 50(3), 444-451.

Kloos, W.E., Zimmerman, R.J. and Smith, R.F. 1976. Preliminary studies on the characterization and distribution of *Staphylococcus* and *Micrococcus* species on animal skin. Appl. Environ. Microbiol. 31, 53-59.

Kolawole, D.O. and Shittu, A.O. 1997. Unusual recovery of animal staphylococci from septic wounds of hospital patients in Ile-Ife, Nigeria. Lett. Appl. Microbiol. 24, 87-90.

Li, D., Wang, Y., Schwarz, S., Cai, J., Fan, R., Li, J., Feßler, A.T., Zhang, R., Wu, C. and Shen, J. 2016. Co-location of the oxazolidinone resistance genes optrA and cfr on a multiresistance plasmid from *Staphylococcus sciuri*. J. Antimicrob. Chemother. 71(6), 1474-1478.

Lüthje, P. and Schwarz, S. 2006. Antimicrobial resistance of coagulase-negative staphylococci from bovine subclinical mastitis with particular reference to macrolide-lincosamide resistance phenotypes and genotypes. J. Antimicrob. Chemother. 57, 966-969.

Marsou, R., Bes, M., Boudouma, M., Brun, Y., Meugnier, H., Freney, J., Vandenesch, F. and Etienne, J. 1999. Distribution of *Staphylococcus sciuri* subspecies among human clinical specimens, and profile of antibiotic resistance. Res. Microbiol. 150, 531-541.

Moodley, A. and Guardabassi, L. 2009. Clonal spread of methicillin-resistant coagulase-negative staphylococci among horses, personnel and environmental sites at equine facilities. Vet. Microbiol. 137, 397-401.

Nagase, N., Sasaki, A., Yamashita, K., Shimizu, A., Wakita, Y., Kitai, S. and Kawano, J. 2002. Isolation and species distribution of staphylococci from animal and human skin. J. Vet. Med. Sci. 64, 245-250.

Nam, H.M., Lim, S.K., Kim, J.M., Kang, H.M., Moon, J.S., Jang, G.C., Wee, S.H., Joo, Y.S. and Jung, S.C. 2010. Antimicrobial susceptibility of coagulase-negative staphylococci isolated from bovine mastitis between 2003 and 2008 in Korea. J. Microbiol. Biotechnol. 20, 1446-1449.

Nemeghaire, S., Argudin, M.A., Fessler, A.T., Hauschild, T., Schwarz, S. and Butaye, P. 2014a. The ecological importance of the *Staphylococcus sciuri* species group as a reservoir for resistance and virulence genes. Vet. Microbiol. 171, 342-356.

Nemeghaire, S., Argudin, M.A., Haesebrouck, F. and Butaye, P. 2014b. Molecular epidemiology of methicillin-resistant *Staphylococcus sciuri* in healthy chickens. Vet. Microbiol. 171, 357-363.

Nemeghaire, S., Vanderhaeghen, W., Argudin, M.A., Haesebrouck, F. and Butaye, P. 2014c. Characterization of methicillin-resistant *Staphylococcus sciuri* isolates from industrially raised pigs, cattle and broiler chickens. J. Antimicrob. Chemother. 69, 2928-2934.

Stepanovic, S., Dakic, I., Djukic, S., Lozuk, B. and Svabic-Vlahovic, M. 2002. Surgical wound infection associated with *Staphylococcus sciuri*. Scand. J. Infect. Dis. 34, 685-686.

Stepanovic, S., Jezek, P., Vukovic, D., Dakic, I. and Petras, P. 2003. Isolation of members of the *Staphylococcus sciuri* group from urine and their relationship to urinary tract infections. J. Clin. Microbiol. 41, 5262-5264.

Ugochukwu, E.I. and Agwu, C.O. 1991. Aerobic bacteria from nasal discharge of goats suffering from clinical PPR: isolation and identification. Microbios. 65(263), 81-85.

Wallet, F., Stuit, L., Boulanger, E., Roussel-Delvallez, M., Dequiedt, P. and Courcol, R. J. 2000. Peritonitis due to *Staphylococcus sciuri* in a patient on continuous ambulatory peritoneal dialysis. Scand. J. Infect. Dis. 32, 697-698.

Weisburg, W.G., Barns, S.M., Pelletier, D.A. and Lane, D.J. 1991. 16S ribosomal DNA amplification for phylogenetic study. J. Bacteriol. 173, 697-703.

13

Cutaneous squamous cell carcinoma in the lateral abdominal wall of local Libyan ewes

S.K. Tmumen[1], S.A. Al-Azreg[2], M.H. Abushhiwa[1,*], M.A. Alkoly[1], E.M. Bennour[3] and S.R. Al-Attar[2]

[1]Department of Surgery and Theriogenology, Faculty of Veterinary Medicine, University of Tripoli, Tripoli, Libya
[2]Department of Pathology and Clinical Pathology, Faculty of Veterinary Medicine, University of Tripoli, Tripoli, Libya
[3]Department of Internal Medicine, Faculty of Veterinary Medicine, University of Tripoli, Tripoli, Libya

Abstract
Gross and histopathological features of surgically excised squamous cell carcinomas (SCC) observed in thirteen local Libyan ewes were reported. The age of the ewes enrolled in the current study ranged from 2 to 3 years. The cases were admitted to private veterinary clinics in south-western region of Tripoli, Libya, during the period between July 2014 and October 2015. All lesions were located in the right and left lateral abdominal wall (caudo-ventrally) with a size range of 8 to 11 cm in diameter. The tumor masses have been removed by surgical excision. The histopathological examination of surgically excised masses has revealed the characteristic cell nests of SCC showing central keratinization and hyalinization with presence of apoptotic bodies, fattened keratinocytes, and a heavy interstitial infiltration of neutrophils and lymphocytes. The follow up of the cases showed no signs of tumor reoccurrence. In conclusion, SCC in Libyan sheep affects mainly the woolless areas and can be successfully removed by surgical excision.
Keywords: Histopathological findings, Lateral abdominal wall, Libyan ewes, Squamous cell carcinoma, Surgical excision.

Introduction

Tumors of skin and subcutaneous tissues are the most frequently recorded tumors in farm animal species (Tmumen, 1992; Hassanein and Mahmoud, 2009; Ahmed and Hassanein, 2012). Squamous Cell Carcinoma (SCC) is a malignant tumor of epidermal cells causing the differentiation of these cells to keratinocytes (Goldschmidt and Hendrick, 2002). SCC is the second most common skin tumor in farm animals. This type of tumor is mostly seen in aged animals, so that it is almost impossible to determine the incidence of SCC in farm animals as a large percentage of these animals slaughtered at an early age (Del Fava et al., 2001; Goldschmidt and Hendrick 2002; Valentine, 2004). The proposed etiologies for SCC include the prolonged exposure to sunlight and photosensitizing-agents containing plants and the lack of skin pigmentation and hair (Valentine, 2004; Hassanein and Mahmoud, 2009). Additionally, the overexpression of p53 has been found to play an important role in the development of SCC in human and animals (Teifke and Löhr, 1996). Papilloma virus has also been mentioned as a possible cause of SCC in sheep (Del Fava et al., 2001).
In sheep, SCC has been reported in different breeds (Hassanein and Mahmoud, 2009; Ahmed and Hassanein, 2012; Najarnezhad and Aslani, 2012) and in various locations throughout the body (Foreyt et al., 1991; Ramadan et al., 1991; Mendez et al., 1997). In a

large scale study investigating the skin tumors in fat-tailed sheep and goats in the Kingdom of Saudia Arabia by Ahmed and Hassanein (2012), it has been found that SCC was much more common in females than males. The locations of SCC in sheep included head, shoulder, back, abdomen, limbs and tail. SCC in the lumbar region in sheep was reported in only one ewe as an unusual site (Najarnezhad and Aslani, 2012).
Metastasis of SCC to local lymph nodes can occur after long time from its appearance and wide surgical excision has been found to be successful to treat SCC prior to spreading to surrounding tissues (Valentine, 2004).
The current study aimed to record and describe thirteen cases of cutaneous SCC in local Libyan ewes in south-western Tripoli as well as the outcome of surgical excision of such lesions.

Materials and Methods
Animals, history and clinical examination
The present study was carried out on thirteen Libyan ewes of 2-3 years old age. These ewes were brought from different geographical localities within the south-western area of Great Tripoli during the period from July 2014 to October 2015. Tumor masses of different sizes erupted since 3-5 months on the lateral abdominal wall. The case history has been taken and a general clinical examination has been performed. In addition, a special examination for the tumor mass location, size and nature of lesion have been performed. Then, the

*Corresponding Author: Dr. Mohamed H. Abushhiwa. Faculty of Veterinary Medicine, University of Tripoli, Tripoli, Libya.
E-mail: mabushhiwa@yahoo.com

affected ewes were subjected to a surgical excision for tumor mass removal and for further diagnosis by histopathological examination.

Surgical procedure

Before the surgical intervention, animals were deprived of food for the period of 24 h. The animal was sedated and a local anesthetic agent was infiltrated at the surgical site. An elliptical skin incision was performed and the tumor mass was excised gently with some healthy tissues by blunt dissection. Then, the surgical wound was closed using non-absorbable suture material. The suture was removed 8-12 days post operation. The tumor masses were finally submitted to histopathological examination. Most of the cases were followed up via clinic visits or phone contact with the owners.

Histopathology examination

For histopathological examination, five tissue specimens were fixed in 10% buffered formalin for later processing and examination. All histopathological procedures were performed according to Bancroft and Cook (1984). The tissue sections were stained with haematoxylin and eosin (H&E) following the standard procedure. The stained tissue sections were examined under light Microscope (ZEISS, Germany). The degree of tumor differentiation was determined according to Goldschmidt and Hendrick (2002).

Results

Clinical examination

The clinical examination showed that all animals were in a good general condition with normal body temperature.

SCC lesions description

Grossly, the tumor masses were firm in consistency with different sizes (8-11cm in diameter) and shapes (Fig. 1). The tumors were located in the caudo-ventral part of the lateral abdominal wall (9 cases at the right side and 4 cases at the left side). The lesion was sometimes associated with exudation, ulceration, feted odor or hemorrhage and surrounded by inflammatory zone.

Histopathological findings

Five biopsies involving the skin and subcutaneous tissue of the abdominal wall were examined. Large irregular subcutaneous mass was extensively ulcerated and necrotized with hemorrhage. Microscopical examination of the biopsies in all cases revealed the characteristic (pathognomonic) cell nests of SCC showing central keratinization and hyalinization with the presence of apoptotic bodies, fattened keratinocytes, and a heavy interstitial infiltration of neutrophils and lymphocytes. The neutrophils and lymphocytes appeared in the sections as they were trying to invade the cell nests, while some has already invaded the centers of cell nests with phagocytic and lytic activities. Hydropic degeneration in some of the

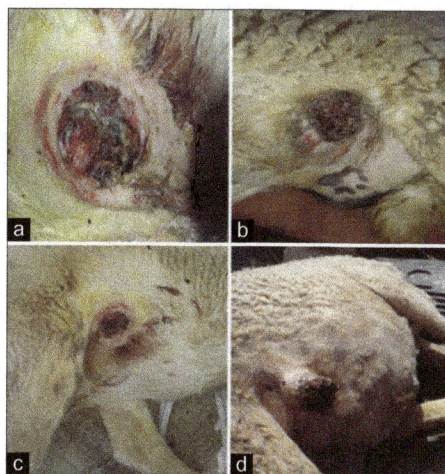

Fig. 1. Gross appearance and location of the SCC in Libyan sheep. (a) Almost round shaped SCC lesion at the left ventral abdominal wall with exudation and hemorrhage. (b) Unevenly shaped SCC lesion at the left ventral abdominal wall. (c) SCC lesion at the right ventral abdominal wall. (d) Projected fingerlike firm SCC lesion with ulceration and hemorrhage at the right ventral abdominal wall.

prickle cells surrounding the keratinized central layer has also been noticed. Numerous mitotic figures in all cases were also existed (Fig. 2a-f). Additionally, based on the histopathological findings, some carcinomas were well-differentiated and some of them were poorly differentiated.

Prognosis of the surgical excision

The follow up of the SCC cases showed no signs of tumor reoccurrence seven months after surgery. This indicated the effectiveness of the surgical intervention as an approach to treat such cases. Furthermore, there were no signs of local metastasis to the regional lymph nodes in any of the cases.

Discussion

Skin tumors, particularly SCC, has been extensively reported in the literature and stated by some authors as relative common skin tumor in sheep (Del Fava et al., 2001; Goldschmidt and Hendrick, 2002; Valentine, 2004; Hassanein and Mahmoud, 2009; Ahmed and Hassanein, 2012).

The current study reported the gross and microscopical characteristics of SCC masses found in the lateral abdominal wall of 13 local Libyan ewes aged between 2 and 3 years.

Cutaneous SCC has been reported to affect sheep in various sites in the hairless areas of the skin including head, shoulder, back, abdomen, limbs and tail (Ahmed and Hassanein, 2012), lumbar region (Najarnezhad and Aslani, 2012) and cervix and vagina (Ferrer et al., 2011). Interestingly, in all sheep recorded in our study, the tumor masses were at the same area, the lateral abdominal wall, and all animals were females which is the first report of such findings, as all findings

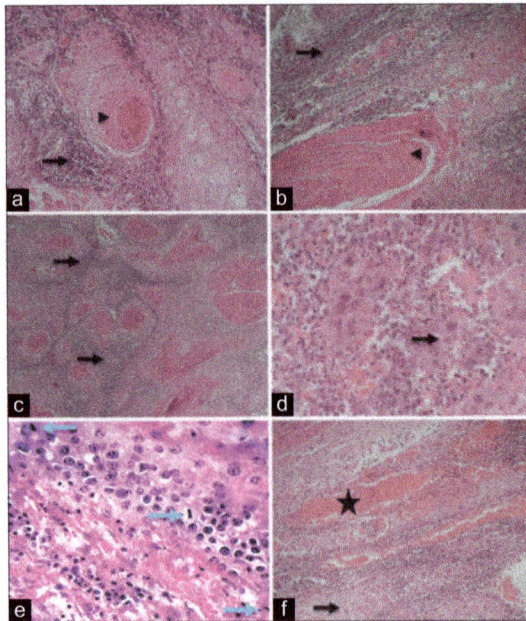

Fig. 2. Histopathological findings of the squamous cell carcinomas. (a&b) Central keratinization and hyalinization (arrowheads) with heavy interstitial infiltration of inflammatory cells (neutrophils and lymphocytes) (arrows). (c) Aggregation of neutrophils around the outer layer of the cell nest. (d) Fattening and hyalinization of the central cell layer. (e) Neoplastic cells with mitotic figures (arrows). (f) Intense inflammatory reaction represented by dilated blood vessels (star) and huge aggregation of neutrophils and lymphocytes. The neutrophils invading some of the structures of cell nest specially the central keratinocytes (arrows). (H&E stain: a&b x100; c&f x50; d&e x400).

reported before showed that the tumor masses located in various parts throughout the body and recorded in both males and females. Although, in a recent report, ewes appeared to be more susceptible to SCC than rams (Ahmed and Hassanein, 2012).

Our findings are largely consistent with most of the previous reports in regard to the age of sheep affected with this kind of tumor. It has been found that the highest prevalence of SCC in sheep is from 4 to 6 years age and rarely recorded in sheep less than 4-year old (Mendez *et al.*, 1997; Valentine, 2004; Ahmed and Hassanein, 2012). On the other hand, it has been stated that SCC is commonly reported in middle-aged to old sheep (Lloyd, 1961; Vandegraaff, 1976; Ladds and Entwistle, 1977; Riet-Correa *et al.*, 1981; Lagadic *et al.*, 1982; Scott, 2007). In the present study, the age of ewes affected with cutaneous SCC was between 2 and 3 years, which is supported by the findings of Scott (2007) and considered quite unique finding showing that this tumor can occur in younger age.

The underline cause of skin tumor is still unclear in general. However, several predisposing factors are

believed to play a role in causing such tumors. One of these factors is the long exposure to sunlight and ultraviolet radiation (Valentine, 2004; Ahmed and Hassanein, 2012). Based on the geographical location of the ewes enrolled in the present study, the long exposure to radiation is likely to be the predisposing factor. Secondarily, the area of the lateral ventral abdomen is very susceptible to irritation by rough ground which might be another reason for having the tumor masses in this area instead of other predicted sites reported in literature.

Conclusion

We could conclude that the local Libyan ewes could be affected with SCC. The tumor affects mainly the right and left lateral abdominal woolless skin. The recorded cases were all females. Histopathological examination of the tumor biopsies revealed the pathognomonic cell nests of SCC. We could also conclude that surgical excision is an efficient treatment of non metastatized or infiltrated SCC without recurrence for several months. Further studies are required to investigate the prevalence of this skin tumor in Libyan sheep as well as its predisposing factors.

Acknowledgment

The authors would like to thank Turkia Aduma and Asma Al-Hammali, the technicians at the Pathology and Clinical Pathology Laboratory, Faculty of Veterinary Medicine, University of Tripoli, for their kindness and technical assistance.

Conflict of interest

For the present work the authors received no financial support and there is no conflict of interest.

References

Ahmed, A.F. and Hassanein, K.M.A. 2012. Ovine and caprine cutaneous and ocular neoplasms. Small Rum. Res. 106, 189-200.

Bancroft, J.D. and Cook, H.C. 1984. Manual of Histological Techniques. Churchill Livingstone, Edinburgh, London, Melbourne, New York.

Del Fava, C., Verissimo, C.J., Rodrigues, C.F.C., Cunha, E.A., Ueda, M., Maiorka, P.C. and Angelino, D.J.L. 2001. Occurrence of squamous cell carcinoma in sheep from a farm in Sao Paulo state, Brazil. Arquivo do Instituto de Biologia de Sao Paulo 68(1), 35-40.

Ferrer, L.M., Lacasta, D., Ramos, J.J., Jalón, J.A., Ruiz De Arcaute, M. and Conde, T. 2011. Squamous cell carcinoma of the vagaina and cervix in sheep- Case report. Acta Vet. Hung. 59, 123-127.

Foreyt, W.J., Hullinger, G. and A.Leathers, C.W. 1991. Squamous Cell Carcinoma in a Free-ranging Bighorn Sheep (Ovis Canadensis californiana). J. Wildl. Dis. 27, 518-520.

Goldschmidt, M.H. and Hendrick, M.J. 2002. Tumors of the skin and soft tissues. Tumors in Domestic

Animals. 4th ed. Iowa State University, pp: 105-107.

Hassanein, K.M.A. and Mahmoud, A.Z. 2009. Pathological studies on tumor incidence in farm animals. Alex. J. Vet. Sci. 28, 105-117.

Ladds, P.W. and Entwistle, K.W. 1977. Observations on squamous cell carcinomas of sheep in Queensland, Australia. Br. J. Cancer 35, 110-114.

Lagadic, M., Wyers, M., Mialot, J.P., ParodI, A.L. 1982. Observation d'une enzootie de cancers de la vulve chez la brebis. Zentralblatt für Veterinärmedizin Reihe A 29, 123-135.

Lloyd, L.C. 1961. Epithelial tumors of the skin of sheep. Br. J. Cancer 15, 780-789.

Mendez, A., Perez, J., Ruiz-Villamor, E., Garcia, R., Martin, M.P. and Mozos, E. 1997. Clinicopathological study of an outbreak of squamous cell carcinoma in sheep. Vet. Rec. 23, 597-600.

Najarnezhad, V. and Aslani, M. R. 2012. Unusual case of cutaneous squamous cell carcinoma in an ewe. Iranian J. Vet. Sci. Technol. 4, 49-53.

Ramadan, R.O., Gameel, A.A. and El Hassan, A.M. 1991. Squamous cell carcinoma in sheep in Saudi Arabia. Rev. Elev. Med. Vet. Pays. Trop. 44, 23-26.

Riet-Correa, F., Cassal, A.B., Scarsi, R.M., Schild, A.L. and Mendez, M.C. 1981. Carcinomas Epidermóides em ovinos em um estabelecimento do Rio Grande do Sul. Pesq. Vet. Bras. 1, 65-68.

Scott, R.P. 2007. The skin. In. Scott, R.P. Sheep Medicine. Manson Publication Ltd. The Veterinary Press, pp: 240-264.

Teifke, J.P. and Löhr, C.V. 1996. Immunohistochemical detection of P53 over expression in paraffin wax-embedded squamous cell carcinomas of cattle, horses, cat and dogs. J. Comp. Pathol. 114, 205-210.

Tmumen, S.K. 1992. Surgical swelling in farm animals. M.V.Sc. Thesis. University of Tripoli. Tripoli, Libya.

Valentine, B.A. 2004. Neoplasia. In: Farm animal surgery. Saunders. Fubini, S.L. and Ducharme, N.G. 1st ed. St Louis: Philadelphia: Saunders, pp: 23-44.

Vandegraaff, R. 1976. Squamous Cell Carcinoma of the Vulva in Merino Sheep. Aust. Vet. J. 52, 21-23.

14

Occipital condylar dysplasia in a Jacob lamb (*Ovis aries*)

Alison M. Lee[*], Nicola F. Fletcher, Conor Rowan and Hanne Jahns

School of Veterinary Medicine, Veterinary Science Centre, University College Dublin, Belfield, Dublin 4, Ireland

Abstract

Jacob sheep (*Ovis aries*) are a pedigree breed known for their "polycerate" (multihorned) phenotype. We describe a four-horned Jacob lamb that exhibited progressive congenital hindlimb ataxia and paresis, and was euthanased four weeks post-partum. Necropsy and CT-scan revealed deformity and asymmetry of the occipital condyles, causing narrowing of the foramen magnum and spinal cord compression. Histopathology demonstrated Wallerian degeneration of the cervical spinal cord at the level of the foramen magnum. These findings are consistent with occipital condylar dysplasia. This condition has been infrequently reported in the literature as a suspected heritable disease of polycerate Jacob sheep in the USA, and is assumed to arise during selection for the polycerate trait. This is the first reported case in European-bred Jacob sheep. Occipital condylar dysplasia should be considered as a differential diagnosis in polycerate Jacob lambs showing ataxia. It is important to raise awareness of this disease due to its suspected heritability and link to the popular polycerate trait.

Keywords: Ataxia, Congenital, Jacob sheep, Occipital condylar dysplasia, Polycerate.

Introduction

Jacob sheep are a popular pedigree/ornamental breed used for meat production and as a source of high-quality wool. There are approximately 8,000 Jacob sheep registered with the European-based Jacob Sheep Society (mainly in the UK and Ireland) with approximately 3,000 new lambs registered annually (Richardson, 2016). In the USA, there were over 10,000 Jacob sheep registered with the Jacob Sheep Breeder's Association in 2006 (Jacob Sheep Breeders Association, 2009).

An important heritable condition in this breed is G_{M2} gangliosidosis (Tay-Sachs disease) and a diagnostic test has recently been developed to facilitate its elimination from affected flocks (Lewis *et al.*, 2014). Another potentially heritable condition of this breed, known as "occipital condylar dysplasia" has been reported in a total of four Jacob sheep in the scientific literature, and (to the authors' knowledge) only in the USA (Johnson *et al.*, 1994; Ellis and Brown, 2014). However, there is anecdotal awareness of this condition among the American Jacob sheep-breeding community (Ellis and Brown, 2014). It is assumed to be a genetic defect (possibly resulting from selective breeding for the polycerate phenotype) as it appears to occur exclusively in four-horned sheep (Ellis and Brown, 2014). This is the first reported case of the condition in Europe. It is important to raise awareness among veterinarians and breeders of the possible existence of another potentially-heritable condition in this increasingly popular breed, in order that it be monitored and controlled if necessary.

Case details

History, clinical findings, treatment

The animal in question was a pedigree, four-horned male Jacob lamb with a history of progressive congenital ataxia. It was a twin lamb born to a primiparous two-year-old ewe, and its female twin and both parents were clinically normal. There was no flock history of ataxia or other neurological signs, and the lamb's dam and grand-dam were home-bred. Its mother's dam produced 11 healthy lambs (seven females of which are still present in this flock, and have never produced lambs with signs of occipital condylar dysplasia).

The sire was used for breeding for the past four years within this flock, and had sired 21 clinically-normal registered lambs at the time of this lamb's birth. Before breeding, the lamb's mother was treated with an intravaginal progesterone-soaked sponge to induce oestrus. The sire was the only ram who had access to her at the time of oestrus, and both were housed together in a well-secured shed. All ewes were routinely supplemented with copper, selenium, cobalt, potassium iodide and vitamins A, D3, E, B1 and B12, and both parents were tested and found to be negative for the causative mutation of G_{M2} gangliosidosis.

The lamb in question displayed mild, bilateral, symmetrical hindlimb ataxia and paresis at birth, which worsened with age until falling and difficulty rising from recumbency were frequently observed. Low head carriage was also noted. The animal remained bright, alert and able to feed. The referring practitioner (a first-opinion mixed-practice veterinarian) performed a

*Corresponding Author: Alison M. Lee. Veterinary Pathobiology Section, School of Veterinary Medicine, Veterinary Sciences Centre, University College Dublin, Belfield, Dublin 4, Ireland. E-mail: *alison.lee@ucdconnect.ie*

limited on-farm neurological examination, and no cranial nerve/postural reaction deficits were noted. Therefore the lesion was presumptively localised to the spinal cord.

The principal clinical differential diagnoses included copper deficiency and spinal abscess or trauma. Less likely differentials (given the genetic status of the lamb's parents and knowledge of endemic infectious diseases) were G_{M2} gangliosidosis, infectious diseases causing congenital skeletal/cerebral malformations (e.g. Schmallenberg virus, Border disease), and other infectious conditions such as enterotoxaemia, toxoplasmosis, or otitis media.

The lamb was treated with copper methionate 20 mg/ml (0.5 ml, Ballinskelligs Vet. Products Ltd), amoxicillin-clavulanic acid 140/35 mg/ml (8.75 mg/kg, Noroclav Injection, Norbrook Laboratories Limited) and dexamethasone 2 mg/ml (1 mg/kg, Colvasone, Norbrook Laboratories Limited) for four consecutive days. Despite treatment, at four weeks of age, the lamb became recumbent and euthanasia was elected on humane grounds. The lamb was submitted for post-mortem examination to the University College Dublin Veterinary Hospital.

Gross post-mortem examination

A routine, complete necropsy examination was carried out. The lamb was in good body condition, with no appreciable external conformational abnormalities. Upon dissection of the skull and spinal column, both occipital condyles were found to be markedly distorted, asymmetrical, and deviated to the right (Fig. 1).

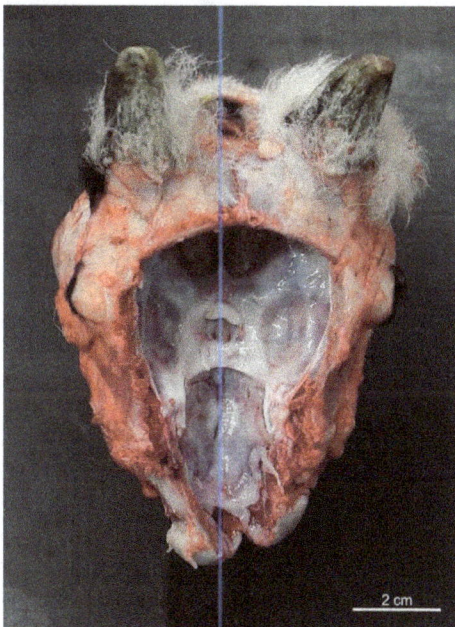

Fig. 1. Dorsal view of skull, crown removed. Vertical line indicates normal orientation of midline. Here, there is marked lateral deviation of the foramen magnum and occipital condyles.

The corresponding articular facets of the atlas were irregular in appearance, with the left facet located slightly caudal to the right. The cartilage of the articular surfaces was multifocally roughened and irregular in thickness.

The brain appeared normal in size and morphology, with no appreciable abnormalities common to teratogenic viral infections, and no macroscopic evidence of inflammation. The cervical spinal cord was narrow and bilaterally compressed in cross-section at the foramen magnum. No other gross abnormalities were present in the remaining vertebral column or spinal cord, or other tissues examined grossly at necropsy.

CT-scan

For better visualisation and accurate measurement of the condylar pathology, a CT-scan of the skull of the lamb was carried out subsequent to dissection using a 4 slice multi-detector (Somatom Sensation 4, Software version A40, Siemens, Germany; Fig. 2).

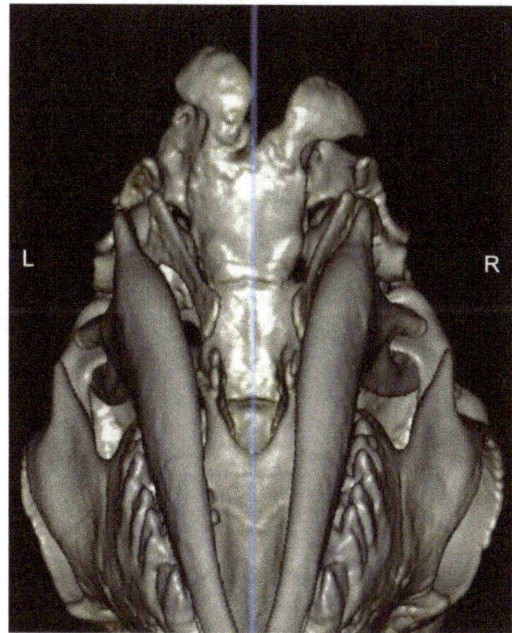

Fig. 2. CT-scan of skull (ventral aspect). Both condyles are asymmetrical, irregular, and deviated to the right.

The left condyle was found to measure 16.16 mm rostral to caudal x 11.4 mm wide x 13.7 mm high and extended caudoventromedially to form an angle of 41° with the nasal septum, 42° with the vertical ramus of the left mandible and 58° with the hard palate. The right condyle (measuring 11.86 mm rostral to caudal x 7.9 mm wide x 9.2 mm high) had a more flattened articular surface and extended caudoventrolaterally to form an angle of 42° with the nasal septum, 50° with the vertical ramus of the right mandible and 45° with the hard palate. At the rostral aspect of the occipital condyles, the foramen magnum measured 16.5 mm wide.

Histopathologic examination

For histopathological evaluation, following routine fixation in 10% neutral buffered formalin, brain, spinal cord and occipital condyles (decalcified) were embedded in paraffin wax and sectioned at 5μm. Sections were stained with Gill®-2 Haematoxylin and Eosin (HE) and Luxol fast blue (Bancroft and Gamble, 2002). On histopathologic examination of the central nervous system, the principal lesions were observed in the cervical spinal cord at the point of compression (the foramen magnum). Here, the central canal appeared compressed and rectangular in cross-section. The ventral medial fissure was deviated laterally by approximately 5° from the vertical in cross-section (Fig. 3).

There was marked dilation (ballooning) of the myelin sheaths with occasional fragmentation, affecting mainly the ventral and lateral funiculi. These dilated sheaths contained multifocal, swollen, irregular, spherical, pale, amorphous eosinophilic degenerate axons (spheroids). Low numbers of myelin sheaths contained one or more microglia with moderate amounts of eosinophilic foamy cytoplasm (Fig. 3, inset). Marked loss of myelin in these areas was seen on Luxol fast blue stain (Fig. 4). These changes are characteristic of Wallerian degeneration. Digestion chambers were observed in longitudinal sections. The spinal cord grey matter was unaffected. Similar, less marked changes were present in the dorsal funiculi. Similar degenerative axonal changes were observed throughout the cervical, thoracic and lumbar spinal cord, becoming progressively less severe towards the caudal aspect of the cord.

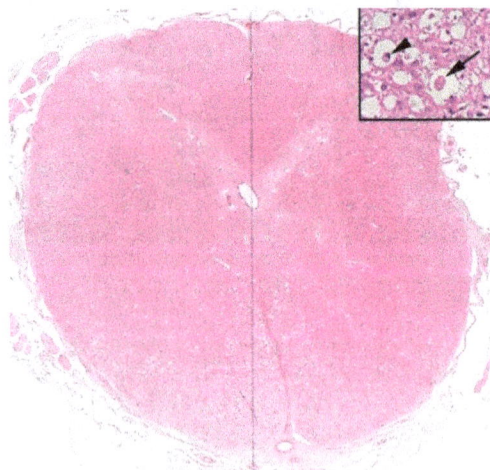

Fig 3 Cross section of cervical spinal cord at the level of the foramen magnum; (4-week-old Jacob lamb with occipital condyle dysplasia,) 5° deviation of the ventral fissure from the midline and marked vacuolation of white matter in the ventral and lateral funiculi, inset; Wallerian degeneration seen as dilated myelin sheets containing spheroids (arrow) and microglia (arrow head), H&E.

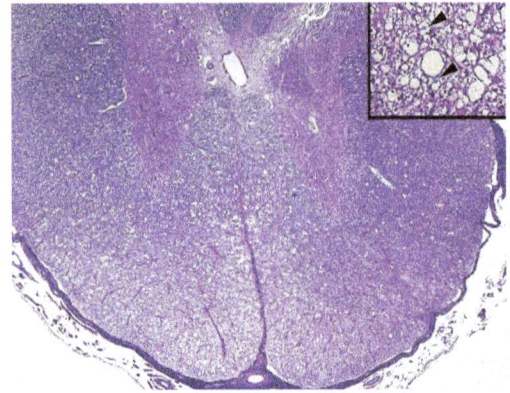

Fig. 4. Cross-section of cervical spinal cord at the level of the foramen magnum; (4-week-old Jacob lamb with occipital condylar dysplasia). On Luxol fast blue stain, myelin fibres appear blue, neuropil appears pink and nerve cells appear purple. Marked loss of myelin in white matter in the ventral and lateral funiculi. Inset; dilated myelin sheaths contain no myelin or only little clumped remnants of myelin (arrowheads). Luxol Fast Blue.

No inflammatory changes or lesions indicative of lysosomal storage disease or copper deficiency were present. Histopathology of the occipital condyles revealed normal endochondral ossification. No pathological changes were found on histologic examination of the brain.

Ancillary tests

Genetic analysis, as described by Torres *et al.* (2010), was conducted on DNA extracted from hepatic tissue by LGC (Herts, UK). The lamb was found to have homozygous G at nucleotide position 1330 of the hexa cDNA and therefore did not show the G_{M2} gangliosidosis mutation. Liver copper values were within normal limits (1.2 mmol/kg; reference range: 0.06 - 2.5 mmol/kg). Routine PCR on frozen lamb liver tissue for pestivirus, Bluetongue virus and Schmallenberg virus were negative.

Based on these findings, a diagnosis of occipital condylar dysplasia was made.

Discussion

The gross condylar lesions described above (asymmetry and distortion) closely resemble previous occipital condylar dysplasia cases (Johnson *et al.*, 1994; Ellis and Brown, 2014). Johnson *et al.* (1994) described the disease in two lambs in Missouri. It was also reported in two lambs in Georgia, in a poster presentation by Ellis and Brown (2014). The main difference between the present case and previous reports was that one of the lambs described by Ellis and Brown (2014) developed clinical signs at four months of age (as opposed to at birth). However, the overall similarities in clinical presentation and pathologic findings suggest a common aetiology and pathogenesis. The atlanto-occipital joint forms part of the craniovertebral junction, consisting of the occiput, atlas, axis and their supporting ligaments. It encloses the structures of the cervicomedullary junction (medulla, spinal cord and lower cranial nerves) (Smoker, 1994).

In general, craniovertebral junctional anomalies occur sporadically in most species, and defects affecting the atlanto-occipital joint in isolation are infrequent (Johnson et al., 1994). There are several well-described familial pathologies of animals affecting the craniocervical junction, including Chiari-like malformation in Cavalier King Charles Spaniels (Loughin, 2016), atlantoaxial instability in toy dogs (Slanina, 2016), occipitoatlantoaxial malformation in Arabian horses (Watson and Mayhew, 1986), and complex vertebral malformations in Holstein calves (Agerholm et al., 2001). Atlanto-axial instability is also a characteristic of humans with Down syndrome (Pueschel et al., 1981; Burke et al., 1985). Reported craniocervical anomalies of sheep include vertebral canal stenosis in Suffolks (Palmer et al., 1981; Jackson and Palmer, 1983), occipitoatlantoaxial malformation in a Suffolk-cross lamb (Schmidt et al., 1993), and dens hypoplasia in a Columbia-cross lamb (Parish et al., 1984). However, occipital condylar dysplasia appears to be specific to Jacob sheep. Occipital condylar dysplasia ("coconut condyle") has only been reported in humans as a single case report (Halanski et al., 2006).

The observed clinical signs (progressive hindlimb ataxia and paresis) were consistent with cervical spinal cord compression and subsequent Wallerian degeneration, and occur non-specifically in many of the craniovertebral junction disorders mentioned previously. Cord compression was observed grossly at the foramen magnum, and histopathological examination revealed lesions typical of compressive spinal injury (Summers et al., 1995).

A number of potential clinical differential diagnoses were considered in this case. One of these was "swayback/enzootic ataxia" (copper deficiency). Clinical signs include progressive paraparesis, hyporeflexia and muscle atrophy, and it is caused by inadequate copper intake by the dam in pregnancy (Thomas, 2016). Congenital swayback can manifest grossly as bilateral, symmetrical cerebral cavitation, or be restricted to histological changes: degeneration of neurons in the red, lateral vestibular, medullary reticular, and dorsal spinocerebellar nuclei in Clarke's column, and in the spinal motor neurons, and also Wallerian degeneration of dorsolateral and ventromedial spinal cord tracts (Cantile, 2016). Again, this diagnosis was unlikely due to the history of copper supplementation, lack of typical gross and/or histological lesions, and the liver copper analysis results. Spinal abscess or trauma were among other clinical differential diagnoses.

However, the lamb failed to respond to antibiotics and anti-inflammatory treatment, rendering this diagnosis less likely. It had been kept indoors since birth due to ataxia, thus reducing the likelihood of tick bites and subsequent abscessation, and precautions were taken to prevent omphalitis. However its tail had been docked by rubber-ring, providing a potential entry portal for pathogens. There was no history of spinal injury and no lesions consistent with injury (e.g. vertebral fracture, penetrating foreign body) or spinal abscess found at post-mortem. A further clinical differential was the lysosomal storage disease, G_{M2} gangliosidosis. This has recently been described in Jacob sheep in the UK and USA (Torres et al., 2010; Porter et al., 2011; Wessels et al., 2014).

G_{M2} gangliosidosis manifests as progressive ataxia in six-to-eight month-old lambs, and progresses over a period of ten days to eight weeks. Clinical signs include fore- and hind-limb abduction, ataxia and recumbency, as seen here. Histologically, neuronal cell bodies throughout the CNS are markedly distended with pale amphophilic granular material or microvacuolar change (Wessels et al., 2014). However, this was not the cause of disease in this case, as both of this lamb's parents and the lamb itself tested negative for carrier mutations, the neurological signs occurred immediately after birth, as opposed to at several months old, and no typical histological lesions were present. Certain teratogenic viruses (e.g. Schmallenberg, Bluetongue, Border disease virus, Akabane disease virus, Wesselsbron virus etc.) can cause congenital neuronal malformations and/or abnormalities in multiple axial and appendicular bones, leading to congenital neurological signs and skeletal defects in affected neonates (Dittmer and Thompson, 2015). However, many of these viruses are exotic to Ireland (e.g. Bluetongue, Akabane disease virus, Wesselsbron virus) so were not considered likely differentials. Schmallenberg virus and Border disease virus are present in Ireland, and both diseases may cause a variety of gross cerebral defects, (e.g. hydrocephalus, hydranencephaly, porencephaly, microcephaly, cerebellar hypoplasia). In the case of Schmallenberg disease, skeletal defects (brachygnathia, arthrogryposis, kyphosis, scoliosis, torticollis, lordosis, cleft palate) are often present (Herder et al., 2012; Dittmer and Thompson, 2015).

However, a single focal lesion at the level of the occipital condyles would be a highly unusual presentation of Schmallenberg virus. Additionally, this animal did not display the characteristic hairy coat or tremors of a lamb with congenital Border disease infection. It is also unlikely that these infectious diseases would only affect one animal in a flock (Dittmer and Thompson, 2015), for the lambs' twin to be clinically normal, and for PCR on liver tissue for

Border disease virus, Schmallenberg virus and Bluetongue virus to be negative. Other infectious diseases that cause neurological signs in young lambs, such as enterotoxaemia, toxoplasmosis and otitis media, were ruled out based on the absence of typical gross and histological findings.

The Jacob breed is polycerate, and to date occipital condylar dysplasia has only been reported in four-horned sheep (Johnson *et al.*, 1994; Ellis and Brown, 2014). In addition, mild condylar asymmetry was observed in six out of eight clinically-unaffected polycerate Jacob skulls (Ellis and Brown, 2014). This suggests that while there appears to be an association with the polycerate gene, which is dominant over the two-horned phenotype (Kijas *et al.*, 2016), the penetrance is variable. In the present case the sire consistently produced clinically-normal lambs for four years, and while the home-bred dam was primiparous, she and the affected lamb's twin sibling were healthy. This suggests occipital condylar dysplasia is not a simple autosomal trait, and more research is needed to ascertain its mode of inheritance. It also raises the possibility that this case was caused by a sporadic mutation with no genetic background, given the lack of family history.

A recent genome-wide association study (GWAS) on the polycerate Jacob and Navajo-Churro sheep breeds has linked this trait to single nucleotide polymorphisms (SNPs) in a non-coding region of chromosome 2, upstream of the Homeobox D (HOXD) gene cluster (Kijas *et al.*, 2016). These genes control anterior-posterior body axis and appendage development (Lemons *et al.*, 2005). Two separate GWASs examining different polycerate sheep breeds drew similar conclusions (Greyvenstein *et al.*, 2016; Ren *et al.*, 2016). It is therefore tempting to speculate that OCD may be linked to alteration of HOXD gene expression by polyceraty-associated SNPs. Indeed, it has been found that HOXD11 mutant mice exhibit supernumerary lumbar vertebrae, indicating that HOXD gene expression anomalies can affect vertebral column development (Davis and Capecchi, 1994). Interestingly, an association has been found between four-horned and polled phenotypes and the presence of "split-eyelid abnormalities", which also sporadically occur in Jacob sheep (Kijas *et al.*, 2016). This indicates that deviations from the "normal" two-horned state may be linked to abnormalities in various anatomical regions.

To the author's knowledge, occipital condylar dysplasia has not been reported in other polycerate sheep breeds and the incidence in Jacob sheep appears low. Given the existence of pro-active breed societies who are tackling the elimination of G_{M2} gangliosidosis, the paucity of occipital condylar dysplasia reports is striking and may be due to low incidence combined with misdiagnosis. Misdiagnosis may be explained by the non-specific clinical signs, similar to other neurologic conditions of lambs and to G_{M2} gangliosidosis. It has been shown that the American Jacob sheep population exhibit a striking genetic divergence from other breeds, and that their inter-breed genetic diversity is low (Kijas *et al.*, 2016). It is thought that G_{M2} gangliosidosis was brought to the USA by a carrier ram from the UK (Wessels *et al.*, 2014), and it is likely that the gene pool of American Jacob sheep is quite small, as the population arose from a relatively low number of sheep imported from Europe (Jacob Sheep Conservancy, 2016). This may explain why occipital condylar dysplasia thus far appears more prevalent in the USA than Europe.

Occipital condylar dysplasia should therefore be considered by breeders, veterinarians and pathologists as a differential diagnosis in Jacob lambs with ataxia. The molecular pathogenesis and prevalence of this condition require further investigation. This will help improve our understanding of rare-breed sheep genetics and guide future breeding decisions. Future investigations may also shed light on aspects of embryology that are relevant to both animals and humans.

Conflicts of Interest

The authors declare that there is no conflict of interest.

Acknowledgements

We thank Bernadette Byrne MVB for her management of this case, Brian Cloak and Alex Fawcett for their technical assistance, and Dr. Catherine d'Helft for carrying out the CT-scan.

References

Agerholm, J.S., Bendixen, C., Andersen, O. and Arnbjerg, J. 2001. Complex vertebral malformation in Holstein calves. J. Vet. Diagn. Invest. 13, 283-289.

Bancroft, J.D. and Gamble, M. 2002. Theory and practice of histological techniques 5th ed. London: Churchill Livingstone.

Burke, S.W., French, H.G., Roberts, J.M., Johnston, C.E., Whitecloud, T.S. and Edmunds Jr, J.O. 1985. Chronic atlanto-axial instability in Down syndrome. J. Bone Joint Surg. 67, 1356-1360.

Cantile, C. 2016. Nervous system. In Jubb, Kennedy and Palmer's pathology of domestic animals, Ed., Grant Maxie, M. St. Louis, MO: Elsevier, pp: 32-329.

Davis, A.P. and Capecchi, M.R. 1994. Axial homeosis and appendicular skeleton defects in mice with a targeted disruption of hoxd-11. Development 120, 2187-2198.

Dittmer, K.E. and Thompson, K.G. 2015. Approach to investigating congenital skeletal abnormalities in livestock. Vet. Pathol. 52, 851-861.

Ellis, A.E. and Brown, C.A. 2014. Occipital condylar dysplasia in Jacob sheep. In the Proceedings of the 2014 Diagnostic Pathology Focused Scientific Session.

Greyvenstein, O.F., Reich, C.M., Marle-Koster, E., Riley, D.G. and Hayes, B.J. 2016. Polyceraty (multi-horns) in Damara sheep maps to ovine chromosome 2. Anim. Genet. 47, 263-266.

Halanski, M.A., Iskandar, B., Nemeth, B. and Noonan, K.J. 2006. The coconut condyle: occipital condylar dysplasia causing torticollis and leading to C1 fracture. J. Spinal Disord. Tech. 19, 295-298.

Herder, V. Wohlsein, P., Peters, M., Hansmann, F. and Baumgärtner, W. 2012. Salient lesions in domestic ruminants infected with the emerging so-called Schmallenberg virus in Germany. Vet. Pathol. 49, 588-591.

Jackson, P.G. and Palmer, A.C. 1983. Quadriplegia in young lambs. Vet. Rec. 112, 65-66.

Jacob Sheep Breeders Association .2009. Jacob Sheep Breeders Association. Available at: www.jsba.org/ (Accessed 25 March 2017).

Jacob Sheep Conservancy. 2016. History of the Jacob Sheep. Available at: http://www.jacobsheepconservancy.com/#!history/c1jm9 (Accessed 25 March 2017).

Johnson, G.C., Turk, J.R., Morris, T.S., O'Brien, D. and Aronson, E. 1994. Occipital condylar dysplasia in two Jacob sheep. Cornell Vet. 84, 91-98.

Kijas, J.W., Hadfield, T., Naval Sanchez, M. and Cockett, N. 2016. Genome-wide association reveals the locus responsible for four-horned ruminant. Anim. Gen. 47, 258-262.

Lemons, D., Pearson, J.C. and McGinnis, W. 2005. Modulating Hox gene functions during animal body patterning. Nat. Rev. Genet. 6, 893-904.

Lewis, C., Wessels, M., Carty, H., Baird, P., Cox, T., Cachon, B., Wang, S., Holmes, P., Mackintosh, A. and Chianini, F. 2014. Testing sheep for GM2 gangliosidosis. Vet. Rec. 175, 260.

Loughin, C.A. 2016. Chiari-like malformation. Vet. Clin. North Am. Small Anim. Pract. 46, 231-242.

Palmer, A.C., Kelly, W.R. and Ryde, P.S. 1981. Stenosis of the cervical vertebral canal in a yearling ram. Vet. Rec. 109, 53-55.

Parish, S., Gavin, P. and Knowles, D. 1984. Quadriplegia associated with cervical deformity in a lamb. Vet. Rec. 114, 196.

Porter, B.F., Lewis, B.C., Edwards, J.F., Alroy, J., Zeng, B.J., Torres, P.A., Bretzlaff, K.N. and Kolodny, E.H. 2011. Pathology of G_{M2} gangliosidosis in Jacob sheep. Vet. Pathol. 48, 807-813.

Pueschel, S.M., Scola, F.H., Perry, C.D. and Pezzullo, J.C. 1981. Atlanto-axial instability in children with Down syndrome. Pediatr. Radiol. 10, 129-132.

Ren, X., Yang, G-L., Peng,W-F., Zhao,Y-X., Zhang, M., Chen, Z-H., Wu, F-A., Kantanen, J., Shen, M. and Li, M-H. 2016. A genome-wide association study identifies a genomic region for the polycerate phenotype in sheep (Ovis aries). Sci. Rep. 7:25322. doi: 10.1038/srep25322.

Richardson, C. 2016. Jacob Sheep Society. Available at: http://www.jacobsheepsociety.co.uk/ (Accessed 25 March 2017).

Schmidt, S.P., Forsythe, W.B., Cowgill, H.M. and Myers, R.K. 1993. A case of congenital occipitoatlantoaxial malformation (OAAM) in a lamb. J. Vet. Diagn. Invest. 5, 458-462.

Slanina, M.C. 2016. Atlantoaxial Instability. Vet. Clin. North Am. Small Anim. Pract. 46, 265-275.

Smoker, W.R. 1994. Craniovertebral junction: normal anatomy, craniometry, and congenital anomalies. Radiographics 14, 255-277.

Summers, B.A., Cummings, J.F. and de Lahunta, A. 1995. Injuries to the Central Nervous System. In Veterinary Neuropathology, Eds., Duncan, L. and McCandless, P.J. St. Louis, MO: Mosby Publishers, pp: 527.

Thomas, W.M. 2016. Nutritional disorders of the spinal column and cord. Available at: http://www.msdvetmanual.com/nervous-system/diseases-of-the-spinal-column-and-cord/nutritional-disorders-of-the-spinal-column-and-cord (Accessed 25 March 2017).

Torres, P.A., Zeng, B.J., Porter, B.F., Alroy, J., Horak, F. and Kolody, E.H. 2010. Tay-Sachs disease in Jacob sheep. Mol. Genet. Metab. 101, 357-363.

Watson, A.G. and Mayhew, I.G. 1986. Familial congenital occipitoatlantoaxial malformation (OAAM) in the Arabian horse. Spine, 11, 334-339.

Wessels, M.E., Holmes, J.P., Jeffrey, M., Jackson, M., Mackintosh, A., Kolodny, E.H., Zeng, B.J., Wang, C.B. and Scholes, S.F.E. 2014. G_{M2} Gangliosidosis in British Jacob Sheep. J. Comp. Pathol. 150, 253-257.

15

First report of cerebellar abiotrophy in an Arabian foal from Argentina

S.A. Sadaba[1,2], G.J. Madariaga[3], C.M. Corbi Botto[1,2], M.H. Carino[1], M.E. Zappa[1], P. Peral García[1], S.A. Olguín[4], A. Massone[3] and S. Díaz[1,*]

[1]IGEVET – Instituto de Genética Veterinaria "Ing. Fernando Noel Dulout" (UNLP-CONICET La Plata), Facultad de Ciencias Veterinarias, Universidad Nacional de La Plata, La Plata, Argentina
[2]Research Fellows from Consejo Nacional de Investigaciones Científicas y Técnicas (CONICET). Av. Rivadavia 1917 (C1033AAJ) CABA, Argentina
[3]Laboratorio de Patología Especial Veterinaria, Facultad de Ciencias Veterinarias, Universidad Nacional de La Plata, La Plata, Argentina
[4]Cátedra de Métodos Complementarios de Diagnóstico, Facultad de Ciencias Veterinarias, Universidad Nacional de La Plata, La Plata, Argentina

Abstract

Evidence of cerebellar abiotrophy (CA) was found in a six-month-old Arabian filly with signs of incoordination, head tremor, wobbling, loss of balance and falling over, consistent with a cerebellar lesion. Normal hematology profile blood test and cerebrospinal fluid analysis excluded infectious encephalitis, and serological testing for *Sarcocystis neurona* was negative. The filly was euthanized. Postmortem X-ray radiography of the cervical cephalic region identified not abnormalities, discounting spinal trauma. The histopathological analysis of serial transverse cerebellar sections by electron microscopy revealed morphological characteristics of apoptotic cells with pyknotic nuclei and degenerate mitochondria, cytoplasmic condensation and areas with absence of Purkinje cells, matching with CA histopathological characteristics. The indirect DNA test for CA was positive in the filly, and DNA test confirmed the CA carrier state in the parents and the recessive inheritance of the disease. To our knowledge this is the first report of a CA case in Argentina.

Keywords: Apoptosis, Arabian horses, Cerebellar abiotrophy, DNA, Purkinje cells.

Introduction

In the Arabian horse, head injuries along with cerebellar abiotrophy (CA) and meningoencephalitis are the most common processes affecting the cerebellum. For differential CA diagnosis, family congenital diseases such as cerebellar hypoplasia, diseases caused by physical head injuries, meningoencephalomyelitis of diverse etiology, toxic diseases (mycotoxins) and neoplasms should be discarded by a series of analysis.

CA is a neurological condition which affects a number of animal species characterized by postnatal degeneration of Purkinje cells (de Lahunta, 1990). Although the symptoms and pathological features of this neurodegenerative condition are the same as in other species, in horses, CA is mainly found in the Arabian horse breed (Fraser, 1966; Blanco *et al.*, 2006), and it has also been described in Swedish Gotland ponies and in an American Miniature Horse colt (Fox *et al.*, 2000).

The occurrence of CA in other horse breeds is not well-known, because breeders are usually reluctant to disclose that their breeding stock has produced foals with a neurological disease (Brault and Penedo, 2011).

New DNA scanning techniques have identified at least one CA carrier in three additional breeds, such as Bashkir Curly Horses, Trakehners and Welsh ponies, with a CA allele frequency between 2.8 and 0.33% (Brault and Penedo, 2011). As pointed out by these authors, CA was introduced into these breeds by Arabian ancestry. Therefore, the CA mutation is present in horse breeds that allow crossbreeding with Arabian horses and in breeds that have used Arabians as foundation stock during their development (Brault *et al.*, 2011b). To our knowledge this is the first report of a CA case in Argentina. Therefore, the risk of producing an affected foal from a particular mating is still unknown.

CA is characterized by postnatal (between six weeks and four months of age) degeneration of cerebellar Purkinje cells. Since Purkinje cells are the most prominently and consistently affected component, their degeneration leads to a concurrent degeneration of cerebellar granule neurons (Dungworth and Fowler, 1966; Fraser, 1966; Palmer *et al.*, 1973) and to a disorganization of the molecular and granular layers, with the remaining Purkinje cells being small and shrunken.

*Corresponding Author: Silvina Díaz. IGEVET, Facultad de Ciencias Veterinarias, Universidad Nacional de La Plata, La Plata, Argentina. Email: sdiaz@igevet.gob.ar

Overall size and thickness of the cerebellum, however, is largely unaffected (Dungworth and Fowler, 1966). Without Purkinje cells, the horse loses spatial and time perception, making it difficult to maintain the equilibrium and the coordination of the body members. Although CA itself is not fatal, the general lack of balance and hyperactivity of affected horses poses a danger to both horses and handlers (Brault and Penedo, 2011). Symptoms include intention head tremors, ataxia, exaggerated or paddling action of the forelegs, a wide-based stance and a lack of menace response (Dungworth and Fowler, 1966; Palmer *et al.*, 1973; DeBowes *et al.*, 1987).

CA-affected horses are often confused with those affected with wobbler, which is a condition of the spinal cord, not of the brain, or are misdiagnosed as animals that have suffered a head injury in an accident. Although symptoms are distinctive, they are similar to other neurological conditions; thus, accurate diagnosis can be a challenge and is often reached only after other possible conditions have been eliminated (Dungworth and Fowler, 1966; Brault *et al.*, 2011b). Until recently, conclusive diagnosis of the disease could only be made postmortem by histopathological exam of the cerebellum after euthanasia.

CA is inherited as an autosomal recessive trait (Brault *et al.*, 2011b). Preliminary data suggest an approximate location for CA on the horse genome, indicating the presence of a gene in this region that may be responsible for CA. A single nucleotide polymorphism (CA allele) has been identified in the horse TOE1 gene which is associated with CA in Arabian horses (Brault *et al.*, 2011a).

A test has now been developed which can be used to identify affected foals; in addition, it would be possible to determine if a horse carries one or two copies of the CA allele, using different tissues. Test results are reported as "N", meaning that the mutation associated with CA is not present, or "CA", indicating the presence of the CA mutation. The test is available in most horse genetics molecular diagnostic laboratories.

This case report describes the presence of ultrastructural signs of apoptosis in Purkinje cells of an Arabian filly affected with CA, and the complementary diagnostic methods employed to accurately determine the CA status for the first time in a foal in Argentina.

Case details

A 6-month-old Arabian filly was presented to the responsible veterinarian with a history of progressive clinical signs of loss of balance, head tremor and wobbling. There was no history of trauma or previous illness. The animal was from a closed breeding herd of Arabian horses with no history of similar cases, exhibiting progressive neurologic abnormalities consistent with cerebellar disease first noticed at weaning. Physical examination revealed the colt to be alert and responsive but exhibiting head tremor and a base-wide stance in the forelimbs. Pulse rate, respiratory rate and temperature were within normal limits. The colt had a tendency to fall to the side or back, and spastic hyperextension of the forelimbs when it was startled. There was no evidence of neuromuscular weakness. Clinical signs were consistent with a cerebellar lesion.

Hematology profile blood test values were normal, and cerebrospinal fluid analysis (CSF) was unremarkable, thus allowing exclusion of infectious encephalitis. Serological reaction tests for *Sarcocystis neurona* were negative. On the other hand, X-rays of the cervical region showed no abnormalities, discounting spinal trauma. The CA-affected filly was euthanized. Postmortem X-ray scan of the cervical cephalic region identified no abnormalities. Dorsoventral (DV) radiographic views showed an unaltered atlanto-occipital space. Both the lateral left-side (LLI) and the DV views showed normal cervical disc spaces, like the vertebral canal, with good spinal alignment and no signs of listhesis.

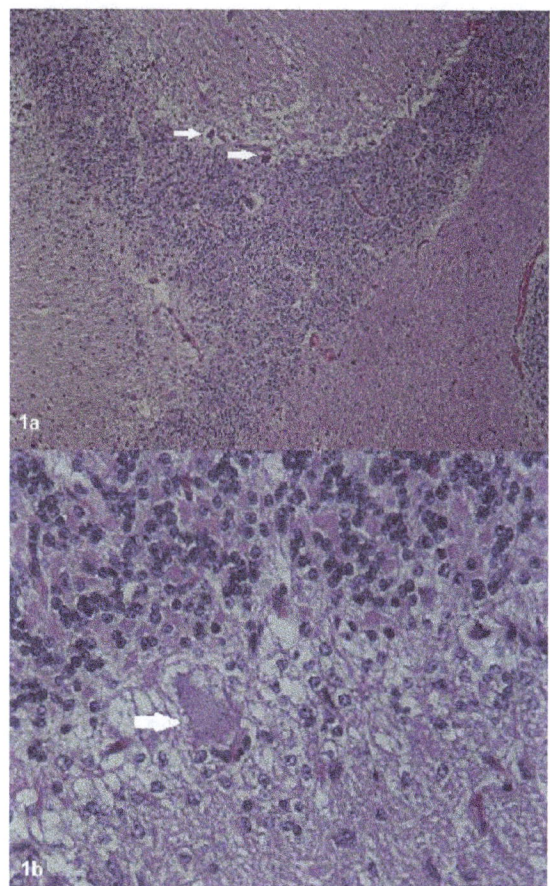

Fig. 1. Histological examination of cerebellar sections after staining with hematoxylin and eosin. **a**: Cerebellum of the CA affected foal 10 x: Almost complete absence of Purkinje cells. The remaining Purkinje cells are shrunken and hyperchromatic. **b**: Cerebellum of the CA affected foal 40 x.

The cerebellum was removed and fixed. Histopathological studies (Fig 1a,b) of serial transverse cerebellar sections and electron microscopy (JEM 1200EX II, Jeol), revealed morphological characteristics of apoptotic cells with pyknotic nuclei and degenerate mitochondria, cytoplasmic condensation and areas with absence of Purkinje cells, allowing us to confirm the CA diagnosis (Fig 2a,b,c). The indirect DNA test for CA was positive in the filly, and DNA testing of the parents confirmed their carrier state and the recessive inheritance of the disease.

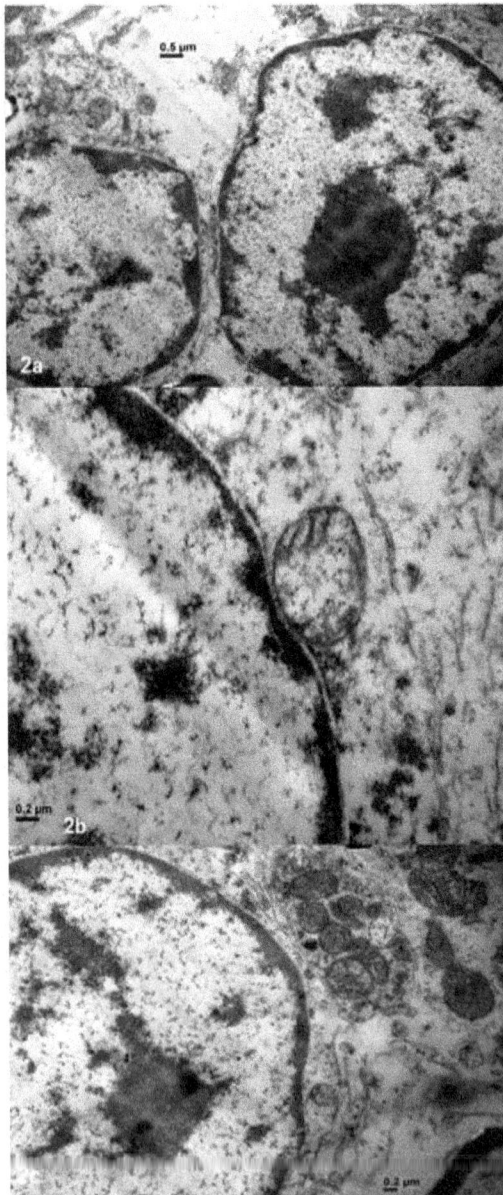

Fig. 2. Electron microscopy (JEM 1200EX II, Jeol) of a cerebellar section from the CA-affected foal (Camera ES500W Erlangshen C). (a): Morphological characteristics of apoptotic cells (0.5 μm). (b-c): degenerate mitochondria, pale, swollen and vacuolated Purkinje cells (0.2 μm).

Discussion

The complementary methods employed in this study to make an accurate diagnosis of CA were effective. Since CA is inherited as a recessive trait, the mating of two carriers may result in an affected foal (Brault *et al.*, 2011b). Thus, for a foal to be born with CA, two copies of the mutated allele must be present, each corresponding to each parent. Only mating between two carriers can produce an affected foal. Carriers of the mutant allele (heterozygous) do not have clinical signs, and the carrier state does not have negative consequences for health and athletic performance. The indirect DNA test for CA was positive in the filly, and DNA testing of both parents confirmed their carrier state, consequently the mating of the two heterozygote parents resulted in an affected foal.

CA diagnosis in the Arab population would be useful for Arabian breeders from our country when choosing their breeding stock (Brault *et al.*, 2011b; Brault and Penedo, 2011). To date it is only relevant whether the animals concerned are known to have produced affected foals, in order to eliminate a genetic disorder. To our knowledge this is the first case reported of a CA case in Argentina. The Arabian filly with CA belongs to a closed breeding herd of Arabian horses with no previous history of similar clinical signs of cerebellar defects. A second foal was CA diagnosed in the same year, but the observed clinical signs were slightly present, and could be confused with other conditions. This second foal descends from the same stallion and a different carrier dam. These two foals were the first cases of the disease in the history of the farm.

Since no CA cases were reported to date in Argentina, the risk of producing an affected foal from a particular mating is still unknown. The complementary diagnosis methods employed here allowed to accurate CA diagnosis, which was confirmed by the DNA test. The molecular test also allowed determining the carrier state of the stallion and the dam, giving the breeder the knowledge for choosing the matings in order to diminish the probabilities of produce affected foals.

Conflict of interest

The authors declare that there is no conflict of interest.

Acknowledgements

The authors wish to acknowledge the Electronic Microscopy Service from the National University of La Plata School of Veterinary Sciences for their assistance in acquiring the 6-month-old foal cerebellum sample. We are also grateful to the Arabian owner and breeder who generously provided the filly and DNA samples of the parents for research purposes. Thanks are also due to A. Di Maggio for manuscript correction.

References

Blanco, A., Moyano, R., Vivo, J., Flores-Acuña, R., Molina, A., Blanco, C. and Monterde JG. 2006.

Purkinje cell apoptosis in Arabian horses with cerebellar abiotrophy. J. Vet. Med. A Physiol. Pathol. Clin. Med. 53, 286-287.

Brault, L.S., Cooper, C.A., Famula, T.R., Murray, J.D. and Penedo, M.C. 2011a. Mapping of equine cerebellar abiotrophy to ECA2 and identification of a potential causative mutation affecting expression of MUTYH. Genomics 97, 121-129.

Brault, L.S., Famula, T.R. and Penedo, M.C. 2011b. Inheritance of equine cerebellar abiotrophy in Arabians. Am. J. Vet. Res. 72(7), 940-944.

Brault, L.S. and Penedo, M.C. 2011. The frequency of the equine cerebellar abiotrophy mutation in non-Arabian horse breeds. Equine Vet. J. 43(6), 727-731.

DeBowes, R.M., Leipold, H.W. and Turner-Beatty, M. 1987. Cerebellar abiotrophy. Vet. Clin. North Am.

Equine Pract. 3(2), 345-352.

de Lahunta, A. 1990. Abiotrophy in domestic animals: a review. Can. J. Vet. Res. 54(1), 65-76.

Dungworth, D.L. and Fowler, M.E. 1966. Cerebellar hypoplasia and degeneration in a foal. Cornell Vet. 56(1), 17-24.

Fox, J., Duncan, R., Friday, P., Klein, B. and Scarratt, W. 2000. Cerebello-olivary and lateral (accessory) cuneate degeneration in a juvenile American Miniature Horse. Vet. Pathol. 37(3), 271-274.

Fraser, H. 1966. Two dissimilar types of cerebellar disorder in the horse. Vet. Rec. 78(18), 608-612.

Palmer, A.C., Blakemore, W.F., Cook, W.R., Platt, H. and Whitwell, K.E. 1973. Cerebellar hypoplasia and degeneration in the young Arab horse: clinical and neuropathological features. Vet. Rec. 93(3), 62-66.

16

First isolation and nucleotide comparison of the *gag* gene of the caprine arthritis encephalitis virus circulating in naturally infected goats from Argentina

Carlos Javier Panei[1,2,*], Maria Laura Gos[2,3], Alejandro Rafael Valera[1], Cecilia Monica Galosi[1,4] and Maria Gabriela Echeverria[1,2]

[1]*Virology Laboratory, Faculty of Veterinary Sciences, National University of La Plata, 60 and 118, CC 296, 1900, La Plata, Argentina*
[2]*National Scientific and Technical Research Council (CONICET), Argentina*
[3]*Immunoparasitology Laboratory, Faculty of Veterinary Sciences, National University of La Plata, 60 and 118, CC 296, 1900, La Plata, Argentina*
[4]*Scientific Research Commission of Buenos Aires Province (CIC-PBA), Argentina*

Abstract

Caprine arthritis encephalitis virus (CAEV) has been reported in different countries worldwide, based on serological and molecular detection. In Argentina, the prevalence of CAEV infections is increasing, with goats showing symptoms associated mostly with cachexia and arthritis. Although in Argentina the virus has been detected by serology, it has never been isolated or characterized. Thus, the objectives of this work were to isolate and analyze the nucleotide sequences of the *gag* gene of Argentine CAEV strains and compare them with those of other SRLVs previously reported. Nucleotide sequence comparison showed homology with CAEV-Co, the CAEV prototype. Phylogenetic analyses showed that the Argentine strains clustered with genotype B, subtype B1. Because the molecular characterization of the *gag* region is suitable for phylogenetic studies and may be applied to monitor the control of SRLV, molecularly characterizing the Argentine CAEV strains may help develop a proper plan of eradication of CAEV infections.

Keywords: CAEV isolate, Caprine arthritis encephalitis virus, *gag* gene.

Introduction

Caprine arthritis encephalitis virus (CAEV) infections in goats have been reported in different countries around the world, based on serology and molecular detection. In Argentina, the last report on the CAEV epidemiological status was based on an enzyme-linked-immunosorbent assay (ELISA) of sera collected from 2010 to 2011. That study evidenced an increase in farm goats positive for CAEV from 19.4% in 2010 to 21.5% in 2011, while the prevalence of positive animals in 2011 was 3.86% (Trezeguet *et al.*, 2013). CAEV infects macrophages and dendritic cells, causing immune-mediated lesions in a variety of organs and leading to lymphocyte accumulation (Blacklaws *et al.*, 1994). Around 30 to 40% of infected animals develop clinical symptoms (Cheevers *et al.*, 1988), associated with interstitial pneumonia, mastitis, encephalitis, and arthritis (Houwers *et al.*, 1988; Narayan and Clements, 1989). Clinical and subclinical mastitis can lead to substantial economic losses in the goat industry (Leitner *et al.*, 2004, 2010). However, the most common clinical manifestation of CAEV infections in goats is the arthritic form (Pugh, 2002). CAEV is genetically and antigenically closely related

to the visna-maedi virus (VMV), also known as the ovine progressive pneumonia virus. Both CAEV and VMV are grouped into small ruminant lentiviruses (SRLVs), where cross-species transmission can cause lentiviral diseases in goats and sheep (Pasick, 1998; Shah *et al.*, 2004; Pisoni *et al.*, 2007).

The genome of SRLVs has the typical proviral genomic organization of the genus *lentivirus*, family Retroviridae and subfamily Orthoretrovirinae (www.ictvonline.org). It consists of two identical single strands of the RNA (+) subunit, and contains the *gag, pol* and *env* structural genes and the *tat, rev,* and *vif* regulatory genes, flanked by non-coding long terminal repeat regions (Gifford, 2012).

The SRLVs are divided into five principal groups (A to E) according to their sequences. Genotypes A, B and E may be further distributed into different subtypes, differing in 15% to 27% of their nucleotide sequences. Thus, genotype A has been divided in several subtypes from A1 to A15, genotype B has been divided into three subtypes, B1-B3, and genotype E has only been divided in two subtypes, E1 and E2 (Shah *et al.*, 2004). These genetic variations of the virus represent challenges in the SRLV diagnosis implementing the use of native

---

*Corresponding Author: Carlos Javier Panei. Faculty of Veterinary Sciences, National University of La Plata, 60 and 118, CC 296, 1900, La Plata, Argentina. Email: *javierpanei@fcv.unlp.edu.ar*

proteins from different viral strains obtained from goats or sheep of a given region or country (De Andres *et al.*, 2005).

Although the circulation of CAEV and the disease in Argentina have been known for more than ten years, the virus has never been isolated or characterized. Therefore, the aims of this work were to isolate and analyze the nucleotide sequences of the *gag* gene of the CAEV strains circulating in Argentina and compare them with those of other SRLVs previously reported.

Materials and Methods

Saanen goats belonging to five flocks from different geographic areas, located in 'Sierras Pampeanas' and 'Pampa Humeda', from Argentina, with history of CAEV infection were considered for SRLV molecular detection due to the occurrence of clinical symptoms of arthritis and cachexia (Fig. 1A and B).

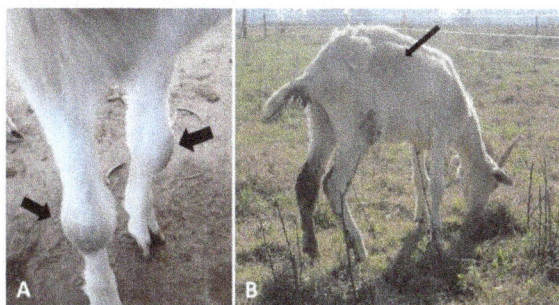

Fig. 1. (A): Saanen goat positive to CAEV with joint carpal arthritis (black arrow). (B): Saanen goat positive to CAEV with cachexia (arrow).

Blood samples with anticoagulant were collected from five goats, each representing its flock, for DNA provirus detection, while synovial fluid from one of them with joint carpal arthritis was collected for virus isolation (Fig. 1A). Peripheral blood leukocytes (PBLs) were separated by centrifugation through Histopaque™ (Sigma–Aldrich) according to the manufacturer's protocols and kept at 4°C until DNA genomic extraction with a commercial kit (DNA Purification Kit, Promega, WI, USA). The synovial fluid from the goat with joint carpal arthritis was extracted with a sterile needle, diluted 1:5 with PBS, filtered with a 0.22-μm pore membrane and co-cultured with CAEV-negative goat synovial membrane (GSM) cells in six-well dishes. One dish was kept without infection as negative control. The cultures were maintained at 37°C in a 5% CO_2 atmosphere with minimum essential medium, supplemented with 10% fetal bovine serum, penicillin (100 U/ml), and streptomycin (100 μg/ml). After several passages, the cultures were stained with Giemsa to display cytopathic effect (CE). For RNA isolation of viral particles from the supernatant of the cell culture with CE, a commercial kit (SV RNA-Isolation System, Kit, Promega, WI, USA) was used.

To amplify the complete *gag* gene (1.3 kb), a hemi-nested PCR was carried out using the primers listed in Table 1. Samples with no amplification were tested by a single round of PCR to amplify a short segment of the *gag* gene (0.645 kb) representing 45% of the gene (Table 1). Primers for the complete *gag* gene were designed by DNAman software according to the CAEV-Cork (CAEV-Co) prototype of CAEV; while the PCR forward primer of the short *gag* region has been reported previously (Valas *et al.*, 1997), the reverse primer was designed by the same software according to the CAEV-Co prototype of CAEV and Icelandic 1514 prototype of VMV sequences.

Table 1: List of primers used to amplify the complete and partial *gag* gene in this study.

Primers	Nucleotide sequence 5'-3'	Location
gagF 331-352	AGTAAGGTAAGTGAC TCTGCT	
gagR 1975-1995	AATCCTTGCAGTTTT ATCCTTCC	Complete *gag* gene
gagR 2008-2028	TTATTCCATTTTTCT CCTTCTAC	
gagF 959-979	GCAGGAGGGAGAAGY TGGAA	Partial *gag* gene (45%)
gagR 1608-1628	YCCTTCKGATCCCAC ATCTC	

The reaction conditions of the first and second round of the hemi-nested PCR were: 1 cycle of the initial denaturation at 94 °C for 5 minutes, 40 cycles of denaturation at 94 °C for 30 seconds, annealing at 56 °C for 30 seconds, and extension at 72 °C for 40 seconds; followed by another extension step at 72 °C for 10 minutes to complete the reaction. The cycle profile for the short *gag* gene amplification was: 1 cycle at 94 °C for 5 minutes, 35 cycles of denaturation at 94 °C for 30 seconds, annealing at 54 °C for 30 seconds, and extension at 72 °C for 40 seconds; followed by another extension step at 72 °C for 7 minutes to complete the reaction. The PCRs were performed in a DNA Thermal Cycler (Perkin-Elmer Cetus, Norwalk, CT, USA) and the PCR reactions carried out with the PCR Master Mix according to the manufacturer's protocols (Promega, WI, USA). The same conditions were used for reverse transcriptase activity with a previous step of 37°C for 60 min.

The amplified products were visualized on 1.5% (w/v) agarose gel and staining with ethidium bromide. Each amplified *gag* gene was subcloned into the pGEM-T easy vector® according to manufacturer's protocol and sent to sequencing in an ABI3130XL Sequencer (Applied Biosystems, USA), Unidad Genómica, INTA Castelar, Argentina. The nucleotide sequences obtained were assembled and analyzed by the Bioedit software and the nucleotide compositions were compared with other strains reported in GenBank. Genetic homology and the neighbor-joining tree of the nucleotide sequences were assessed using MEGA software version 4.0

Results and Discussion

The first isolate of CAEV in Argentina was obtained from the synovial fluid extracted of the joint carpal arthritis from a goat with clinical symptoms of CAEV infection (Fig. 1). CE coincident with syncytia was observed after two passages using GSM cells (Fig. 2).

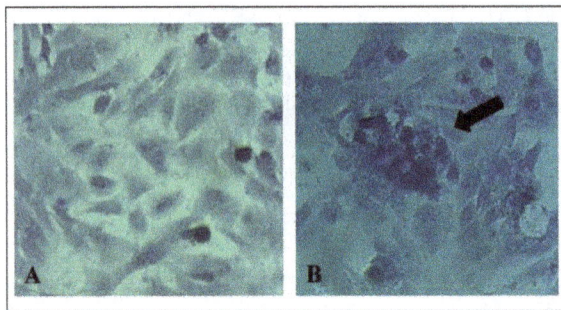

Fig. 2. Culture of goat synovial membrane (GSM) cells. (A): Non-infected cells as negative control. (B): Infected cell with synovial fluid from goat with carpal arthritis; the black arrow shows cytopathic effect (CE) coincident with syncytium after two passages (25X).

The presence of viral particles in the supernatant of the cell culture was quickly confirmed by reverse transcriptase activity by hemi-nested PCR amplifying the complete *gag* gene of 1.3 kb. In contrast, the amplification of the CAEV from the remaining four goats was obtained from DNA genomic provirus detected in PBLs.

Because it was not possible to amplify the complete *gag* gene of the virus in these goats, probably due to the variability in nucleotide composition, we amplified a product of 0.645 kb corresponding to 45 % of the *gag* gene. The variability in the nucleotide sequences characteristic of lentiviruses may result in a high rate of mutation, capable of forming many different strains or quasispecies (Santry *et al.*, 2013). Thus, new primers should be designed to succeed in the amplification of the strains circulating in Argentina.

Because a *gag* region is suitable for phylogenetic studies and may be applied to monitor SRLV eradication programs (Santry *et al.*, 2013), the five nucleotide sequences obtained were aligned and compared with the SRLV sequences reported in GenBank. The percentage of major homology found between the complete and short region of the *gag* gene showed an average of 90.5% of identity compared with CAEV-Co sequences. Moreover, the nucleotide composition of the Argentine strains showed a range of 86 to 92% identity compared to each other.

In addition, the phylogenetic trees were built using

alignments of the complete (Fig. 3A) and partial *gag* genes (Fig. 3B).

Our analysis was carried out by neighbor-joining algorithm to obtain the differentiation and the branching order of groups to classify the genotypes and subtypes proposed by Shah *et al.* (2004). In both cases, the Argentine strains were clustered together with the isolate classified as genotype B, subtype B1. Regarding the partial *gag* gene, the Argentine strains clustered with the reference strain CAEV-Co isolated from a goat of North America, representative of the prototype caprine lentivirus (Cork *et al.*, 1974).

These clades were the same as those for CAEV-Philippines, Gansu-China and a strain reported in Brazil (Ravazzolo *et al.*, 2001) (Fig. 3B). Based in these results obtained and compared with the phylogenetic distance in relation to the Icelandic 1514 strain, prototype of VMV (genotype A), the SRLV detected in this work and circulating in Argentina were identified as CAEV.

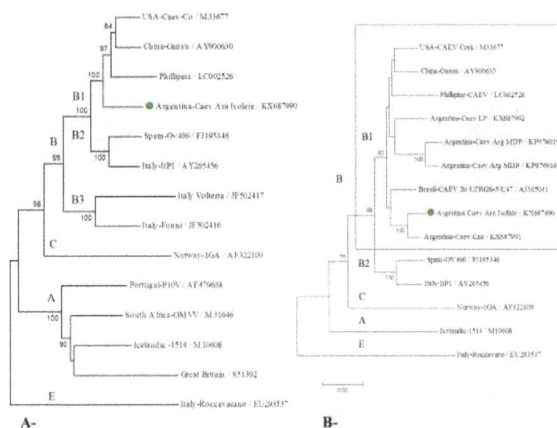

Fig. 3. (A): Neighbor-joining phylogenetic tree using the complete *gag* sequence (1313 bp). (B): Neighbor-joining phylogenetic tree using the partial *gag* sequence (645 bp). Bootstrap values are based on 1000 repetitions. SRLVs representative of each genotype and subtype according to the classification by Shah *et al.* (2004) were used. The sequence of the Argentine isolate is shown with a green circle. Each SRLV sequence is denoted by country and GenBank access number. Sequences of genotype B1 are shown with a box.

Subtype B1 has been reported to have undergone cross-species transmission from goats to sheep (Pisoni *et al.*, 2005) and although antibodies of SRLV have also been detected in sheep flocks in Argentina (Trezeguet *et al.*, 2013), the virus has never been characterized in this species to determine whether another genotype is circulating.

The success in preventing SRLV infection spread depends largely on early detection of infected animals in the flocks (Ramirez *et al.*, 2013). For that, and due to the last report of prevalence in Argentina, studies should also be conducted to investigate the presence of SRLV strains circulating in sheep, especially in the case where they coexist in the same herd with goats.

In this work, we were able to isolate CAEV for the first time from naturally infected goats circulating in our country. The genetic characterization of the virus is necessary to obtain more information to implement a control method and eradication plan of CAEV infections in Argentina.

Acknowledgements

The technical assistances of Mr. Claudio Leguizamón and Mrs. Adriana Conde are highly acknowledged.

Conflict of interest

The authors declare that there is no conflict of interest.

References

Blacklaws, B.A., Bird, P., Allen, D. and McConnell, I. 1994. Circulating cytotoxic T lymphocyte precursors in maedi-visna virus-infected sheep. J. Gen. Virol. 75, 1589-1596.

Cheevers, W.P., Knowles, D.P., McGuire, T.C., Cunningham, D.R., Adams, D.S. and Gorham, J.R. 1988. Chronic disease in goats orally infected with two isolates of the caprine arthritis-encephalitis lentivirus. Lab. Invest. 58, 510-517.

Cork, L.C., Hadlow, W.J., Craeford, T.B., Gorham, J. R. and Piper, R.C. 1974. Infectious leukoencephalomyelithis of young goats. J. Infec. Dis. 129, 134-141.

De Andres, D., Klein, D., Watt, N.J., Berriatua, E., Torsteinsdottir, S., Blacklaws, B.A., and Harkiss, G.D. 2005. Diagnostic tests for small ruminant lentiviruses. Vet. Microbiol. 107, 49-62.

Gifford, R.J. 2012. Viral evolution in deep time: Lentiviruses and mammals. Trends Genet. 28, 89-100.

Houwers, D.J., Pekelder, J.J., Akkermans, J.W., Van der Molen, E.J., and Schreuder, B.E. 1988. Incidence of indurative lymphocytic mastitis in a flock of sheep infected with maedi-visna virus. Vet. Rec. 122, 435-437.

Leitner, G., Krifuck, O., Weisblit, L., Lavi, Y., Bernstein, S. and Merin-Lerondelle, U. 2010. The effect of caprine arthritis encephalitis virus infection on production in goats. Vet. J. 183, 328-331.

Leitner, G., Merin, U. and Silanikove, N. 2004. Changes in milk composition as affected by subclinical mastitis in goats. J. dairy Sci. 87, 1719-1726.

Narayan, O. and Clements, J.E. 1989. Biology and pathogenesis of lentiviruses. J. Gen. Virol. 70, 1617-1639.

Pasick, J. 1998. Maedi-visna virus and caprine arthritis-encephalitis virus: distinct species or quasispecies and its implications for laboratory diagnosis. Can. J. Vet. Res. 62, 241-244.

Pisoni, G., Quasso, A., Moroni, P. 2005. Phylogenetic analysis of small-ruminant lentivirus subtype B1 in mixed flocks: evidence for natural transmission from goats to sheeps. Virology 339, 147-152.

Pisoni, G., Bertoni, G., Puricelli, M., Macacalli, M. and Moroni, P. 2007. Demostration of coinfection with the recombinant by caprine arthritis encephalitis virus and maedi-visna virus in naturally infected goats. J. Virol. 81, 4949-4955.

Pugh, D.G. 2002. Sheep and goat medicine. W. B. Saunders Company. Philadelphia, pp: 126, 239-240, 296, 388.

Ramirez, H., Reina, R., Amorena, B., De Andrés, D. and Martínez, H.A. 2013. Small Ruminant Lentiviruses: Genetic Variability, Tropism and Diagnosis. Viruses 5, 1175-1207.

Ravazzolo, A.P., Reischak, D., Peterhans, E. and Zanoni, R. 2001. Phylogenetic analysis of small ruminant lentiviruses from Southern Brazil. Virus Res. 79, 117-123.

Santry, L.A., De jong, J., Gold, A.C., Walsh, S.R., Menzies, P.I. and Wootton S.K. 2013. Genetic characterization of small ruminant lentivirus circulating in naturally infected sheep and goats in Ontario, Canada. Virus. Res. 175, 30-44.

Shah, C., Huder, J.B., Boni, J., Schonmann, M., Muhlherr, J., Lutz, H. and Schupbach, J. 2004. Direct evidence for natural transmission of small ruminant lentiviruses of subtype A4 from goats to sheeps and vice versa. J. Virol. 78, 7518-7522.

Trezeguet, M.A., Suarez, M.F., Barral, L.E., Periolo, F., Maidana, C.E., Farías, P.C., Rodríguez, C.E., Debenedetti, R.T., Marcos, A. and Cosentino, B. 2013. Epidemiological situation of maedi-visna and caprine arthritis encephalitis in Argentine. Servicio Nacional de Sanidad y Calidad Agroalimentaria (SENASA). 1, 1-11.

Valas, S., Benoit, C., Guionaud, C., Perrin, G. and Mamoun R.Z. 1997. North American and French caprine arthritis-encephalitis viruses emerge from ovine-visna viruses. Virology 237, 307-318.

17

Comparison and validation of ELISA assays for plasma insulin-like growth factor-1 in the horse

Courtnay L. Baskerville[1], Nicholas J. Bamford[1], Patricia A. Harris[2] and Simon R. Bailey[1,*]

[1]Faculty of Veterinary and Agricultural Sciences, The University of Melbourne, Werribee, Victoria, Australia
[2]Equine Studies Group, WALTHAM Centre for Pet Nutrition, Melton Mowbray, Leicestershire, UK

Abstract
Insulin-like growth factor-1 (IGF-1) plays several important physiological roles, and IGF-related pathways have been implicated in developmental osteochondral disease and endocrinopathic laminitis. This factor is also a downstream marker of growth hormone activity and its peptide mimetics. Unfortunately, previously used assays for measuring equine IGF-1 (radioimmunoassays and ELISAs) are no longer commercially available, and many of the kits on the market give poor results when used on horse samples. The aim of the present study was to compare three different ELISA assays (two human and one horse-specific). Plasma samples from six Standardbreds, six ponies and six Andalusians were used. The human IGF-1 ELISA kit from Immunodiagnostic Systems (IDS) proved to be the most accurate and precise of the three kits; the other two assays gave apparently much lower concentrations, with poor recovery of spiked recombinant human IGF-1 and unacceptably poor intra-assay coefficients of variation (CV). The IDS assay gave an intra-assay CV of 3.59 % and inter-assay CV of 7.31%. Mean percentage recovery of spiked IGF-1 was 88.82%, and linearity and dilutional parallelism were satisfied. The IGF-1 plasma concentrations were 123.21 ±8.24 ng/mL for Standardbreds, 124.95 ±3.69 ng/mL for Andalusians and 174.26 ±1.94 ng/mL for ponies. Therefore of the three assays assessed, the IGF-1 ELISA manufactured by IDS was the most suitable for use with equine plasma samples and may have many useful applications in several different research areas. However, caution should be used when comparing equine studies where different analytical techniques and assays may have been used to measure this growth factor.
Keywords: Equine, Insulin-like growth factor, Ponies.

Introduction

Insulin-like growth factor (IGF-1) is a 70 amino acid peptide, produced by the liver, which plays a role in cell growth and turnover in several different mammalian tissues. Receptors for this growth factor are found in skeletal muscle, bone, cartilage and some epithelial cells, and increased concentrations of this mediator have been associated with developmental osteochondral lesions in growing horses (Verwilghen et al., 2009).

Investigators have suggested that IGF-1 plays a critical role in the expression and synthesis of collagen type II as well as protecting chondrocytes from apoptosis. Therefore, changes in concentrations of IGF-1 could modulate the biological mechanisms that regulate joint and bone development (Lejeune et al., 2007). Serum IGF-1 concentrations appear to peak in horses at 10 months of age correlating with the beginning of reproductive maturity and then begin to decrease, reaching a steady adult concentration at approximately 450 days old (Fortier et al., 2005).

The biological activity of circulating IGF-1 is modulated by a family of IGF-binding proteins, which may promote its interaction with the receptor as well as prolonging its half-life (Kostecka and Blahovec, 1999). Furthermore, the major stimulus for the secretion of IGF-1 from the liver is growth hormone; therefore an 'IGF-1/GH axis' has been described (De Palo et al., 2001).

The measurement of plasma IGF-1 concentration can be useful clinically as an indicator of growth hormone deficiency in humans (Faust et al., 2012), and in horses measuring IGF-1 concentrations has been found to be a reliable indicator to monitor plasma GH concentrations (Fortier et al., 2005). This is helped by the fact that plasma IGF-1 concentrations typically remain relatively stable throughout the day. Certain performance enhancing agents including some peptides may mimic the effects of growth hormone, and so an accurate IGF-1 ELISA assay for use in equine blood samples may be useful in testing performance horses as well as monitoring age related orthopaedic disorders (Popot et al., 2001). Furthermore, the role of the IGF-1 signalling pathway is being investigated in equine laminitis (de Laat et al., 2013).

Currently the most sensitive means for detecting IGF-1 in equine plasma is LC electrospray ionisation mass spectrometry (Popot et al., 2008). However, cost,

*Corresponding Author: Prof. Simon Bailey. Faculty of Veterinary and Agricultural Sciences, University of Melbourne, Corner of Park Drive and Flemington Road, Parkville 3052, Victoria, Australia. Email: bais@unimelb.edu.au

sample preparation time and the availability of equipment may limit the use of this technique. Radioimmunoassays (RIAs) have also been widely used to measure IGF-1.

Comparisons across species have shown that the equine IGF-1 nucleotide sequence is highly homologous to that of other mammals including humans, suggesting that human IGF-1 immunoassays should be appropriate for use in the horse (Ropp et al., 2003). De Kock et al. (2001) determined the effect of GH administration on IGF-1 concentrations in the horse, validating an RIA assay.

In a study by Noble et al. (2007), IGF-1 was measured in a large population of 1,880 Thoroughbred horses, also by RIA. The mean concentration was 310 ng/mL, with a similar magnitude between geldings and mares but increased magnitude in intact males.

Unfortunately these RIAs, as well as a number of previously-used ELISA assays, are no longer commercially available. There are a number of IGF-1 ELISA assays on the market (mostly developed as human IGF-1 assays, with human specific reagents). However, many of these assays give poor results when used for horse samples. There is currently no standard recommended assay for equine IGF-1 that is widely used and this makes it difficult to compare values obtained between different studies.

It is therefore important to validate and compare available assays to determine the most acceptable assay to use in the horse. Also, since there are breed differences in metabolism associated with different concentrations of the important related peptide hormone insulin (Bamford et al., 2014), it may be important to consider different breeds when measuring IGF-1.

The aim of this study was to compare three different ELISA assays (two human and one horse-specific).

Materials and Methods

A total of eighteen horses were used in this study: six Standardbreds (mean age: 9.8 years; range 6-16 years), six ponies of various breed (10.2 years; 6-17 years) and six crossbreed Andalusians (10.0 years; 7-14 years). EDTA and heparinised blood samples were collected from each subject via aseptic venipuncture using 10-mL BD Vacutainer tubes with 20 gauge needles. After collection, samples were placed on ice immediately and transported to the laboratory. Plasma was separated and stored in 1-mL aliquots at -80°C and was not thawed until assayed (within 3 months).

Three assays were evaluated: Assay A: Human IGF-1 ELISA kit (ab100545; Abcam Inc, Massachusetts, USA) (developed for measuring human IGF-1), Assay B: Horse insulin-like growth factor 1 (somatomedin C; IGF-1) ELISA kit (Cusabio Biotech, Hubei Province, China) (equine specific), and Assay C: IGF-1 ELISA-Immunoenzymometric assay for the quantitative determination of Insulin-like growth factor 1 (IGF-1) in human serum or plasma (Immunodiagnostic Systems (IDS), Boldon, UK) (developed for measuring human IGF-1 in serum or plasma).

Reagents and standards were prepared according to the manufacturers' instructions. The manufacturers' instructions in regards to assay procedures were also followed; however, the addition of an IGF-1 extraction step for Assay B was also implemented to dissociate IGF-1 from the insulin-like growth factor binding proteins (IGFBPs). All assays were read using an automated microplate reader (Synergy H1 Hybrid Reader, BioTek, Vermont, USA), with Gen5 Microplate Reader Software (BioTek, Vermont, USA). Assay A was a commercially available sandwich ELISA kit based on a human IGF-1 antibody-coated plate. Samples were treated with acid-ethanol extraction solution prepared as per the manufacturer's instructions and incubated for 30 minutes. Samples were then centrifuged and 100 µL of supernatant was added to 200µL of Tris-buffer (pH 7.6). Following this, 300µL of sample diluent was added to each tube and 100µL of each sample was pipetted into appropriate wells. Samples were then washed, treated with 100µL of biotinylated antibody and incubated for 1 hour. The sample plate was then washed again and treated with 100µL of streptavidin. TMB was added and the reaction was stopped after 30 minutes incubation and read immediately at 450nm.

Assay B was a commercially available competitive ELISA kit without extraction based on an equine specific IGF-1 fragment. In addition to performing the assay without extraction, an acid-ethanol extraction was performed to dissociate IGF-1 from the IGFBPs; 120µL of commercially purchased acid-ethanol solution was added to 30µL of sample in 3mL polyethylene centrifuge tubes, the samples were then vortexed and incubated at room temperature for 30 minutes. Samples were centrifuged for 5 minutes at 10,000 rpm after which 100µL of supernatant was removed and placed in fresh centrifuge tubes and mixed with 200µL of neutralising solution (2M Tris buffer, pH 7.6).

All samples were then processed as per the manufacturer's instructions. Briefly, samples were diluted with sample diluent and 50µL was added to appropriate wells, 50µL of HRP-conjugate solution was then added and incubated for 40 minutes. The samples were then washed, 90µL of TMB substrate was added to each well and the reaction was stopped after 20 minutes incubation. Absorbance was read immediately at 450nm.

Assay C was a commercially available sandwich ELISA, based on a human IGF-1 antibody-coated plate, and suitable for assay of either human serum or plasma samples.

Rather than an acid-ethanol extraction solution, Assay C employs a proprietary releasing reagent that inactivates IGFBPs. All samples were processed as per the manufacturer's instructions. Briefly, 25µL of sample was added to plastic tubes and incubated with 100µL of releasing agent for 10 minutes. Sample diluent was then added to each tube and 50µL of the diluted sample was added, with 200µL of enzyme conjugate added before a two-hour incubation. The samples were washed and 200µL of TMB substrate was added to each well and stopped after a 30-minute incubation. Absorbance was read immediately at 450nm with a reference wavelength of 650nm.

The coefficient of variation (CV) was determined for each assay using pooled samples from each breed group. Each heparinised plasma sample was processed three times within the same analytical run for each assay to determine intra-assay variation. EDTA plasma samples were also processed for comparison with heparinised plasma.

The target acceptance measure for intra-assay variation was <10%. Inter-assay variation was subsequently determined where an acceptable intra-assay CV was obtained; the acceptable target was also <10%. The accuracy of each assay was determined by investigating parallelism of the standard curve with serial dilutions. Pooled samples from each breed group were diluted (1:2, 1:4, 1:8 and 1:16) with phosphate-buffered saline (PBS) in 3mL polyethylene centrifuge tubes. Expected concentrations of IGF-1 were calculated from the mean concentrations observed for each breed previously and the ratio of observed vs expected concentrations was determined for each dilution. Linearity was determined by plotting observed vs expected concentrations, and linear regression was used to calculate the r^2 value for these plots.

Pooled plasma samples from each breed group were assayed for IGF-1 after they had been spiked with human recombinant IGF-1. The amount of recombinant IGF-1 added to each sample was based on the detection range for each assay so that the expected final concentration did not exceed the working range (Assay A: 18.2 ng/mL, Assay B: 40ng/mL and Assay C: 190ng/mL). Samples were incubated overnight with the recombinant IGF-1 to allow equilibration with binding proteins and then processed as described above. Percentage recovery was then calculated.

Results and Discussion

Assay C proved to be the most accurate and precise of the three kits (Table 1), giving concentrations in the 100-200 ng/mL range for normal plasma, plus it gave the best recovery and validation characteristics. Assay A in comparison gave very low IGF-1 concentrations in the samples and poor recovery. Assay B was slightly better; however, the intra-assay coefficients of variation for both Assays A and B were unacceptably poor.

Assay A yielded the lowest IGF-1 concentrations in the plasma samples of 1.0 ±1.25 ng/mL (mean ±SD) for Standardbreds and 1.05 ±1.69 ng/mL for Andalusians. Ponies showed slightly higher concentrations (2.25 ±3.90 ng/mL). Assay B gave a mean concentration of 11.97 ±2.10 ng/mL for Standardbreds, 15.71 ±7.84 ng/mL for Andalusians and 17.25 ±9.14 ng/mL for ponies. In the absence of an extraction step, all concentrations were below 9 ng/mL in this assay.

Assay C recovered much higher concentrations in the samples, with a mean concentration of 123.21 ±8.24 ng/mL for Standardbreds, 124.95 ±3.69 ng/mL for Andalusians and 174.26 ±1.94 ng/mL for ponies.

The intra-assay coefficient of variation obtained from the three kits ranged from 1.14% - 173.21%, with Assay C being the only kit to have a mean CV less than the acceptable 10% range (3.59 ±1.63 %; Table 1). Percentage recovery from the spiked samples was the lowest for Assay A with a mean of only 28.86% and Assay B had a mean percentage recovery of 79.97%. Assay C had the highest mean % recovery of 88.82%. Dilutional parallelism could only be satisfied for Assays B and C. Since Assay C was the only one of the kits to give IGF-1 plasma concentrations approaching those obtained in previous studies using RIAs (Noble *et al.*, 2007), and was the only one with an acceptable intra-assay coefficient of variation, further investigation and validations were only performed for this kit. Firstly, assay characteristics were repeated for Assay C using EDTA plasma samples for comparison with heparinised plasma. Ponies were again found to have the highest IGF-1 concentration of 121.12 ±14.82 ng/mL, followed by Andalusians with 94.30 ±4.15 ng/mL and then Standardbreds with an IGF-1 concentration of 70.36 ±0.60 ng/mL. The mean CV of 5.83% was again acceptable and the mean % recovery was found to be 87.10%. Parallelism performed on pooled samples was found to be linear (Fig. 1). Values obtained for heparinised plasma conducted at the same time were found to be comparable to the previous values with a mean IGF-1 concentration for ponies of 201.95 ±14.6 ng/mL, Andalusians 146.16 ±3.64 ng/mL and Standardbreds 138.74 ±5.24 ng/mL. Again parallelism was satisfied and % recovery was 90.65%. Therefore values obtained from heparinised plasma were consistently higher than values from the same animals using EDTA plasma, even though recovery appeared to be similar. The inter-assay variation across analytical runs on different days (and on different plates) was also determined for Assay C only, and found to be 7.31%. This study evaluated the performance of three ELISA assays for the measurement of IGF-1 in the horse, using plasma samples obtained from three different breeds/types; namely ponies (of mixed breed), Andalusian horses and Standardbred horses.

Table 1. Comparison between different assay kits for the measurement of IGF-1 in heparinised equine plasma from ponies, Andalusian horses and Standardbred horses. Intra-assay coefficients of variation (CV) were calculated from the standard deviation (SD) expressed as a % of the mean; recovery was calculated by using spiked samples and linearity was determined by linear regression from plots of observed vs expected values.

	Mean (ng/mL)	SD	CV %	% Recovery	Linearity (r^2)	Parallelism (yes/no)
Assay A (Abcam)						
Pony	2.25	3.90	173.21	43.20	0.77	No
Andalusian	1.05	1.69	160.99	18.68	0.47	No
Standardbred	1.00	1.25	124.90	24.70	0.84	No
Mean			153.00	28.86		
SEM			14.50	7.38		
Assay B (Cusabio)						
Pony	17.25	9.14	52.98	72.98	0.99	Yes
Andalusian	15.71	7.84	49.90	81.93	0.97	Yes
Standardbred	11.97	2.10	17.57	73.01	0.99	Yes
Mean			40.15	75.97		
SEM			11.30	2.98		
Assay C (IDS)						
Pony	174.26	1.94	1.14	90.40	0.99	Yes
Andalusian	124.95	3.69	2.95	82.92	0.99	Yes
Standardbred	123.21	8.24	6.69	93.13	0.99	Yes
Mean			3.59	88.82		
SEM			1.63	3.05		

Table 2. Comparison between EDTA and heparinised plasma samples. IGF-1 concentrations were measured in EDTA and heparinised plasma samples from ponies and horses. Intra-assay coefficients of variation (CV) were calculated from the standard deviation (SD) expressed as a % of the mean; recovery was calculated by using spiked samples and linearity was determined by linear regression from plots of observed vs expected values.

	Mean (ng/mL)	SD	CV %	% Recovery	Linearity (r^2)	Parallelism (yes/no)
EDTA plasma						
Pony	121.12	14.82	12.24	83.69	0.99	Yes
Andalusian	94.30	4.15	4.40	90.85	-	No
Standardbred	70.36	0.60	0.85	86.75	-	No
Mean			5.83	87.10		
SEM			3.36	2.07		
Heparin plasma						
Pony	201.95	14.16	7.01	93.25	1.00	Yes
Andalusian	146.16	3.64	2.49	90.79	0.99	Yes
Standardbred	138.74	5.24	3.77	87.92	1.00	Yes
Mean			4.42	90.65		
SEM			1.35	1.54		

These types were selected because Standardbreds represent most typical athletic breeds of horse, while ponies and Andalusian horses tend to demonstrate metabolic characteristics including hyperinsulinaemic responses to dietary carbohydrates, regional obesity and also an increased risk of laminitis (Bamford et al., 2014). Assay A was found to be totally unsuitable for use in the horse, since it gave a recovery of less than 30% of spiked human recombinant IGF-1 in equine plasma, and parallelism could not be satisfied. Clearly there were substances in the plasma which interfered with the detection of the target peptide that resulted in very low apparent concentrations of IGF-1 in the assay of normal equine plasma samples. The factors interfering with IGF-1 detection are unknown. The IGFBPs may well be involved, although the acid-ethanol extraction method used in this assay to dissociate IGF-1 from its binding proteins is typical of many other kits, both ELISAs and RIAs. An acid-ethanol extraction method was also used in Assay B, although recovery was much improved compared with Assay A.

a.

b.

c.

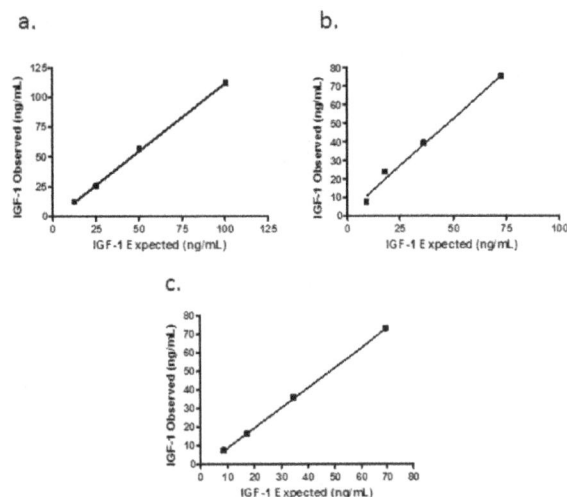

Fig. 1. Observed vs. expected concentrations of IGF-1 measured by Assay C, following dilution of pony (a), Andalusian (b) and Standardbred (c) heparinised plasma. R^2 values were 0.99 in all cases. The plasma assayed for each breed group was a pooled sample containing 6 individual animals.

However, recovery from spiked samples was still not optimal even though parallelism appeared to be satisfied, and relatively low values were also measured in the normal plasma samples. The intra-assay coefficient of variation was certainly not acceptable, and therefore either the extraction of IGF-1 from binding proteins or the degree of binding to the capture antibody may have been very variable from sample to sample or well to well.

Of the three IGF-1 assays evaluated, Assay C was the most suitable for measuring IGF-1 concentrations in the horse. This assay had an excellent coefficient of variation, both intra- and inter-assay, showed good dilutional parallelism and the plots of expected to observed concentrations in the diluted samples clearly demonstrated a linear relationship. The assay results in normal equine plasma were in the range of approximately 100-200 ng/mL which was at least an order of magnitude higher than the other two assays. The percentage recovery after spiking samples (88.42%) was slightly lower than the recovery reported by the manufacturer (95%), and this was acceptable although still not ideal. The improved recovery compared with the other two kits may have been related to the extraction method, since the other kits used the acid-ethanol technique; however, acid-ethanol extraction has been considered as an acceptable method in previous assays, including the very useful and sensitive RIAs (Noble *et al.*, 2007). The range of normal concentrations for IGF-1 in equine plasma reported using radioimmunoassay techniques is around 300 ng/mL (Noble *et al.*, 2007). That study measured concentrations in Thoroughbreds, which presumably

would have IGF-1 concentrations similar to Standardbreds, which had the lowest IGF-1 concentrations of the breeds in our study. Therefore assuming the RIA is accurate, ELISA assay C may tend to under-report the true plasma concentration, and this might be associated with the recovery being less than 100%. However, in the studies by Noble *et al.* (2007) and Ropp *et al.* (2003), it is notable that they measured IGF-1 in samples of serum rather than plasma. It could be argued that plasma samples might be more appropriate for the measurement of IGF-1, because platelets contain significant quantities of IGF-1 (bound to IGFBP-3) within their alpha granules (Chan and Spencer, 1998). This additional IGF-1 would be released during the clotting process, accounting for a considerably higher apparent concentration. Therefore the concentrations found in the present study, using heparinised plasma, may represent more accurately the actual circulating concentration of this hormone. Serum samples were not available in the present study for comparison. Heparinised plasma consistently gave higher values than EDTA plasma. It should be noted that EDTA has occasionally been found to interfere with some types of ELISA (Assink *et al.*, 1983).

It was interesting to note that the plasma IGF-1 concentrations recorded in samples from ponies appeared to be higher than those observed in the horse breeds, although this was not the primary objective of the current study. Further studies would be necessary to confirm whether there are breed differences. If there are, then this would not appear to be related to the hyperinsulinaemia and insulin resistance seen in ponies, because the IGF concentrations in Andalusian horses (which also show this tendency) were not different to Standardbreds (Bamford *et al.*, 2014). These findings confirm the suitability of the IGF-1 ELISA-Immunoenzymometric assay manufactured by IDS for use in the horse and this kit seems to provide a convenient, straightforward and cost effective method for measuring this growth factor.

It may have applications for detecting the use of growth hormone or its mimetics and in the investigation of developmental osteochondral disease and endocrinopathic laminitis. Caution should be used when comparing equine studies where different analytical techniques have been used to measure concentrations of IGF-1.

Conflict of interest

The authors declare that there is no conflict of interest.

Acknowledgements

The authors would like to thank Miss Samantha Potter and Ms Lianne Salerno for their technical assistance and care of the animals in this project. This study was supported by the Australian Research Council (project number LP100200224) and The WALTHAM Centre for Pet Nutrition.

References

Assink, H.A., Brouwer, H.J., Blijenberg, B.G. and Leijnse, B. 1983. The influence of the label on the quality of a solid-phase immunoassay: evaluation of a commercial ELISA kit for serum ferritin. J. Clin. Chem. Clin. Biochem. 21(11), 695-702.

Bamford, N.J., Potter, S.J., Harris, P.A. and Bailey, S.R. 2014. Breed differences in insulin sensitivity and insulinemic responses to oral glucose in horses and ponies of moderate body condition score. Domest. Anim. Endocrinol. 47, 101-107.

Chan, K., and Spencer, E.M. 1998. Megakaryocytes endocytose insulin-like growth factor (IGF) I and IGF-binding protein-3: a novel mechanism directing them into alpha granules of platelets. Endocrinol. 139(2), 559-565.

De Kock, S.S., Rodgers, J.P., Swanepoel, B.C. and Guthrie, A.J. 2001. Administration of bovine, porcine and equine growth hormone to the horse: effect on insulin-like growth factor-I and selected IGF binding proteins. J. Endocrinol. 171, 163-171.

de Laat, M.A., Pollitt, C.C., Kyaw-Tanner, M.T., McGowan, C.M. and Sillence, M.N. 2013. A potential role for lamellar insulin-like growth factor-1 receptor in the pathogenesis of hyperinsulinaemic laminitis. Vet. J. 197(2), 302-306.

De Palo, E.F., Gatti, R., Lancerin, F., Cappellin, E. and Spinella, P. 2001. Correlations of growth hormone (GH) and insulin-like growth factor I (IGF-I): effects of exercise and abuse by athletes. Clin. Chim. Acta. 305(1-2), 1-17.

Faust, M., Åkerblad, A.C., Buchfelder, M., Johannsson, G., Jonsson, P., Kann, P., Touraine, P. and Koltowska Häggström, M. 2012. Growth hormone replacement in adults with severe growth hormone deficiency is effective even if baseline IGF-1 levels are in the normal range. Exp. Clin. Endocrinol. Diabetes 120, P4.

Fortier, L.A., Kornatowski, M.A., Mohammed, H.O., Jordan, M.T., O'Cain, L.C. and Stevens, W.B. 2005. Age-related changes in serum insulin-like growth factor-I, insulin-like growth factor-I binding protein-3 and articular cartilage structure in Thoroughbred horses. Equine Vet. J. 37, 37-42.

Kostecka, Y., and Blahovec, J. 1999. Insulin-like growth factor binding proteins and their functions (minireview). Endocr. Regul. 33(2), 90-94.

Lejeune, J.P., Franck, T., Gangl, M., Schneider, N., Michaux, C., Deby-Dupont, G. and Serteyn, D. 2007. Plasma Concentration of insulin-like growth factor I (IGF-I) in growing Ardenner horses suffering from juvenile digital degenerative osteoarthropathy. Vet. Res. Comm. 31, 185-195.

Noble, G.K., Houghton, E., Roberts, C.J., Faustino-Kemp, J., de Kock, S.S., Swanepoel, B.C. and Sillence, M.N. 2007. Effect of exercise, training, circadian rhythm, age, and sex on insulin-like growth factor-1 in the horse. J. Anim. Sci. 85(1), 163-171.

Popot, M.A., Bobin, S., Bonnaire, Y., Delahaut, P.H. and Closset, J. 2001. IGF -I plasma concentrations in non-treated horses and horses administered with methionyl equine somatotropin. Res. Vet. Sci. 71(3), 167-173.

Popot, M.A., Woolfitt, A.R., Garcia, P. and Tabet, J.C. 2008. Determination of IGF-I in horse plasma by LC electrospray ionisation mass spectrometry. Anal. Bioanal. Chem. 390(7), 1843-1852.

Ropp, J.K., Raub, R.H. and Minton, J.E. 2003. The effect of dietary energy source on serum concentration of insulin-like growth factor-I, growth hormone, insulin, glucose, and fat metabolites in weanling horses. J. Anim. Sci. 81, 1581-1589.

Verwilghen, D.R., Vanderheyden, L., Franck, T., Busoni, V., Enzerink, E., Gangl, M., Lejeune, J.P., van Galen, G., Grulke, S. and Serteyn, D. 2009. Variations of plasmatic concentrations of Insulin-like Growth Factor-1 in post-pubescent horses affected with developmental osteochondral lesions. Vet. Res. Comm. 33, 701-709.

18

Effect of melatonin on maturation capacity and fertilization of Nili-Ravi buffalo (*Bubalus bubalis*) oocytes

G. Nagina[1,*], A. Asima[1], U. Nemat[2] and A. Shamim[1]

[1]PMAS Arid Agriculture University, Rawalpindi, Pakistan
[2]University of Animal and Veterinary Sciences Lahore, Pakistan

Abstract

This study evaluated the effect of melatonin supplementation of *in vitro* maturation media on *in vitro* maturation (IVM) and *in vitro* fertilization (IVF) rate of buffalo oocytes. Cumulus oocytes complexes (COCs) were aspirated from follicles of 2-8 mm diameter. In experiment I, COCs were matured in IVM medium supplemented with 0 (control), 250, 500, and 1000 µM melatonin for 22-24 hours in CO_2 incubator at 38.5°C with 5% CO_2 and at 95% relative humidity. The maturation rate did not differ in media supplemented with melatonin at 250 µM, 500 µM, 1000 µM and control (0 µM). In experiment II, the matured oocytes were fertilized in 50 µl droplets of Tyrode's Albumin Lactate Pyruvate (TALP) medium having 10 ug/ml heparin for sperm (2 million/ml) capacitation. The fertilization droplets were then kept for incubation at 5% CO_2 39°C and at 95% relative humidity for 18 hours. The fertilization rate was assessed by sperm penetration and pronuclear formation. Fertilization rate was improved when maturation medium was supplemented with 250 µM melatonin compared to control. In conclusion, melatonin supplementation to serum free maturation media at 250 µM improved the fertilization rate of buffalo oocytes.

Keywords: Buffalo, *In vitro* fertilization, *In vitro* maturation, Melatonin.

Introduction

Buffalo is important for ecologically disadvantaged agricultural systems as it not only provides meat, milk and working power but is also essential as a livestock source. Due to low maintenance requirements and good ability of feed conversion, buffaloes are considered ideal for low input systems and for the low cost production systems (Zicarelli, 1994). In spite of these qualities, the production potential of our dairy buffalo is low compared to dairy cattle in developed countries. Therefore consistent efforts are being made to improve the genetic potential of buffalo through assisted reproductive technologies. Artificial insemination that utilizes the superior male germplasm has been developed and is in use to some extent. Embryo transfer that utilizes superior male and female germplasm simultaneously is at the verge of experimentation in Pakistan. The efficiency of *in vitro* embryo production (IVEP) is lower in buffalo compared to cattle (Nandi *et al.*, 2002). The low number of primordial and antral follicles as well as high incidence of follicular artresia is the major impediment for the *in vitro* embryo production in this species (Palta *et al.*, 1998).

When cultured *in vitro*, oocytes are exposed to light, increased oxygen concentrations, increased or decreased concentrations of metabolites and substrates during handling of oocytes that causes oxidative stress (Agarwal *et al.*, 2006). Naturally, free radical-scavenging antioxidants exist within the follicular and oviductal fluid that is able to protect the oocytes against oxidative stress (Wang *et al.*, 2002), however, this system becomes insufficient under *in vitro* conditions. Melatonin and its metabolites have the ability to scavenge directly the free radicals and indirectly to act as powerful antioxidant (Adriaens *et al.*, 2006; Kang *et al.*, 2009). It has been reported that melatonin directly protects the oocytes of human and mouse from oxidative stress (Tamura *et al.*, 2008). In bovine oocytes, melatonin stimulated the re-initiation of meiosis but it was unable to complete the meiosis or cleavage of oocytes after their maturation and fertilization in the laboratory (Sirotkin and Schaeffer, 1997). Present study was designed to assess the role of melatonin in *in vitro* maturation media on *in vitro* maturation (IVM) and *in vitro* fertilization (IVF) of buffalo oocytes.

Materials and Methods

This study was conducted at Physiology Laboratory, Faculty of Veterinary and Animal Sciences, Pir Mehr Ali Shah Arid Agriculture University, Rawalpindi.

Reagents and chemicals

The reagents and chemicals used in the study were purchased from Sigma (St. Louis MO, USA), or mentioned when purchased from other source.

Collection of ovaries

Nili-Ravi buffalo ovaries were collected immediately after slaughtering from local slaughterhouse at Sihala (Islamabad), and transported to laboratory within two hours in a thermos having sterilized saline solution held at 37 °C (Mehmood, 2007). In the laboratory, ovaries were washed with 70% ethanol for 30 seconds followed by three times rinse in saline solution (Jamil, 2007).

Retrieval of oocytes

A 10 ml syringe attached to a needle (18 guage) was used to retrieve cumulus oocyte complexes from follicles having diameter of 2-8 mm. The follicular fluid was collected in a conical tube and kept for 10-15 minutes. After discarding the supernatant, the sediment was collected in 60 mm petri dish and oocytes were searched under stereo microscope.

Classification of oocytes

The cumulus oocytes complexes were graded as: A Grade: having evenly granulated homogenous ooplasm with cumulus cells of three or more compact layers, B Grade: having homogenous ooplasm with two to three layers of cumulus cells, C Grade: having irregular ooplasm with less compact cumulus cells and D Grade: having irregular dark ooplasm and highly expanded cumulus cells (Singhal et al., 2009).

Maturation of oocytes

Total number of buffalo ovaries used in the present study was 1179 and the numbers of oocytes recovered were 1300. Only grade A (n= 315) and B (n=290) oocytes were used for INM. The oocytes were washed twice with oocytes wash media and once with IVM media (pH 7.3-7.4). The oocytes were placed in IVM medium (Jamil et al., 2007) with some modifications (MM; TCM-199 supplemented with BSA 6 mg/mL, 10 IU/mL LH, 0.5 ug/mL FSH, 1 ug/mL estradiol-17β and 50 ug/mL gentamicin) alone or with melatonin supplemented at 250 μM, 500 μM and 1000 μM in four experimental groups covered with mineral oil. The maturation dishes containing oocytes were placed for 22-24 hours in an incubator with 5% CO_2, at 39 °C and at humidity of about 95%.

Sperm preparation

Swim up technique was used to separate the most motile spermatozoa in medium known as Tyrode's albumin lactate pyruvate (Sperm TALP) (Jamil et al., 2007). Briefly, 3 mL of TALP medium (pH 7.3-7.4) was taken in each of the four 15 ml tubes and incubated for two hours in an incubator at 39°C temperature and 5% CO_2. Cryopreserved buffalo semen was thawed at 37°C for 30 seconds. About 70 μl of thawed semen was transferred into four 15 ml tubes containing sperm TALP, placed at an angle of 45° and incubated at 39°C, 5% CO_2 and 95% humidity. The supernatant containing the most motile spermatozoa was transferred to a 15 ml falcon tube for centrifugation at 1600 rpm for 10 minutes. The sperm pellet was suspended in fertilization TALP having 10μg/mL heparin for capacitation. Neubauer hemocytometer was used for measuring sperm concentration (Hafez and Hafez, 2000) and sperm concentration was adjusted to 1×10^6/mL by adding fertilization media.

In vitro fertilization

Following maturation, oocytes were washed three times in the fertilization TALP and then 5-10 oocytes were incubated in 50 μl droplets of fertilization TALP (mTALP) having sperm under mineral oil at 5% CO_2, 95% humidity and 39 °C for 18 hours.

Evaluation of in vitro maturation

Cumulus cell expansion

After 24 hour of incubation, the degree of cumulus expansion was assessed using stereo microscope as; not expanded oocytes without loosened, partially expanded with slightly loosened or fully expanded oocytes with cumulus cells completely loosened.

Stage of nuclear maturation

After IVM, oocytes were vortexed in 1 ml M-199 containing 300 μl/mL hyaluronidase for 2 minutes to completely denude the oocytes. The denuded oocytes were washed with simple maturation media, placed on grease-free slide and cover slipped with 4 droplets of Vaseline/Paraffin (40:1) mixture. Oocytes were slightly compressed and fixative (acetic acid and ethanol in the ratio of 1:3 v/v) was used for fixing oocytes for 5 minutes. Acetoorcein stain (1% orcein in 45% acetic acid) was used for staining of oocytes. After 3-5 minutes, excess stain was removed from oocytes by a de-staining solution composed of acetic acid: distilled water: glycerol (1:3:1) in the same manner as staining of oocytes. Phase contrast microscope (400X) was used to determine the stage of maturation (Hewitt et al., 1998). Oocytes were classified at germinal vesicle (GV; prophase I having a prominent nucleolus), germinal vesicle breakdown (GVBD; condensation of chromosomes by resolution of nuclear membrane), metaphase I (M-I; arrangement of chromosomes at equator but without a polar body) and metaphase II (M-II; when polar body was extruded).

Assessment of in vitro fertilization

After 18 h of insemination, oocytes were stained as described earlier. Oocytes with penetrating head, with male pronucleus (MPN) and female pro-nucleus (FPN) were considered as normal fertilized. Oocytes with three or more pro-nuclei were considered as polyspermic.

Statistical analysis

The data on maturation rate of oocytes and IVF rate of in vitro matured oocytes were analyzed by chi square analysis. Statistically significant confidence interval was taken as $P<0.05$.

Results

Recovery of oocytes

Oocytes were classified into four different grades on the basis of homogenous ooplasm and the compactness of the cumulus cells as shown in the Fig. 1. Data on the recovery of different grade oocytes from the ovaries is given in the Table 1. Total oocytes recovered from buffalo ovaries (n=1179) were 1300 in number which were retrieved from follicles of 2-8 mm by aspiration method. Out of these oocytes grade C oocytes were higher (28.07%) followed by grade D (25.38%), grade A (24.23%) and grade B (22.30%).

Oocytes maturation in IVM media supplemented with melatonin

Expansion of Cumulus Cells

The data on degree of cumulus expansion of buffalo oocytes with the supplementation of melatonin in IVM media are given in the Table 2 and Fig. 2 as well. Fully expanded oocytes were 33.04, 42.85, 38.88 and 32.50% in control, 250 µM, 500 µM, and 1000 µM melatonin supplemented maturation media, respectively.

Degree of maturation of oocytes

The data on the number of oocytes at different stages of maturation after 24 hours of incubation are given in the Table 3 and Fig. 3. The oocytes that remained at GV stage were 5.12% and 3.03% in control and 500 µM melatonin supplemented media. While no oocyte was found at GV stage in the media supplemented with 250 µM and 1000 µM of melatonin. The oocytes reaching GVBD were 12.82% in control, while 6.06%, 9.09% and 6.25% in media supplemented with 250 µM, 500 µM and 1000 µM melatonin. The oocytes at M-I stage were 30.76%, 24.24%, 24.24% and 28.12% in control, 250 µM, 500 µM and 1000 µM melatonin supplemented media, respectively. The MII stage oocytes were recorded as, 51.28% 69.69%, 63.63% and 65.62% in control, 250 µM, 500 µM and 1000 µM melatonin supplemented media, respectively. Oocytes

at M-II were considered to be matured, the percentage of which in the media supplemented with different concentrations of melatonin was found slightly higher compared to control, however the difference remained non-significant (P>0.05).

Fertilization of oocytes (IVF)

The data on the effect of IVM media supplemented with different concentrations of melatonin on fertilization of buffalo oocytes after 18 hours of insemination are given in the Table 4 and Fig. 4. The oocytes that were penetrated remained 2.3% in control and 10.25% when the oocytes were matured in 1000 µM melatonin supplemented IVM media. Oocytes with 2PN were recorded as 25.58%, 46.15%, 43.58%, and 23.07% in control, 250 µM, 500 µM and 1000 µM melatonin supplemented groups. A small number of polyspermic oocytes (10.25%) were found when the oocytes were matured in media supplemented with 1000 µM melatonin. The number of oocytes that remained unidentified was 2.3%, 10.25%, 15.4% and 15.38%, in control, 500 µM, 250 µM and 1000 µM melatonin supplemented media.

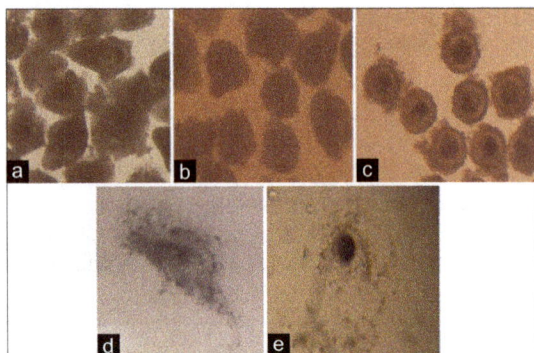

Fig. 1. Recovery of different grades oocytes from buffalo ovaries by aspiration. (a) Grade A oocyte with cumulus cells of 3-4 layers. (b) Grade B oocyte with cumulus cells of 2-3 layers. (c) Grade C oocytes cumulus cells maximum 1 layer. (d) Grade D oocyte highly denuded (e) or denuded (f). (400x by stereo microscope).

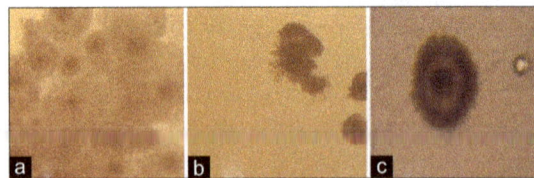

Fig. 2. Degree of expansion of oocytes complexes after 24 hours of IVM. (a) Fully expanded cumulus layer. (b) Partially expanded cumulus layer. (c) Not expanded cumulus layer. (400x by stereo microscope).

Table 1. Frequency distribution of different grades of Oocytes recovered from buffalo ovaries (n=1179) by aspiration method.

Oocytes	Recovery rate	
	Total	Per ovary (%)
Oocytes recovered	1300	1.1
Usable oocytes (A, B)	605	0.51
Grade A (%)	315 (24.2)	0.26
Grade B (%)	290 (22.3)	0.25
Grade C (%)	365 (28.1)	0.31
Grade D (%)	330 (25.4)	0.28

Table 2. Effect of supplementation of melatonin in media for IVM on degree of cumulus expansion of buffalo oocytes after 24 hours of maturation.

IVM Media	No. of oocytes	Degree of cumulus expansion n (%)		
		Not expanded	Partially expanded	Fully expanded
Maturation media (MM)	115	34 (29.6)	43 (37.4)	38 (33.0)
Mm+250 µM melatonin	112	32 (28.6)	32 (28.6)	48 (42.8)
Mm+500 µM melatonin	108	31 (28.7)	35 (32.4)	42 (38.9)
Mm+1000 µM melatonin	120	42 (35.0)	39 (32.5)	39 (32.5)

Chi-square analysis, p>0.05

Table 3. Effect of supplementation of melatonin in media for IVM on nuclear maturation of buffalo oocytes after 24 hours of in vitro maturation.

Treatments	No. of Oocytes	n (%)			
		GV	GVBD	M1	M2
Maturation media (MM)	39	2 (5.1)	5 (12.8)	12 (30.8)	20 (51.3)
MM+250 µM melatonin	33		2 (6.1)	8 (24.2)	23 (69.7)
MM+500 µM melatonin	33	1 (3.0)	3 (9.1)	8 (24.2)	21 (63.7)
MM+1000 µM melatonin	32		2 (6.3)	9 (28.1)	21 (65.6)

Chi-square analysis, p>0.05

Table 4. Effect of supplementation of melatonin in media for IVM on in vitro fertilization of buffalo oocytes after 18 hours of insemination.

Treatments	No. of ocytes						
	Inseminated	Fertilized	With 2PN	Penetrated	Polyspermic	Not fertilized	Not identified
Maturation media (MM)	43	12 (27.9) [b]	11 (25.6)	1 (2.3)		30 (69.8)	1 (2.3)
MM+250 µM melatonin	39	18 (46.2) [a]	18 (46.2)			15 (38.5)	6 (15.4)
MM+500 µM melatonin	39	17 (43.6) [b]	17 (43.6)			20 (51.3)	4 (10.3)
MM+1000 µM melatonin	39	17 (43.6) [b]	9 (23.1)	4 (10.3)	4 (10.3)	22 (56.4)	6 (15.4)

MM: Maturation media; PN: Pro-nucleus; Chi-square analysis, p<0.05

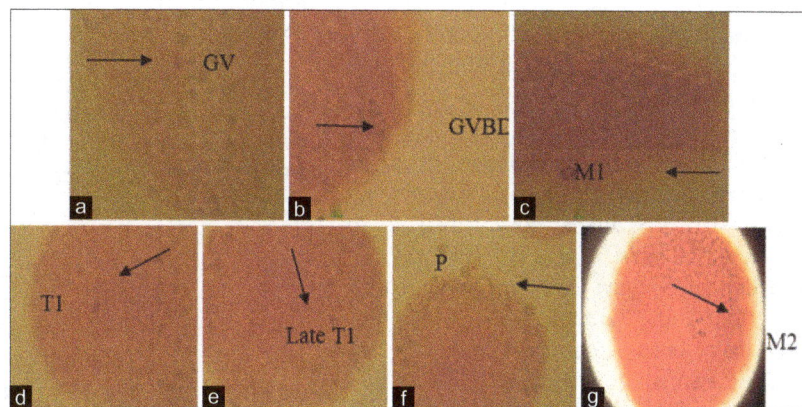

Fig. 3. Different stages of nuclear maturation after 24 hours of IVM. (a) Germinal vesicle (GV), showing nucleolus. (b) Germinal vesicle breakdown (GVBD), showing condensation of chromosomes. (c) Metaphase I (MI), showing chromosomes at meiotic plate without any polar body. (d) Telophase (T1) stage. (e) Late Telophase (T1). (f) Metaphase 2 (M2), stage showing extrusion of first polar body. (g) Metaphase 2. (400x by phase contrast microscopy).

The overall percentage of fertilized oocytes in control and in the media supplemented with 250 µM, 500 µM and 1000 µM were 27.90%, 46.15%, 43.58% and 43.58% respectively. The percentage of fertilized oocytes in the media supplemented with 500 µM and 1000 µM melatonin did not differ significantly from the control (MM+BSA). However, percentage of fertilized oocytes was higher (P<0.05) when the oocytes were matured in media supplemented with 250 µM melatonin compared to control.

Discussion

Maturation involves important events which an oocyte needs to complete for successful fertilization and early embryogenesis. Appropriate maturation is the basis for implantation, initiation of pregnancy, and fetal development (Brevini and Gandolfi, 2001; Sirard et al., 2006). Generally, maturation involves accumulation of mRNA, proteins, substrates, and nutrients that are required to achieve oocyte's developmental competence that fosters embryonic developmental competence (Brevini and Gandolfi, 2001; Krisher, 2004; Sirard et al., 2006).

The oocytes are more exposed to light, air and chemicals during in vitro handling that is responsible for generation of reactive oxygen species (ROS). Buffalo oocytes were found much sensitive to stress caused by

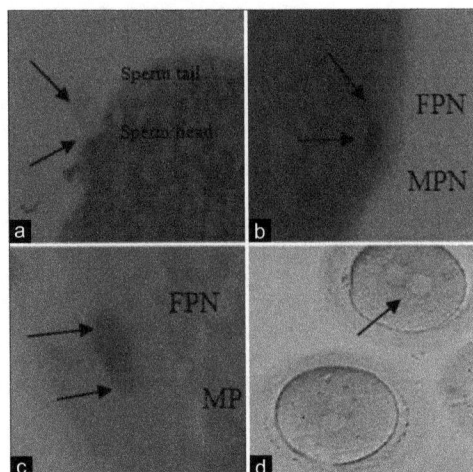

Fig. 4. Different stages of *in vitro* fertilization (IVF) of buffalo oocytes after 18 hours of insemination. (a) Penetrated oocytes showing sperm head and tail. (b&c) Fertilized oocytes showing fused male (MPN) and female pro-nucleus (FPN). (d) Fertilized oocyte with two nuclei. (400x by phase contrast microscopy).

reactive oxygen species during culturing in laboratory (Boni *et al.*, 1992). The oocyte developmental competence was reported to be improved by increasing the antioxidant capacity of oocytes during IVM, as the high lipid content makes buffalo oocytes/embryos sensitive to oxidative damages (Boni *et al.*, 1992).

Melatonin has the ability to scavenge oxygen radical, and is effective in reducing apoptosis in different cell types (Allegra *et al.*, 2003; Juknat *et al.*, 2005). Melatonin reduces oxidative stress of ovarian follicles and helps in protection of oocytes from free radical damage (Takasaki *et al.*, 2003; Tamura *et al.*, 2008). Melatonin receptors have been reported on cumulus cells and when supplemented in maturation media, it reduced apoptosis of cumulus cells in mouse (Na *et al.*, 2005). Further, improvement in maturation and cleavage rates with the supplementation of melatonin in IVM and IVF medium was reported in mice (Na *et al.*, 2005), bovine (Dimitriadis *et al.*, 2005) and humans (Parka *et al.*, 2006). Similarly, positive effect of melatonin was reported during in *vitro* embryo development in mouse (Ishizuka *et al.*, 2000), pig (Rodriguez *et al.*, 2007, Kang *et al.*, 2009, Shi *et al.*, 2009) and buffalo (Manjunatha *et al.*, 2009).

The overall recovery rate of oocytes in our study was lower as the study was conducted in the low breeding season that affects the overall production of progesterone and estradiol required for follicular growth and development. In present study, the percentage of fully expanded COCs decreased progressively with increasing melatonin concentration but difference in the degree of cumulus expansion between different concentrations of melatonin and control was not

significant (P>0.05). The dose dependent effect of melatonin on cumulus cells expansion has previously been reported in mouse (Adriaens *et al.*, 2006).

The rate of nuclear maturation did not differ significantly with melatonin supplementation (250 µM, 500 µM and 1000 µM) of IVM and control (0 µM) in the present study (P>0.05) as reported earlier that higher concentrations of melatonin mighthave negativeeffect onsurvival of follicles leading to lower rates of maturation (Adriaens *et al.*, 2006). In contrast to our study, useful effects of melatonin have been reported during porcine IVM (Kang *et al.*, 2009). Similarly, increase in the maturation rate and transformable embryo yield was reported earlier in buffalo when melatonin was supplemented in IVM media (Manjunatha *et al.*, 2009). Furthermore, as the melatonin receptors are present in bovine cumulus cells and its lower concentrations (0.1 pM to 1000 nM) may positively affect cytoplasmic and nuclear maturation (Raey *et al.*, 2011), however, it was not observed in present study.

In present study, the IVF rate of oocytes was independent of maturation rate and was significantly improved in the group treated with 250 µM of melatonin. The beneficial effects of melatonin on *in vitro* embryo development have already been reported in mouse (Gao *et al.*, 2012) and in buffalo (Zhang *et al.*, 1995). However, in bovine, melatonin supplementation of IVM media did not improve the cleavage and blastocyst rates (Tsantarliotou *et al.*, 2007). The supplementation of melatonin in IVM and IVF medium simultaneously, improved maturation and cleavage rates in mice (Na *et al.*, 2005), bovine (Dimitriadis *et al.*, 2005) and humans (Parka *et al.*, 2006). This study showed that increasing melatonin concentrations beyond 250 µM does not have any significant effect on maturation rates of buffalo oocytes. Melatonin at higher concentrations may be toxic and may result in cell injury and lower blastocyst rates due to its toxicity (Rodriguez *et al.*, 2007). So, it is concluded that addition of melatonin at 250 µM improved the fertilization rates of buffalo oocytes, although it did not show improvement IVM rate of buffalo oocytes.

References

Adriaens, I., Jacquet, P., Cortvrindt, R., Janssen, K. and Smitz, J. 2006. Melatonin have dose-dependent effects on mouse folliculogenesis, oocyte maturation capacity and steroidogenesis. Toxicology 228, 333-343.

Agarwal, A., Tamer, S., Mohammed, A.B., Jashoman, B. and Juan, B.A. 2006. Oxidative stressing assisted reproductive techniques. Fertil. Steril. 86, 503-512.

Allegra, M., Reiter, R.J., Tan, D.X., Gentile, C., Tesoriere, L. and Livrea, M.A. 2003. The chemistry of melatonin's interaction with reactive species. J. Pineal Res. 34, 1-10.

Boni, R., Santella, L., Dale, B., Roviello, S., Palo, D.R. and Barbieri, V. 1992. An ultrastructural study of maturation in buffalo oocytes. Acta Med. Vet. 38, 153-l61.

Brevini, T.A. and Gandolfi, F. 2001. The maternal legacy to the embryo cytoplasmic components and their effects on early development. Theriogenology 55, 1255-1276.

Dimitriadis, I., Paapanikolau, T., Vainas, E., Amiridis, G.S., Valasi, I., Samrtzi, F. and Rekkas, C.A. 2005. Effects of melatonin on *in vitro* maturation of bovine oocytes. Annual Conference of the European Society for Domestic Animal Reproduction (ESDAR) Murcia, Spain, pp: 397.

Gao, C., Han, H.B., Tian, X.Z., Tan, D.X. and Wang, L. 2012. Melatonin promotes embryonic development and reduces reactive oxygen species in vitrified mouse 2-cell embryos. J. Pineal Res. 52, 305-311.

Hafez, B. and Hafez, E.S.E. 2000. Appendix IV: Technique for Determining Spermatozoal Concentration Using a Hemacytometer, in Reproduction in Farm Animals, 7th Edition, Lippincott Williams & Wilkins, Baltimore, Maryland, USA. doi: 10.1002/9781119265306.app4.

Hewitt, D.A., Watson, P.E. and England, G.C.W. 1998. Nuclear staining and culture requirements for *in vitro* maturation of domestic bitch oocytes. Theriogenology 49, 1083-1101.

Ishizuka, B., Kuribayashi, Y., Murai, K., Amemiya, A. and Itoh, M.T. 2000. The effect of melatonin on *in vitro* fertilization and embryo development in mice. J. Pineal Res. 28, 48-51.

Jamil, H. 2007. Studies on *in vitro* maturation, sperm preparation and fertilization of Nili-Ravi buffalo follicular oocytes. PhD Thesis, University of Agriculture, Faisalabad.

Jamil, H., Samad, H.A., Rehman, N.U., Qureshi, Z.I. and Lodhi, L.A. 2007. *In vitro* Maturation and Fertilization of Riverine Buffalo Follicular Oocytes in Media Supplemented with Oestrus Buffalo Serum and Hormones. Acta Vet. Brno. 76, 399-404.

Juknat, A.A., Mendez, M.V., Quaglino, A., Fameli, C.I., Mena, M. and Kotler, M.L. 2005. Melatonin prevents hydrogen peroxide-induced Bax expression in cultured rat astrocytes. J. Pineal Res. 38, 84-92.

Kang, J.T., Koo, O.J., Kwon, H.J., Park, H.J., Jang, G., Kang, S.K. and Lee, S.C. 2009. Effects of melatonin on *in vitro* maturation of porcine oocyte and expression of melatonin receptor RNA in cumulus and granulosa cells. J. Pineal Res. 46, 22-28.

Krisher, R.L. 2004. The effect of oocyte quality on development. J. Anim. Sci. 82, 14-23.

Manjunatha, B.M., Devaraj, M., Gupta, P.S.P., Ravindra, J.P. and Nandi, S. 2009. Effect of taurine and melatonin in the culture medium on buffalo *in vitro* embryo development. Reprod. Domest. Anim. 44, 12-16.

Mehmood, A. 2007. Development of homologus *in vitro* fertilization test to predict fertility of buffalo semen. PhD Thesis University of arid agriculture, Rawalpindi, pp: 43.

Na, K., Kim, J., Lee, J., Yoon, T., Cha, K. and Lee, D. 2005. Effect of melatoninon the maturation of mouse GV oocytes and apoptosis of cumulus cells *in vitro*. Fertil. Steril. 84, 103.

Nandi, S., Raghu, H.M., Ravindranatha, B.M. and Chauhan, M.S. 2002. Production of buffalo (*Bubalusbubalis*) embryos *in vitro*: Premises and promises. Reprod. Domest. Anim. 37, 65.

Palta, P., Banzai, N., Prakash, B.S., Manik, R.S. and Madan, M.L. 1998. Endocrinological observation of atresia in individual buffalo ovarian follicles. Indian J. Anim. Sci. 68, 444-447.

Parka, E., Leea, D., Choa, J., Hana, J., Chaa, K. and Yoona, T. 2006. Addition of melatonin in *in vitro* maturation (IVM) medium increases maturation and fertilization of immature human oocytes. Fertil. Steril. 8, 168.

Raey, E.M., Geshi, M., Somfai, T., Kaneda, M., Hirako, M., Ghaffar, A.A.E., Sosa, G.A., Roos, E.M.E. and Nagai, T. 2011. Evidence of melatonin synthesis in the cumulus oocyte complexes and its role in enhancing oocyte maturation in vitro in cattle. Mol. Reprod. Dev. 78, 250-262.

Rodriguez, O.N., Kim, I.J., Wang, H., Kaya, A. and Memilli, E. 2007. Melatonin increases cleavage rate of porcine pre implantation embryos *in vitro*. J. Pineal Res. 43, 283-288.

Shi, J.M., Tian, X.Z., Zhou, G.B., Wang, L., Gao, C., Zhu, S.E., Zeng, S.M., Tian, J.H. and Liu, G.S. 2009. Melatonin exists in porcine follicular fluid and improves *in vitro* maturation and parthenogenetic development of porcine oocytes. J. Pineal Res. 47, 318-323.

Singhal, S., Prasad, S., Singh, B., Prasad, J.K. and Gupta, H.P. 2009. Effect of including growth factors and antioxidants in maturation medium used for *in vitro* culture of buffalo oocytes recovered *in vivo*. Anim. Reprod. Sci. 113, 44-50.

Sirard, M.A., Richard, F., Blondin, P. and Robert, C. 2006. Contribution of the oocyte to embryo quality. Theriogenology 65, 126-136.

Sirotkin, A.V. and Schaeffer, H.J. 1997. Direct regulation of mammalian reproductive organs by serotonin and melatonin. J. Endocrinol. 154, 1-5.

Takasaki, A., Nakamura, Y., Tamura, H., Shimamura, K. and Morioka, H. 2003. Melatonin as a new drug for improving oocytes quality. Reprod. Med. Biol. 2, 139-144.

Tamura, H., Takasaki, A., Miwa, I., Taniguchi, K., Maekawa, R., Asada, H., Taketani, T., Matsuoka, A., Yamagata, Y., Shimamura, K., Morioka, H., Ishikawa, H., Reiter, R.J. and Sugino, N. 2008.

Oxidative stress impairs oocyte quality and melatonin protects oocytes from free radical damage and improves fertilization rate. J. Pineal Res. 44, 280-287.

Tsantarliotou, M.P., Altanasio, L., Rosa, A.D., Boccia, L., Pellerano, G. and Gasparrini, B. 2007. The effect of melatonin on bovine *in vitro* embryo development. Ital. J. Anim. Sci. 6, 488-489.

Wang, X., Falcone, T., Attaran, M., Goldberg, J.M., Agarwal, A. and Sharma, R.K. 2002. Vitamin C and vitamin E supplementation reduce oxidative stress-induced embryo toxicity and improve the blastocyst development rate. Fertil. Steril. 78(6), 1272-1277.

Zhang, L., Jiang, S., Wozniak, P.J., Yang, X. and Godke, R.A. 1995. Cumulus cell function during bovine oocytes maturation, fertilization and embryo development *in vitro*. Mol. Reprod. Dev. 40, 338-344.

Zicarelli, L. 1994. Management under different environmental condition. Buffalo J. 2, 17-38.

19

Uterine involution and progesterone level during the postpartum period in Barbary ewes in North Libya

M.S. Medan[1,2,*] and T. EL-Daek[1]

[1]*Department of Theriogenology, Faculty of Veterinary Medicine, Omar AL-Mukhtar University, AL-Bayda, Libya*
[2]*Department of Theriogenology, Faculty of Veterinary Medicine, Suez Canal University, Ismailia, Egypt*

Abstract

The objectives of the present study were to determine the time of uterine involution and ovarian activity using ultrasound examination and progesterone assay. Weekly progesterone levels were measured starting one week postpartum until two weeks after the 1st postpartum estrus in Barbary ewes lambed during winter in AL-Bayda city, north of Libya. A total of 15 Barbary ewes were used in the present study distributed in three groups according to the month of lambing as group 1 (lambed in January), group 2 (lambed in February) and group 3 (lambed in March). Ewes were examined weekly by trans-rectal ultrasound to check involution of the uterus starting one week after lambing until complete uterine involution. Blood samples were collected from the jugular vein, and serum was separated and stored at -20 °C until measuring progesterone using ELISA. Results showed that uterine involution completed at day 35 postpartum in groups 1 and 2, while it occurred at day 28 in group 3. The mean progesterone level was basal (less than 1 ng/ml) for a long period and started to increase at days 119, 99 and 77 postpartum in group 1, 2 and 3, respectively. One ewe did not show estrus at all during the period of study in group 2 and there were no growing follicles on their ovaries. The obtained results indicate that, uterine involution as determined by ultrasound completed earlier in ewes lambed in March than those lambed in February or January. Also, progesterone level and ultrasound examination showed that there was no ovarian activity for a longtime after parturition indicating that reproduction in Barbary ewes tends to be seasonal in AL-Bayda city, north Libya.

Keywords: Ewes, Ovarian activity, Postpartum uterine involution, Ultrasound.

Introduction

The postpartum period is characterized by uterine involution and restoration of ovarian functions, since both should occur to establish a new pregnancy. The completion of uterine involution was defined as the day when the diameter of the uterus returned to the original non-pregnant size as observed during the normal estrous cycle (Takayama *et al.*, 2010).

Uterine involution occurs in a decreasing logarithmic scale with the greatest change occurring during the first few days after parturition (Noakes *et al.*, 2009). Completion of uterine involution and resumption of sexual activity following parturition in ruminants normally depend on several factors such as nutrition, nursing of offspring and season of parturition (Delgadillo *et al.*, 1998; Yavas and Walton, 2000).

Previously, techniques such hormone measurements (Ishwar, 1995), radiography (Kene, 1991; Tian and Noakes, 1991) and laparotomy (Ishwar, 1995; Rubianes *et al.*, 1996) were used to study the dynamics of uterine involution in small ruminants. However, these techniques are not practical under field conditions (Goddard, 1995).

The use of B-mode trans-rectal ultrasonography for imaging the reproductive tract provides real time, functional and clinical information such the number of follicles (Vinoles *et al.*, 2004), pregnancy (Medan and Abd El-Aty, 2010) and uterine pathology (Yilmaz *et al.*, 2008). Moreover, trans-rectal ultrasonography can be used under field conditions to determine uterine involution in different animals (Lohan *et al.*, 2004; Hajurka *et al.*, 2005 and Yilmaz and Ucar, 2012). Ultrasonography plays a key role to differentiate the normal or abnormal postpartum uterus and in early diagnosis of any abnormal condition related to uterus (Feldman and Nelson, 1996).

In sheep, the interval between parturition and the resumption of ovarian activity has been shown to be influenced by some factors such as suckling intensity (Schirar *et al.*, 1989) or season of parturition (Pope *et al.*, 1989; Delgadillo *et al.*, 1998). Pope *et al.* (1989) reported that there are large breed differences on the extent of the postpartum anestrus prior to a fertile estrus, reflecting a strong genetic component in addition to seasonal influences.

The aim of the present study was to determine the time required for uterine involution in Barbary ewes by mean of ultrasonography and start of ovarian activity through progesterone measurement.

Materials and Methods

This study was carried out on 15 pluriparous Barbary ewes at AL-Bayda city, north Libya (latitude 21.22 N

Corresponding Author: Dr. Mohamed Sabry Medan. Current Address: Department of Theriogenology, Faculty of Veterinary Medicine, Omar AL-Mukhtar University, AL-Bayda, Libya. Email: *medan69@hotmail.com*

and longitude 32 E). The selected ewes had normal lambing during winter and giving birth to singleton. Ewes were distributed on 3 groups according to the date of lambing as group 1 (n=5; lambed in January), group 2 (n=5; lambed in February) and group 3 (n=5; lambed in March). Age of the animals ranged between 4 to 6 years and their body weight ranged between 45-55 kg. Each ewe had fed on 1.5 kg concentrates, divided into two times daily beside roughage. Water was available ad libitum and mineral salt licks were also available during the whole period of the study.

Estrus behavior was monitored two times a day starting one week after parturition up to the end of study, using an intact active ram. A female was recorded as being in estrus when she accepted mounting attempt by the male.

Examination of the postpartum uterus:

Uterine involution was checked through trans-rectal ultrasound examination weekly starting from one week after delivery through complete uterine involution and continued until start of ovarian activity using B-mode ultrasound machine (Landwind, C30 Vet) equipped with a multifrequency 5-10 MHz probe. For ultrasonic examination, the ewe was restrained in a standing position with the help of an assistant. The rectum was evacuated from feces and air with the aid of the lubricated fingers. Thereafter, the lubricated transducer (fixed to an extension rod) was introduced into the rectum. The transducer was moved medially and laterally to get the best view of the uterine horn and maximum diameter was recorded. Uterine involution was considered to be complete when there was no further reduction in the uterine diameter for two successive examinations (Zdunczyk et al., 2004).

Blood sampling and hormonal assay:

Blood samples (10 ml) were collected weekly from each ewe from the jugular vein into vacutainer tubes without anticoagulant, starting one week after lambing until 2 weeks after the appearance of the first postpartum estrus. The tubes were centrifuged at 3000 rpm for 15 minutes. Blood serum was separated and deep-frozen at -20 °C until assessment of progesterone concentration using Enzyme-linked Immunosorbent Assay (ELISA) method.

Statistical analysis:

Results were expressed as means ± SE (standard errors). The analysis of variance (ANOVA) was used to test the significance of differences between means. Significance was assigned at P<0.05. Duncan's multiple range test was applied for post hoc comparison using SPSS software, (SPSS, version 21, 2012).

Results

Uterine involution:

Postpartum gravid horn diameter, as estimated by trans-rectal ultrasonography in the three groups was shown in Table 1. Uterine involution occurred at day 35 postpartum in group 1 and 2, while it occurred at day 28 postpartum in group 3. The results showed that uterine involution in the third group is completed in a shorter time compared with the first group and second group. Uterine horn diameter decreased sharply (P<0.05) in all groups within the first 4 weeks after parturition.

Table 1. Mean (± SEM) of postpartum uterine horn diameters as determined by trans-rectal ultrasonography in ewes lambed in January, February and March.

Day of examination	Uterine horn diameter (cm)		
	Group 1 (n=5) January lambing	Group 2 (n=5) February lambing	Group 3 (n=5) March lambing
7	5.62 0.38[a]	5.28 ± 0.32[a]	5.24 ± 0.37[a]
14	4.44 ± 0.37[b]	3.92 ± 0.24[b]	3.86 ± 0.35[b]
21	3.42 ± 0.29[c]	3.06 ± 0.22[c]	2.84 ± 0.30[c]
28	2.68 ± 0.17[d]	2.36 ± 0.20[d]	1.98 ± 0.17[d]
35	2.10 ± 0.07[de]	2.04 ± 0.15[de]	1.78 ± 0.09[d]
42	1.80 ± 0.06[e]	1.88 ± 0.14[de]	1.74 ± 0.12[d]
49	1.78 ± 0.07[e]	1.76 ± 0.06[e]	1.70 ± 0.09[d]
56	1.78 ± 0.07[e]	1.76 ± 0.07[e]	1.70 ± 0.11[d]
63	1.74 ± 0.05[e]	1.76 ± 0.08[e]	1.68 ± 0.10[d]

Values with different superscripts in the same column are significantly different (P<0.05).

Ultrasonography of the postpartum ovaries:

Trans-rectal ultrasound examination of postpartum ovaries in the present study did not show any follicle > 3 mm in diameter for about 25 days postpartum in all animals. Small follicles (size 3- 5 mm in diameter) were recorded on the ovaries after 25 days postpartum, while follicles > 5 mm in diameter were detected after 50 days postpartum (data not shown). On the other hand, ovulation and corpora lutea formation detected only after estrus.

Progesterone concentration during the postpartum period:

The mean progesterone level in studied groups remained basal (< 1 ng/ml) for a long period after lambing as shown in Fig. 1. Progesterone levels started to elevate at day 119 postpartum in group 1. In group 2, progesterone levels elevated at day 99 postpartum, while in group 3, it started to increase at day 77 postpartum. Figs. 2, 3 and 4 show progesterone level in the individual ewes in groups 1, 2 and 3, respectively. As shown in Fig. 2, one ewe showed an elevated progesterone level at day 91 postpartum without showing estrus. In addition, progesterone level was basal during the whole period of study in one ewe in group 2. The ovaries of that ewe were smooth and did not shown any growing follicles as determined by trans-rectal ultrasonography and also it did not show estrus.

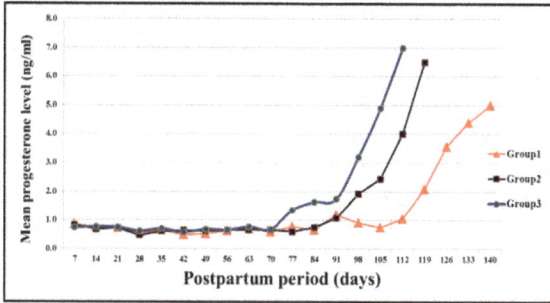

Fig. 1. Mean progesterone levels in postpartum ewes lambed in January (Group 1); February (Group 2); March (Group 3).

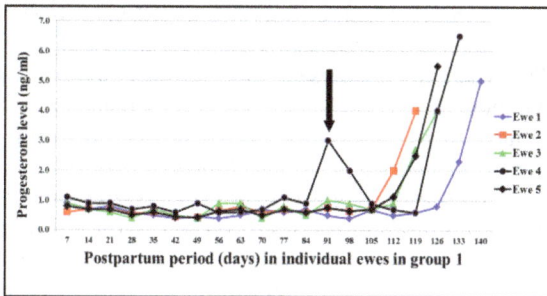

Fig. 2. Progesterone level in individual ewes lambed in January (Group 1). Arrow indicates a rise in progesterone level in one ewe without showing estrus before elevation.

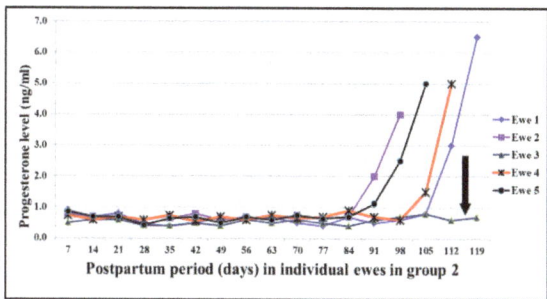

Fig. 3. Progesterone level in individual ewes lambed in February (Group 2). Arrow indicates one ewe that did not show estrus at all.

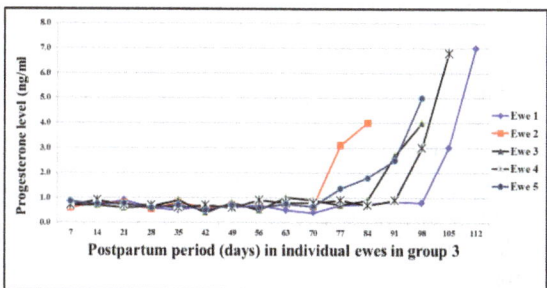

Fig. 4. Progesterone level in individual ewes lambed in March (Group 3).

As shown in Table 2, the first postpartum ovulation and formation of corpora lutea as determined by elevated progesterone (> 1 ng/ml) level occurred at

day 117.00 ± 3.73, 94.25 ± 4.49 and 78.60 ± 4.28 in groups 1, 2 and 3, respectively. The period from parturition until estrus and ovulation was significantly longer in group 1 (lambed in January) than group 2 (lambed in February) and group 3 (lambed in March), however, ovulation rate was nearly similar (Table 2).

Table 2. The day of postpartum estrus and ovulation rate in ewes lambed in January (group1), February (group 2) and March (group 3).

Groups	Day of postpartum estrus	Ovulation rate
Group 1	117.00 ± 3.73[a]	1.4
Group 2	94.25 ± 4.49[b]	1.5
Group 3	78.60 ± 4.28[b]	1.4

Values with different superscripts in the same column are significantly different (P<0.05).

Discussion

There are no data or literature information about postpartum uterine involution in Barbary ewes in Libya and so, the present study is considered very important and necessary to provide information that can be useful for improving reproductive efficiency. The ability to achieve maximum reproductive efficiency in ewes depends upon understanding postpartum changes of uterus and ovaries (Lewis and Blot, 1983).

The uterus experiences considerable distension and distortion of tissues and intensive glandular development to accommodate and nourish the developing fetus to term. The uterus must undergo gross anatomical changes together with extensive remodeling and changes in tissue mass and function during the postpartum period before rebreeding and pregnancy can be established (Hunter, 1980; Sanchez et al., 2002).

The present study on Barbary ewes lambed in January, February and March indicated that uterine involution occurred mostly between day 28 and 35 after parturition. This is in agreement with the results reported in sheep by O'Shea and Wright (1984) and Zdunczyk et al. (2004). Van Niekerk (1976) recorded that uterine involution and regeneration of the epithelium in ewes may not be completed until day 26 during the breeding season, while during anestrous involution was delayed until day 30.

Another study demonstrated that uterine involution was completed within 21 days postpartum in sheep (Fernandes et al., 2013). Tian and Noakes (1991), using radio-opaque markers, recorded that uterine involution was completed around day 29 after lambing. The results of the present study showed that uterine involution in the third group is completed in a shorter time compared with the first group and second group indicating that the date of lambing affects uterine involution. A previous study on sheep showed that uterine involution was completed in 35 days postpartum in the majority of examined cases (Zdunczyk *et al.*, 2004). However, Hauser and Bostedt (2002) mentioned that uterine involution in sheep was delayed in cases of dystocia and cesarean section and retention of placenta. Puerperal complications such as retained placenta and/or acute puerperal endometritis to metritis usually delay uterine involution (Hajurka *et al.*, 2005). In sheep, there is considerable variation in the annual anestrous season depending on the geographical region and day length. Sexual activity in sheep is primarily controlled by the ratio of daylight to dark. In temperate regions, estrus becomes more frequent as the daylight becomes shorter. Longer daylight decreases gonadotropin secretion and causes ovarian cycles to cease.

In contrast, a shift from long to short daylight results in increased gonadotropin secretion and onset of ovarian cycles. The reason is that photoperiod is transduced to a signal influencing gonadotropin-releasing hormone (GnRH) release and communicate directly with GnRH neurons in the hypothalamus (Hileman *et al.*, 2011). In the present study, the mean interval from parturition to the resumption of the ovarian activity differed according to the month of lambing. It was 117.00±3.73 days in ewes lambed in January, which is considered significantly longer than those lambed in February (94.25±4.49 days) and March (78.60±4.28 days).

These results indicate that the time of the year is a major factor controlling the duration of postpartum ovarian activity, which is in agreement with results obtained in ewes by other workers (Santiago-Moreno *et al.*, 2000; Hileman *et al.*, 2011).

Blood concentration of progesterone is a good indicator of luteal function during the postpartum period since progesterone is the major steroid synthesized by the corpus luteum. It is well known that systemic progesterone concentrations greater than 1 ng/ml are associated with presence of a corpus luteum or a luteinized follicle (Berardinelli *et al.*, 2001). The interval from parturition until the first ovulation in ewes is greatly influenced by season (Hileman *et al.*, 2011). The postpartum anestrous interval is longest when ewes lamb during the winter as length of the photoperiod is increasing. The interval is shorter when lambs are born during the summer (Wettemaan, 1980). Moreover, there are large breed differences on the extent of the postpartum anestrus prior to a fertile estrus, reflecting a strong genetic component in addition to seasonal influences (Pope *et al.*, 1989). In the present study, all examined ewes showed a state of ovarian inactivity during the first 70 days after parturition, as indicated by the low serum progesterone level. Prolonged postpartum luteal activity might be a result of the high prolactin hormone observed in the first few weeks postpartum (Lamming *et al.*, 1974). Also, delayed onset of the ovarian activity might be due to a negative energy or protein balance. Ewes nursing lambs were often in negative energy balance during the first month of lactation (Robinson *et al.*, 1979).

One ewe in the group 1 showed a higher progesterone level at day 91 postpartum without showing estrus before that elevation or follicular activity as determined by ultrasound. This elevation may be due to luteinization of small follicles which cannot be detected by ultrasonography. Moreover, one ewe in group 2 did not show estrus at all or follicular growth as determined by ultrasound. This is also confirmed by its basal progesterone level during the period of study. The results of the present study demonstrate that the duration of postpartum anestrus in Barbary ewes is influenced by the time of the year when parturition occurs. In addition, it appeared that ovarian activity in Barbary ewes tends to be seasonal since ewes lambed in January, February and March started ovarian activity at the start of the following breeding season.

Conclusion

The obtained results indicate that, uterine involution as determined by ultrasound was completed earlier in ewes lambed in March than those lambed in February or January. Also, progesterone level and ultrasound examination showed that there was no ovarian activity for a long time after parturition indicating that reproduction in Barbary ewes tends to be seasonal in AL-Bayda city, north Libya.

References

Berardinelli, J.G., Wenig, J., Burfening, P.J. and Adair, R. 2001. Effect of excess degradable intake protein on early embryonic development, ovarian steroid and blood urea nitrogen on days 2, 3, 4 and 5 of the estrus cycle in mature ewes. J. Anim. Sci. 79, 193-199.

Delgadillo, J.A., Flores, J.A., Villareal, M.J., Hoyos, G., Chemineau, P. and Malpaux, B. 1998. Length of postpartum anestrous in goats in subtropical Mexico: effect of season of parturition and duration of nursing. Theriogenology 49, 1209-1218.

Feldman, E.C. and Nelson, R.W. 1996. Canine and Feline Endocrinology and Reproduction, 2nd ed. WB Saunders Company, Toronto, pp: 785. ISBN 0-7216-3634-9.

Fernandes, C.E., Cigerza, C.F., Pinto, G.D.S., Miazi, C. Barbosa-ferreira, M. and Martins, C.F. 2013. Parturition characteristics and uterine involution in native sheep from Brazilian pantanal. Ci. Anim. Bras. Goiânia 14(2), 245-252.

Goddard, P.J. 1995. Veterinary ultrasonography. CAB International, Willington, UK.

Hajurka, J., Macak, V. and Hura, V. 2005. Influence of health status of reproductive organs on uterine involution in dairy cows. Bull. Vet. Inst. Pulawy 49, 53-58.

Hauser, B. and Bostedt, H. 2002. Ultrasonographic observations of the uterine regression in the ewe under different obstetrical conditions. J. Vet. Med. Series A, 49, 511-516.

Hileman, M.S., McManus, C.J., Goodman, R.L. and Jansen, H.T. 2011. Neurons of the lateral preoptic area/rostral anterior hypothalamic area are required for photoperiodic inhibition of estrous cyclicity in Sheep. Biol. Reprod. 85, 1057-1065.

Hunter, R.H.F. 1980. Physiology and Technology of Reproduction in Female Domestic animals. Academic Press, London, UK. pp: 348-351.

Ishwar, A.K. 1995. Pregnancy diagnosis in sheep and goats: a review. Small Rumin. Res. 17, 37-44.

Kene, R.O.C. 1991. Radiographic investigation of dystocia in the West Africa Dwarf Goat. Br. Vet. J. 147, 283-289.

Lamming, G.H., Moeley, S.R., and McNeilly, J.R. 1974. Prolactin release in the sheep. J. Reprod. Fert. 40, 151-168.

Lewis, G.S. and Blot, D.J. 1983. Effect of suckling on postpartum changes in 13, 14-Dihdro-15-Keto-PGF$_2\alpha$ and progesterone induced release of gonadotropins in autum lambing ewes. J. Anim. Sci. 57, 673-682.

Lohan, I.S., Malik, R.K. and Kaker, M.L. 2004. Uterine involution and ovarian follicular growth during early postpartum period of Murrah buffaloes (Bubalus bubalis). Asian-Aust. J. Anim. Sci. 17 (3), 313-316.

Medan, M.S. and Abd El-Aty, A.M. 2010. Advances in ultrasonography and its applications in domestic ruminants and other farm animals reproduction: a review. J. Advanced Res. 1, 123-128.

Noakes, D.E., Parkinson, T.J. and England, G.C.W. 2009. Veterinary Reproduction and Obstetrics. 9th Ed., WB Saunders Elsevier; pp: 194-202.

O'Shea, J.D. and Wright, P.J. 1984. Involution and regeneration of the endometrium following parturition in the ewe. Cell Tissue Res. 236, 477-485.

Pope, W.F., McClure, K.E., Hogue, D.E. and Day, M.L. 1989. Effect of season and lactation on postpartum fertility of Polypay, Dorset, St. Croix and Targhee ewes. J. Anim. Sci. 67, 1167-1174.

Robinson, J.J., McHattie, I., Calderon, C.J.F. and Thompson, J. 1979. Further studies on the response of lactating ewes to dietary protein. Anim. Prod. 29, 257-269.

Rubianes, E., Ungerfeld, R., Vinoles, C., Carbajal, B., de Castro, T. and Ibarra, D. 1996. Uterine involution time and ovarian activity in weaned and suckling ewes. Can. J. Anim. Sci. 76, 153-155.

Sanchez, M.A., Garcia, P., Menendez, S., Sanchez, B., Gonzalez, M. and Flores, J.M. 2002. Fibroblastic growth factor receptor (FGF-R) expression during uterine involution in goat. Anim. Reprod. Sci. 69, 25-35.

Santiago-Moreno, J., López-Sebastián, A., González-Bulnes, A., Gómez-Brunet, A. and Chemineau, P. 2000. Seasonal changes in ovulatory activity, plasma prolactin, and melatonin concentrations, in mouflon (Ovis gmelini musimon) and Manchega (Ovis aries) ewes. Reprod. Nutr. Dev. 40(5), 421-430.

Schirar, A., Cognie, Y. Louault, F. Poulin, N. Levasseur, M.C. and Martinet, J. 1989. Resumption of estrus behavior and cyclic ovarian activity in suckling ewes and non-suckling ewes. J. Reprod. Fertil. 87, 789-794.

SPSS Inc. 2012. SPSS (Statistical Package for the Social Sciences, 21) for windows. Statistical package for the social. Sciences. Chicago, USA.

Takayama, H., Tanaka, T. and Kamomae, H. 2010. Postpartum ovarian activity and uterine involution in non-seasonal Shiba goats, with or without nursing. Small Rumin. Res. 88, 62-66.

Tian, W. and Noakes, D.E. 1991. A radiographic method for measuring the effect of exogenous hormone therapy on uterine involution in ewes. Vet. Rec. 129, 436-466.

Van Niekerk, C.H. 1976. Limitation to female reproductive efficiency. Proc. Inter. Cong. Sheep Breeding, pp: 299-309.

Vinoles, C., Meikle, A. and Forsberg, M. 2004. Accuracy of evaluation of ovarian structures by transrectal ultrasonography in ewes. Anim. Reprod. Sci. 80, 69-79.

Wettemaan, R.P. 1980. Postpartum endocrine function of cattle, sheep and swine. J. Anim. Sci. 51, 2-15.

Yavas, Y. and Walton, J.S. 2000. Postpartum acyclicity in suckled beef cows: A review. Theriogenology 54, 25-55.

Yilmaz, O., Ucar, M., Sahin, O., Sevimli, A. and Demirkan, I. 2008. A diffuse uterine macroabscess formation with unilateral pyometra in a pointer bitch. Indian Vet. J. 85, 309-311.

Yilmaz, O. and Ucar, M. 2012. Ultrasonography of postpartum uterine involution in a bitch. Kocatepe Vet. J. 5(2), 55-58.

Zdunczyk, S., Milewski, S., Baranski, W., Janowski, T., Szczepanski, W., Jurczak, A., Ras, A. and Lesnik, M. 2004. Postpartum uterine involution in primiparous and pluriparous polish longwool sheep monitored by ultrasonography. Bull. Vet. Inst. Pulawy 48, 255-257.

20

Investigation on papillomavirus infection in dromedary camels in Al-Ahsa, Saudi Arabia

Abdelmalik Ibrahim Khalafalla[1,2,*], Ramadan Omer Ramadan[3], Annabel Rector[4] and Seif Barakat[5]

[1]Camel Research Centre, King Faisal University, Al Ahsa, Saudi Arabia
[2]Department of Microbiology, Faculty of Veterinary Medicine, University of Khartoum, Sudan
[3]Department of Clinical Studies, College of Veterinary Medicine, King Faisal University, Al Ahsa, Saudi Arabia
[4]KU Leuven, Department of Microbiology and Immunology, Laboratory of Clinical & Epidemiological Virology, B-3000 Leuven, Belgium
[5]Department of Pathology, College of Veterinary Medicine, King Faisal University, Saudi Arabia

Abstract
We investigated two outbreaks of papillomatosis between 2013 and 2015 in Al Ahsa region of eastern Saudi Arabia involving fourteen dromedary camels. The disease affected both young and adult animals and occurred in coincidence with demodectic mange infestation. Diagnosis was made based on gross and histopathological characteristics of the wart lesion and was confirmed by PCR. Rolling circle amplification followed by degenerate primer PCR and sequencing of the amplicons revealed the presence of both Camelus dromedarius papillomavirus types 1 and 2, previously identified in infected dromedaries in Sudan.
Keywords: Al Ahsa, Dromedary camels, Infection, Papillomavirus, Saudi Arabia.

Introduction

Papillomas (warts) are benign epithelial proliferations of the skin and mucous membranes caused by papillomaviruses (PVs) and are seen worldwide in man and a number of animals. PVs constitute a diverse group of small (52–55 nm), non-enveloped, circular double-stranded DNA viruses, classified in the *Papillomaviridae* family. These viruses are known as species-specific and, in experimental conditions, do not infect another host than their natural one (Campo, 2006).

The first report of papillomatosis associated with PV in dromedaries was published in 1990 (Munz *et al.*, 1990) and showed that dromedary camels in central Somalia aged 6 months to 2 years were primarily affected. Later, cases of papillomatosis in young dromedary camels have also been reported from Kenya (Dioli and Stimmelmayr, 1992), United Arab Emirates (Wernery and Kaaden, 1995) and Sudan (Khalafalla *et al.*, 1998; Ure *et al.*, 2011).

PVs were found associated with a 2 kg wart-like growth on the right fetlock joint of a dromedary camel in India (Sadana *et al.*, 1980) and a corneal papilloma mass in the left eye of a 15-year old dromedary male with a history of chronic severe keratoconjuctivitis (Kilic *et al.*, 2010). Papillomatosis has also been shown in South American camelids in llamas and alpacas (Schulman *et al.*, 2003). The majority of the described camel papillomatosis cases is usually seen in young animals and occurs in the late rainy season, coinciding with

outbreaks of camel contagious ecthyma and camel pox (Munz *et al.*, 1990; Khalafalla *et al.*, 1998).

Currently, the genomes of two Camelus dromedaries PV types (type 1, CdPV1, and type 2, CdPV2) have been fully characterized and genetically grouped within the genus Deltapapillomavirus (Ure *et al.*, 2011). The two genotypes were isolated from a cauliflower-like nodule and a round, oval raised nodule, respectively, observed in 3 and 7 months old dromedary camels in Sudan.

Here, we describe the clinic-pathological features of cases of papillomatosis, as well as the genetic identification of the associated CdPVs from Saudi Arabia.

Material and Methods

Ethical statement
Skin specimens were collected according to the Guidelines for Ethical Conduct for Use and Care of Animals in Research of King Faisal University (KFU), Saudi Arabia and approved by the KFU Ethics Care Committee.

Case description of camel papillomatosis in Al-Ahsa
Group I:
In November 2013, two young dromedary camels (aged 14 months) of the Maghateer breed (Table 1) were referred to the Veterinary teaching hospital of KFU for hernia surgery in one of them.

Group II:
In October 2014, an outbreak of skin warts occurred in a camel farm of KFU in Al-Ahsa province of eastern

---

*Corresponding Author: Abdelmalik Ibrahim Khalafalla. Current address: Veterinary Laboratories Division, Animal Wealth Sector, Abu Dhabi food Control Authority, 52150 Abu Dhabi, United Arab Emirates. Email: *abdokhlf@yahoo.co.uk*

KSA. This farm includes 68 dromedary camels of different breeds; two were at one month of age, ten were less than two years of age, 18 were at 2-4 years of age and the rest were adults (more than four years of age). The farm is located about 2 km away from the Veterinary hospital and perform zero grazing with no access to the pasture or contact with other camel herds. History of the disease, including age and breed of affected animals as well as the type and number of wart lesions is shown in Table 1.

Specimen collection

Specimens of six warts, one from each affected camel, were surgically removed and divided into two parts. One part was processed for DNA extraction and the other was fixed in 10% buffered formalin for histopathology.

Histopathology

For histopathological examination the specimens were trimmed and put in vacuum infiltrating tissue processing machine (Tissue- Tik VIP 5Jr. Japan) and then embedded in paraffin wax by SLEE MPS/C machine, Germany. Specimens were then waxed in blocks and sectioned at 5 µm by LEICA RM 2235 microtome, Germany. Specimens were then mounted on glass slides and stained with Haematoxylin and Eosin (H&E) for histopathological examination (Kiernan, 1999).

DNA extraction

Wart tissues were cut into 2-3 mm pieces by a pair of sterile scissors and a 20% suspension of the minced tissues was made in tris-EDTA (TE) buffer (pH 7.4). Specimens were then homogenized using a mechanical homogenizer (TissueRuptor, Qiagen, Germany) and centrifuged at 1500 g for 10 min at 4°C. Total viral DNA was extracted from 200µl of each specimen's supernatant using GF-1 Viral Nucleic Acid Extraction Kit (Vivantis Technologies, Malaysia) according to manufacturer instructions.

PCR

As the differential diagnosis for camel papillomatosis includes camelpox and contagious ecthyma, all 6 DNA samples were screened using a multiplex gel-based PCR (Khalafalla et al., 2015), which uses the FAP59/64 consensus primers originally designed from L1 gene conserved region of PV (Forslund et al., 1999). Additionally, DNA samples were screened using PV specific degenerate primer pair AR-E1F2/AR-E1R3 (371 bp) in accordance with Rector et al. (2004a).

Rolling circle amplification

Multiply primed rolling circle amplification (RCA) was performed with an Illustra TempliPhi amplification kit (GE Healthcare Life Sciences) following a protocol that was optimized for the amplification of papillomaviral complete genomic DNA (Rector et al., 2004b; Stevens et al., 2010). One microliter of sample (extracted DNA or water as a negative control) was added to 5 µl of TempliPhi sample buffer, containing exonuclease protected random hexamers. The sample was than denatured at 95°C for 3 minutes and afterwards placed on ice. A premix consisting of 5 µl of TempliPhi reaction buffer, 0.2 µl of TempliPhi enzyme mix containing φ29 DNA polymerase, and 0.2 µl of extra deoxynucleotides (dNTPs, each 25 mM) was prepared and added to each sample (5 µl). The reaction was incubated overnight (approximately 16 hours) at 30°C. Reactions were then put on ice, and subsequently heated to 65°C for 10 minutes to inactivate the φ29 DNA polymerase.

To investigate whether papillomaviral DNA was amplified, 2 µl of the RCA product was digested with a restriction enzyme panel consisting of BamHI, EcoRI, SalI, HindIII and HincII. The digestion products were run on a 0.8% agarose gel to check for the presence of a DNA band consistent with full-length PV DNA (~8kb), or multiple bands with sizes adding up to this length.

Table 1. History of dromedary Papillomatosis in two herds in Al Ahsa, eastern Saudi Arabia.

Animal group	Animal No.	Age	Breed	Type of wart lesion (number)	Total number of wart lesions; site (number per site)
I	Rm1	14 months	Maghateer	Cauliflower-like (3)	3: upper lip (1), lower lip (2)
I	Rm2	14 months	Maghateer	Cauliflower-like (2)	2: upper lip (2)
II	CRC1	6 years	Majaheem	Cauliflower-like (8); nodular (12)	20: upper lip (10), lower lip (6), eyelid (4)
II	CRC2	5 years	Majaheem	Cauliflower-like (2); nodular (4)	6: upper lip (3), lower lip (3)
II	CRC3	3 years	Majaheem	Cauliflower-like (1)	1: upper lip
II	CRC4	6 years	Majaheem	Cauliflower-like (4); nodular (3)	7: nostril (3), upper lip (2), lower lip (2)
II	CRC5	7 years	Majaheem	Nodular (19)	19: upper lip (12), lower lip (7)
II	CRC6	4 years	Majaheem	Cauliflower-like (2)	2: upper lip (1), mandible (1)
II	CRC7	14 months	Majaheem	Cauliflower-like (3); nodular (2)	5: upper lip (2), mandible (2), nostril (1)
II	CRC8	2 years	Maghateer	Nodular (2)	2: lower lip
II	CRC22	6 years	Maghateer	Cauliflower-like (1); nodular (7)	3: upper lip (7), mandible (1)
II	CRC28	22 months	Maghateer	Cauliflower-like (1)	1: upper lip
II	CRC42	13 months	Maghateer	Nodular (40)	40: upper lip
II	CRC77	13 months	Majaheem	Nodular (28)	28: upper (22) and lower lips (6)

Degenerate primer PCR and sequencing

Degenerate papillomavirus-specific primers were used to screen RCA products. The following primer pairs were used:FAP59/FAP64 (Forslund *et al.*, 1999), AR-L1F1/AR-L1R3 (Rector *et al.*, 2004a), and AR-E1F2/AR-E1R3 (Rector *et al.*, 2004a).

Previously unpublished primer pairs AR-L1F11/AR-L1R10 and AR-E1F14/AR-E1R12, developed in conserved L1 and E1 regions of ungulate PVs, were also tested (Table 2).

Amplification was performed with the Qiagen OneStep RT-PCR kit following manufacturer's instructions, using a concentration of 2.4 µM of forward and reverse primer, and 1 µl of RCA product as sample in a final reaction volume of 25 µl.

PCR products were checked on agarose gel and further sequenced bi-directionally on an ABI Prism 3100 Genetic Analyzer (Applied Biosystems, Life Technologies). Sequences were analyzed by similarity searches using NCBI BLAST.

Table 2. Degenerate primers of amplification of Papilloma viral E1 and L1 sequences.

Primer	Sequence (5'-3')
FAP59	TAACWGTNGGNCAYCCWTATT
FAP64	CCWATATCWVHCATNTCNCCATC
AR-L1F1	TTDCAGATGGCNGTNTGGCT
AR-L1R3	CATRTCHCCATCYTCWAT
AR-L1F11	GGDGAYATGATGGAHATWGG
AR-L1R10	CCATTRTTCATDCCCTGDGC
AR-E1F2	ATGGTNCAGTGGGCNTATGA
AR-E1R3	TTNCCWSTATTNGGNGGNCC
AR-E1F14	CTTTGACACAYAYCTCAGAAAY
AR-E1R12	AGVTCTAANCGYYCCCATARCCTT

Results

Gross morphology of lesions

The two animals in group I, belonging to a dromedary camel farm in Riyadh region of central Saudi Arabia, showed numerous nodular and cauliflower-like proliferations on the lips and nostrils, which had first been noticed 4 weeks prior to sampling. In group 2, the disease occurred in epizootics form involving 14 (Table 1) out of 81 dromedary camels, giving a morbidity rate of 17.3%. The number of warts per animal varied from one to 20, with a size ranging from 0.3 to 2.2 cm. They were particularly located on the lips, eyelids, nostrils and mandible (Fig. 1). The lesions first appeared as rosy hyperemic elevations of the skin and developed into solid cauliflower-like exophytic growth taking the skin or a darker colour in the majority of the animals. The cauliflower-like papillary masses were dark in color with approximate size of 2 cm in diameter (Fig. 2).

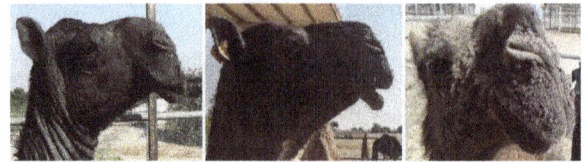

Fig. 1. Papillomatosis in dromedary camels in Al Ahsa, Saudi Arabia. Cauliflower-like and multiple nodular Papillomas on the face that vary in number and size.

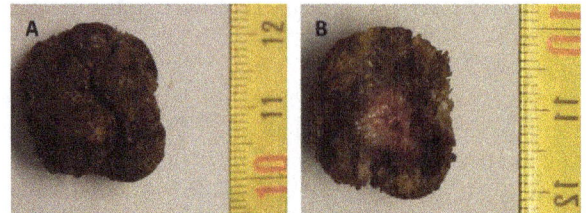

Fig. 2. Gross appearance of the papilloma wart showing cauliflower protruded dark in color. The diameter was 2 cm.

Some animals however showed rounded raised nodules instead. Data on the age of camels, breed, clinical type and numbers of warts are summarized in Table 1. The disease, which began in October 3 continued through October and ended in early November 2014. Later in March 2016, two young dromedaries aged 13 months and from the non-affected pens in the same farm developed typical papilloma lesions.

Histopathological findings

Sections of all the biopsy samples collected from camels with wart-like lesions showed identical histopathological features characterized by multiple papillary proliferation, hyperkeratosis and acanthosis (Fig. 3 and 4).

Diagnostics by PCR and Rolling circle amplification

Pan PV PCR amplification was positive in eight animals, including Rm1, Rm2, CRC3, 5, 7, 8, 22, 42 and CRC 77 (Table 3).

Possible PV genomic amplification by RCA was observed for samples Rm1 and Rm2. These RCA products were submitted to degenerate primer PCR, and PV specific sequences could be amplified for all these samples (Table 3).

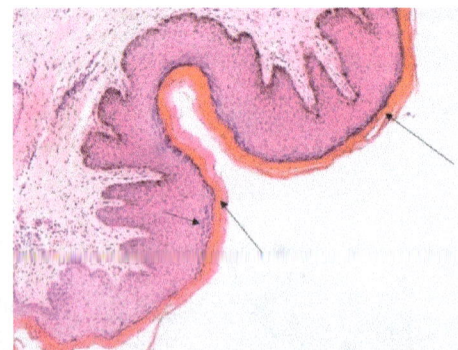

Fig. 3. Skin section of camel, showing hyperkeratosis (long arrows), hydropic degeneration of keratinocytes, acanthosis (short arrow), and mild infiltration of inflammatory cells.

Table 3. Sequence data generated from Papilloma lesions collected from dromedary camels in Saudi Arabia.

Sample	Sequence	# nt*	Most similar to papillomavirus type	% nt identity
Rm1	ARL1F1/ARL1R3	530	Camelus dromedarius papillomavirus 1	97%
	ARL1F11/ARL1R10	328	Camelus dromedarius papillomavirus 1	97%
	ARE1F14/ARE1R12	205	Camelus dromedarius papillomavirus 1	99%
Rm2	ARL1F1/ARL1R3	537	Camelus dromedarius papillomavirus 1	98%
	ARL1F11/ARL1R10	289	Camelus dromedarius papillomavirus 1	98%
CRC 77	FAP59/FAP64	434	Camelus dromedarius papillomavirus 2	98%
CRC 3	FAP59/FAP64	437	Camelus dromedarius papillomavirus 1	98%

*length of the amplicon.

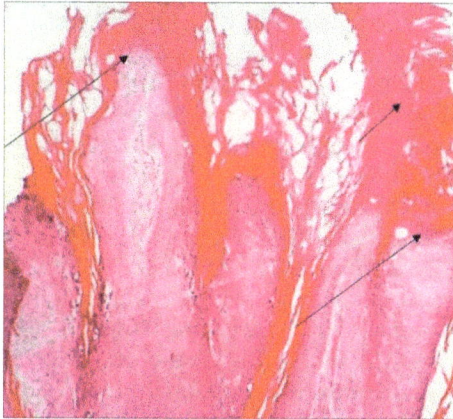

Fig. 4. Skin section of camel (Epidermis), showing multiple papillary proliferations (long arrows), and the epidermis is irregularly thickened and covered by a thick layer of hyperkeratosis (short arrow).

Discussion

We investigated PV infection in two groups of dromedary camels in Al-Ahsa province of eastern Saudi Arabia during 2013 and 2015. The diagnosis was done based on clinical findings, histopathology and PCR testing. While we were limited to gather enough information with group I, we could collect more data from group II.

Of interest, the disease affected predominantly camels severely infested with mange. Further parasitological investigations (data not shown) revealed that the mange mites were of the *Demodex* species. The preferred site of the burrowing mite of the genus *Demodex* is at the hair follicles and sebaceous glands of the skin. Camel mange is an extremely contagious skin disease, characterized by scab formation, pruritic dermatitis, thickening and corrugation of skin and hair loss, and caused by the parasitic mite (Mochabo *et al.*, 2005). Camels in the five other pens did not develop papillomatosis. We therefore suggest that mange was the major predisposing factor for the PV infection in dromedary camels. However, it is also possible that some animals in this herd had other underlying defects predisposing them to more severe infections with several pathogens, such as mange mites and PV. In a previous epidemiological study, we observed that most

cases of PV infections in the Sudan were associated with contagious ecthyma virus infection (Khalafalla *et al.*, 1998). Dioli and Stimmelmayr (1992) in Kenya also observed association between papillomatosis and camelpox virus (CMLV) infection. In line with this, co-infection of PV, ortho- and parapoxviruses in cattle has been described in Italy (Scagliarini *et al.*, 2016).

Our observations raise many questions in the understanding of risk factors of PV infection in camels. It is well documented that transmission of PVs is usually horizontal and occurs via contact, abrasions or micro-lesions of the skin and mucosa, but vertical and iatrogenic transmissions have also been reported, as well as mechanical by arthropods (Campo and Bastianello, 2004).

Breaks in the integrity of the epidermis are likely to facilitate entry of the virus to the basal layers of the skin, hereby allowing infection of the epithelial stem cell which results in permanent viral replication in the epidermis.

Another finding of interest is the development of cutaneous papillomatosis in both adult and young camels while in most previous reports the affected groups were young dromedary camels [3-7 months (Ure *et al.*, 2011), 3-14 months (Khalafalla *et al.*, 1998) and 18-24 months (Oryan *et al.*, 2011)]. All PV sequences showed high degrees of similarity to previously identified PV types. A new PV type is defined as a cloned full-length papillomaviral genome, whose L1 nucleotide sequence is at least 10% dissimilar from that of any other PV type (de Villiers *et al.*, 2004; Bernard *et al.*, 2010). Although no complete L1 ORFs were sequenced in this study, the partial L1 sequences retrieved from the camel samples showed at least 96% identity to Camelus dromedarius papillomavirus types 1 and 2, indicating the presence of subtypes or variants thereof, rather than new papillomavirus types.

Partial papillomaviral L1 sequences were obtained from 4 samples in the present study. Three animals were infected with Camelus dromedarius papillomavirus type 1 and one was infected with Camelus dromedarius papillomavirus type 2. As these two genotypes were previously detected in dromedary camels of Sudan, our results points to a wide distribution of these genotypes that also involve camels of the Arabian Peninsula. In contrast, the study of Ure *et al.* (2011) revealed the presence of two different PV species in only two samples taken from an affected herd, leading the authors to speculate that a wide diversity of PVs exists in dromedaries (Ure *et al.*, 2011). It is noteworthy that in our present study only the same two previously identified Camelus dromedaries papillomavirus types were found. This might point towards a prevalence of these types, but does not exclude the possibility that dromedary camels can be infected by a wide diversity of papillomavirus types, as it has been demonstrated in most animal species that were intensively studied. In cattle, for instance, 15 bovine papillomaviruses (BPVs) have been completely genetically characterized (Papillomavirus Genome database, https://pave.niaid.nih.gov) but only BPV1 and BPV2 are broadly present while the other types are only found occasionally (Grindatto *et al.*, 2015). In order to unravel the complete genomic diversity of camel dromedary PVs, further investigation of a large number of samples, preferably taken from different herds, is necessary.

Of interest, Camelus dromedarius papillomavirus type 2 was detected in a young camel, which showed the disease 13 months after the initial outbreak in farm II. While we only detected genotype 1 in the initial outbreak of this herd, it remains difficult to determine whether this genotype 2 was already circulating at that time but remained undetected or whether it represents a novel infection.

Conclusions

We investigated cases of warts or papillomatosis in camels in Saudi Arabia. Clinical findings, gross and histopathological features suggested papillomavirus infection while PCR and partial genome sequencing confirmed the diagnosis. Both genotypes 1 and 2, previously detected in Sudan, were responsible for these outbreaks.

Acknowlegemets

We thank Dr. Marzook Al-Eknah, Director, Camel Research Center, King Faisal University for support during sample collection and Dr Sophie Duraffour, Bernhard-Nocht Institute for Tropical Medicine, Hamburg, Germany for reading the manuscript.

Conflict of interest

The authors declare that there is no conflict of interests.

References

Bernard, H.U., Burk, R.D., Chen, Z., van Doorslaer, K., zur Hausen, H. and de Villiers, E.M. 2010. Classification of papillomaviruses (PVs) based on 189 PV types and proposal of taxonomic amendments. Virology 401, 70-79.

Campo, M.S. 2006. Bovine papillomavirus: old system, new lessons? In: Papillomavirus Research from Natural History to Vaccines and Beyond. Campo MS, editor. Caister Academic Press, Norwich, UK, pp: 373-383.

Campo, S. and Bastianello, S.S. 2004. Papillomavirus infections In: J.A.W. Coetzer & R.C Tustin (eds.), Infectious Diseases of Livestock, with Special Reference to Southern Africa (second ed.), Oxford University Press Southern Africa, Cape Town, South Africa.

de Villiers, E.M., Fauquet, C., Broker, T.R., Bernard, H.U. and zur Hausen, H. 2004. Classification of papillomaviruses. Virology 324, 17-27.

Dioli, M. and Stimmelmayr, R. 1992. Important camel diseases. In: The One Humped Camel in Eastern Africa, A. Pictorial Guide to Diseases, Health Care and Management. H. J. Schwarts and M. Dioli, editors. Verlag Josef Margrat Scientific Books, pp: 155-164.

Forslund, O., Antonsson, A., Nordin, P., Stenquist, B. and Hansson, B.G. 1999. A broad range of human papillomavirus types detected with a general PCR method suitable for analysis of cutaneous tumours and normal skin. J. Gen. Virol. 80, 2437-2443.

Grindatto, A., Ferraro, G., Varello, K., Crescio, M.I., Miceli, I., Bozzetta, E., Goria, M. and Nappi, R. 2015. Molecular and histological characterization of bovine papillomavirus in North West Italy. Vet. Microbiol. 180, 113-117.

Khalafalla, A.I., Abbas, Z. and Mohamed, M.E.H. 1998. Camel papillomatosis in the Sudan. J. Camel Pract. Res. 5, 157-159.

Khalafalla, A.I., Al-Busada, K.A. and El-Sabagh, I.M. 2015. Multiplex PCR for rapid diagnosis and differentiation of pox and pox-like diseases in dromedary Camels. Virol. J. 7(12), 102-109.

Kiernan, J.A. 1999. Histological and histochemical methods: Theory and practice. 3rd ed. Butterworth Heinemann, Oxford, UK, pp: 502.

Kilic, N., Toplu, N., Aydog, A., Yaygingu, R. and Ozsoy SY. 2010. Corneal papilloma associated with papillomavirus in a one-humped camel (*Camelus dromedarius*). Vet. Ophthalmol. 13(Suppl. 1), 100-102.

Mochabo, K.O., Kitala, P.M., Gathura, P.B., Ogara, W.O., Catley, A., Eregae, E.M. and Kaitho, T.D. 2005. Community perception of important camel diseases in Lapur division of Turkana district, Kenya. Trop. Anim. Health Prod. 37, 187-204.

Munz, E., Moallin, A. S., Mahnel, H. and Reimann, M., 1990. Camel papillomatosis in Somalia. Zentralbl Veterinarmed B 37, 191–196.

Oryan, A., Hashemnia, M., Mohammadalipour, A. and Gowharinia, M. 2011. Gross and histopathological characteristics of fibropapilloma in camels (*Camelus dromedarius*). J. Camel Pract. Res. 18, 65-68.

Rector, A., Bossart, G.D., Ghim, S.J., Sundberg, J.P., Jenson, A.B. and Van Ranst, M. 2004a. Characterization of a novel close-to-root papillomavirus from a Florida manatee by using multiply primed rolling-circle amplification: Trichechus manatus latirostris papillomavirus type 1. J. Virol. 78, 12698-12702.

Rector, A., Tachezy, R. and Van Ranst, M. 2004b. A sequence-independent strategy for detection and cloning of circular DNA virus genomes by using multiply primed rolling-circle amplification. J. Virol. 78, 4993-4998.

Sadana, J.R., Mahajan, S.K. and Satija, K.C. 1980. Note on papilloma in a camel. Indian J. Anim. Sci. 50, 793-794.

Scagliarini, A., Casà, G., Trentin, B., Gallina, L., Savini, F., Morent, M., Lavazza, A., Puleio, R., Buttaci, C., Cannella, V., Purpari, G., Di Marco, P., Piquemal, D. and Guercio, A. 2016. Evidence of zoonotic Poxviridae coinfections in clinically diagnosed papillomas using a newly developed mini-array test. J. Vet. Diagn. Invest. 1, 59-64.

Schulman, F.Y., Krafft, A.E., Janczewski, T., Reupert, R., Jackson, K. and Garner, M.M. 2003. Camelid mucocutaneous fibropapillomas: clinicopathologic findings and association with papillomavirus. Vet. Pathol. l40, 103-107.

Stevens, H., Rector, A. and Van Ranst, M. 2010. Multiply primed rolling-circle amplification method for the amplification of circular DNA viruses. Cold Spring Harbor protocols 2010, pdb prot5415.

Ure, A.E., Elfadl, A.K., Khalafalla, A.I., Gameel, A.A.R., Dillner, J. and Forslund, O. 2011. Characterization of complete genomes of Camelus dromedarius papillomavirus 1 and 2. J. Gen. Virol. 8, 1769-1777.

Wernery, U. and Kaaden, O.R. 1995. Infectious Diseases of Camelids. Blackwell Wissenschafts-Verlag, Berlin.

21

Reactivity of commercially available monoclonal antibodies to human CD antigens with peripheral blood leucocytes of dromedary camels (*Camelus dromedarius*)

Jamal Hussen[1,*], Turke Shawaf[2], Abdulkareem Imran Al-herz[3], Hussain R. Alturaifi[3] and Ahmed M. Alluwaimi[1]

[1]*Department of Microbiology and Parasitology, College of Veterinary Medicine, King Faisal University, Al Ahsaa, Saudi Arabia*
[2]*Department of Clinical Studies, College of Veterinary Medicine, King Faisal University, Al Ahsaa, Saudi Arabia*
[3]*Immunology Unit, Diagnostic Laboratory and Blood Bank, King Fahad Hospital Hufof, Al Ahsaa, Saudi Arabia*

Abstract

Monoclonal antibodies (mAbs) to cell surface molecules have been proven as a key tool for phenotypic and functional characterization of the cellular immune response. One of the major difficulties in studying camel cellular immunity consists in the lack of mAbs that dtect their leukocyte differentiation antigens. In the present study two-parameter flow cytometry was used to screen existing commercially available mAbs to human leukocyte antigens and major histocompatibility molecules (MHC) for their reactivity with camel leukocytes. The comparison of patterns of reactivity obtained after labelling human and camel leukocytes have shown that mAbs specific to human cluster of differentiation (CD) 18, CD11a, CD11b and CD14 are predicted to be cross-reactive with homologous camel antigens.
Keywords: Antibodies, Cross-reactivity, Dromedary camel, Flow cytometry.

Introduction

The immune system consists of a complex network of cellular and non-cellular components, which interact with each other to protect the animal against invading pathogens like bacteria, fungi, parasites and viruses. In comparison to several other veterinary species like cattle (Hussen *et al.*, 2013; Duvel *et al.*, 2014), pigs (Gerner *et al.*, 2015), sheep (Hopkins *et al.*, 1993) and horses (Lunn *et al.*, 1998), the immune system of camels remains to a great extent poorly studied. Although considerable progress has been made in the characterization of camel immunoglobulins (Hamers-Casterman *et al.*, 1993; Muyldermans, 2013), few data are available on the cellular immunity of camels in health or disease (Zidan *et al.*, 2000a,b; Al-Mohammed Salem *et al.*, 2012).

Monoclonal antibodies (mAbs) to leukocyte antigens are highly important tools for phenotypic and functional analysis of cellular immunology. The lack of mAbs that define camel immune cells represents one of the major difficulties in studying the camel cellular immune response.

As the production of mAbs is very costly, attempts are made to study the cross-reactivity of commercially available mAbs to leukocyte antigens of one species with leukocytes of other species.

Comparative studies with mAb to leukocyte antigens of ruminants, swine, horses, and dogs have shown that the pattern of expression of many molecules is conserved cross species (Davis *et al.*, 1995). These findings suggests that it would be useful to use comparative studies for the identification of mAbs that recognize conserved epitopes on leukocyte differentiation antigens in poorly studied species.

The identification of cross-reactive mAbs could reduce the need to develop reagents for some important molecules and would provide an opportunity to compare the immune systems of camel with that of other species.

The objective of the present study was to screen existing mAbs to human leukocyte antigens and major histocompatibility molecules (MHC) for their reactivity with camel leukocytes. This would help in identifying mAbs that could be used to study the immune response of camels to infectious pathogens and as well as their response to vaccination.

Materials and Methods

Animals

Blood was collected from four camels (*Camelus dromedaries;* males aged between 6 and 8 years) at Omran slaughterhouse, Al Ahsaa, Eastern Province, Saudi Arabia.

The camels included in the study were apparently healthy and had no vaccination history. Blood was obtained by venepuncture of the vena jugularis externa into vacutainer tubes containing EDTA (Becton Dickinson, Heidelberg, Germany).

Mononuclear cells and whole leukocytes Separation

Separation of camel mononuclear cells (PBMC) was performed according to a method used for separating

*Corresponding Author: Dr. Jamal Hussen. Department of Microbiology and Parasitology, College of Veterinary Medicine, King Faisal University, Al Ahsaa, Saudi Arabia. E-mail: *jhussen@kfu.edu.sa*

bovine blood cells with modification (Hussen *et al.*, 2016). Blood was layered on Ficoll-Isopaque (Sigma-Aldrich, Germany) and centrifuged at 10°C for 30 min at 3000 rpm. The interphase containing PBMC was washed 3 times in PBS (2000, 1500 and 1000 rpm) and finally suspended in MIF buffer (PBS containing bovine serum albumin (5 g/L) and NaN_3 (0.1 g/L)). For the separation of human PBMC, human blood was layered on Ficoll-Isopaque and centrifuged at 10°C for 30 min at 3000 rpm. The interphase containing PBMC was washed 3 times in PBS (2000, 1500 and 1000 rpm) and finally suspended in MIF buffer. Whole camel and human leukocytes were separated by hypotonic lysis of erythrocytes. Blood was suspended in distilled water for 20 sec and double concentrated PBS was added to restore tonicity. This was repeated (usually twice) until complete erythrolysis. Separated cells were finally suspended in MIF buffer at 5 x 106 cells/ml. Cell purity of separated PBMC and leukocytes was assessed by flow cytometry according to their forward scatter (FCS) and sideward scatter (SSC) properties and always exceeded 90%. The mean viability of separated cells, as determined by exclusion of propidium iodide (2 µg/ml, Calbiochem, Germany) ranged 92% ± 4% (Fig. 1).

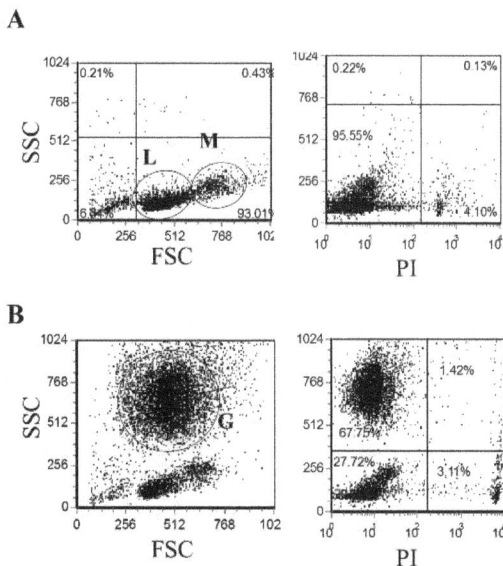

Fig. 1. Separation of camel blood PBMC and leukocytes and gating strategies. Camel PBMC were isolated by density gradient separation using Ficoll-Isopaque **(A)**. Whole camel leukocytes were separated by hypotonic lysis of erythrocytes **(B)**. Cell purity and viability of separated PBMC and leukocytes was assessed by flow cytometry according to their forward scatter (FCS) and sideward scatter (SSC) properties of the cells. The mean viability of separated cells was determined by exclusion of propidium iodide (PI). Gates were placed on granulocytes (G), monocytes (M) and lymphocytes (L) (as displayed in dot plot profile, side light scatter vs forward light scatter).

Monoclonal antibodies

The full list of mAbs (52 commercially available antibodies) used in this study are shown in Table 1.

Table 1. List of anti-human monoclonal antibodies.

Antigen	Antibody clone	Source	Isotype
CD2	S5.2	BD	mIgG2a
CD3	SK7 (Leu-4)	BD	mIgG1
CD4	SK3	BD	mIgG1
CD5	L17F12	BD	mIgG2a
CD7	M-T701	BD	mIgG1
CD7	4H9	BD	mIgG2a
CD8	SK1	BD	mIgG1
CD9	M-L13	BD	mIgG1
CD10	HI10a	BD	mIgG1
CD11a	G43-25B	BD	mIgG2a
CD11b	ICRF44	BD	mIgG1
CD11c	S-HCL-3	BD	mIgG2b
CD11c	KB90	Dako	mIgG1
CD13	L138	BD	mIgG1
CD14	M5E2	BD	mIgG2a
CD14	TÜK4	Biorad	mIgG2a
CD14	MφP9	BD	mIgG2b
CD15	MMA	BD	mIgM
CD16	B73.1	BD	mIgG1
CD16	KD1	BD	mIgG2a
CD18	42557	BD	mIgG1
CD19	4G7	BD	mIgG1
CD19	SJ25C1	BD	mIgG1
CD20	L27	BD	mIgG1
CD20	B9E9	Coulter	mIgG2a
CD20	2H7	Abcam	mIgG2b
CD22	S-HCL-1	BD	mIgG2b
CD33	P67.6	BD	mIgG1
CD38	HB7	BD	mIgG1
CD38	HIT2	BD	mIgG1
CD45	2D1	BD	mIgG1
CD55 (DAF)	JS11KSC2.3	Coulter	mIgG1
CD56	NCAM16.2	BD	mIgG2b
CD58 (LFA-3)	1C3	BD	mIgG2a
CD62L	DREG-56	BD	mIgG1
CD64	42379	BD	mIgG1
CD79a	HM47	Coulter	mIgG1
CD79b	CB3.1	BD	mIgG1
CD95	DX2	Dako	mIgG1
CD99	TÜ12	BD	mIgG2a
CD126	M5	BD	mIgG1
CD182	6C6	BD	mIgG1
TCR-αβ	WT31	BD	mIgG1
TCR-γ/δ	11F2	BD	mIgG1
IgM	G20-127	BD	mIgG1
Ig-lambda chain	1-155-2	BD	mIgG1
Ig-Kappa chain	TB28-2	BD	mIgG1
MHC-II	L243	BD	mIgG2a
MHC-II	G46.2.6	BD	mIgG1
bcl-2	Bcl-2/100	BD	mIgG1
Kappa chain	TB28-2	BD	mIgG1
Lambda chain	1-155-2	BD	mIgG1

Ig: Immunoglobulin; m: mouse; MHC-II: Major Histocompatibility Complex class II.

Immunofluorescence and flow cytometry

Camel or human cells (PBMC or leucocytes; 4×10^5) were incubated with mAbs specific for human CD antigens (Table 1) in PBS containing bovine serum albumin (5 g/l) and NaN_3 (0.1 g/l). After 30 minutes incubation (4°C), cells were washed twice and analyzed on the flow cytometer. A Becton Dickinson FACSCalibur equipped with Cell Quest software (FACSCalibur (Becton Dickinson Biosciences, San Jose, California, USA) was used to collect the data. At least 100 000 cells were collected and analyzed with the FCS Express software Version 3 (De Novo Software, Thornton, Ontario).

In order to exclude signals due to non-specific binding of mouse antibodies, negative isotype controls for mouse IgG1, IgG2a, IgG2b (from BD) and IgM (from Beckmann Coulter) were also included as part of the study.

Results

Flow cytometry was used to determine the reactivity of camel leukocytes with commercially available mAbs to human leukocyte markers. PBMC were isolated by density gradient centrifugation using Ficoll-Isopaque as standard method for studying the phenotype of PBMC without interfering effects of granulocytes (Fig. 1A). Whole leukocytes were separated by hypotonic lysis of erythrocytes (Fig. 1B). Separated camel or human cells were incubated with mouse mAbs specific for human leukocyte antigens or with mouse isotype control antibodies (Table 1) and were analyzed by flow cytometry. For the analysis of population-specific pattern of expression, gates were done for lymphocytes (L), monocytes (M) and granulocytes (G) (Fig.1). The profiles obtained for each mAb were then compared to the labeling pattern of reactivity obtained with human leukocytes.

Reactivity of mAbs to human leukocyte antigens with camel PBMC

The mAb 555923 (clone 6.7; from BD) is a FITC-labelled mouse antibody against human CD18. The expression pattern of CD18 on human and camel PBMC is shown in Fig.2. The mAb 555923 stained all human and camel PBMC, although the expression on lymphocytes was comparatively lower than monocytes. Also for both species, a minor subpopulation of lymphocytes remained negative for mAb 555923.

The mAb 555380 (clone G43-25B; from BD) is a PE-labelled mouse antibody directed against human CD11a. The expression pattern of CD11a on human and camel PBMC is shown in Fig.3. Although it stained all population of human leucocytes widely, mAb 555380 indicated a higher expression of CD11a on human monocytes and a subset of human lymphocytes. For camel cells, the mAb 555380 stained all cell populations weekly than human cells.

PBMC

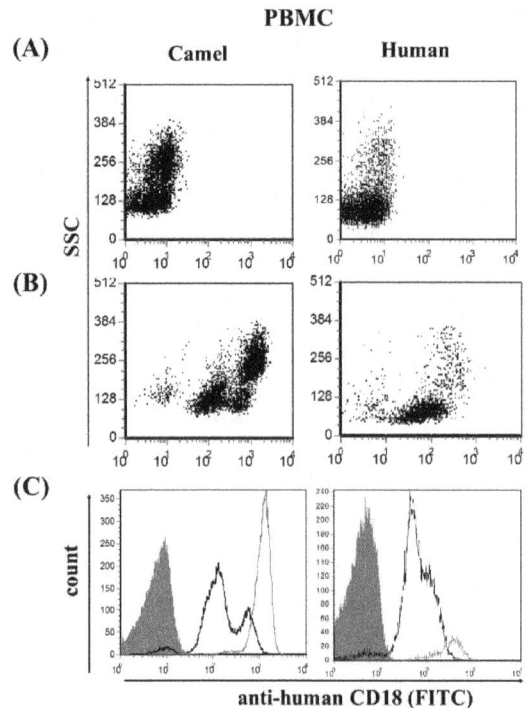

Fig. 2. Analysis of the expression pattern of CD18 on camel and human PBMC. Ficoll-separated camel or human PBMC were incubated with FITC-labelled mouse isotype control antibody **(A)** or the FITC-labelled monoclonal antibody 555923 (clone 6.7) specific for human CD18 **(B)** and analysed on the flow cytometer. The expression pattern of CD18 on camel or human PBMC was analysed by plotting SSC against CD18 expression. After gating lymphocytes and monocytes according to their forward and side scatter characteristics, the expression density of CD18 was shown in an overlapping histogram **(C)**.

However a higher expression could be seen for camel monocytes and a subset of lymphocytes.

The mAb 557743 (clone ICRF44; from BD) is a PE-Cy7-labelled mouse antibody directed against human CD11b. The expression pattern of CD11b on human and camel PBMC is shown in Fig.4. For both human and camel PBMC the mAb 557743 stained only monocytes and a minor subpopulation of lymphocytes, whereas the majority of lymphocytes was negative for this antibody.

The mAbs, 555398 (clone M5E2; from BD) and MCA1568PE (clone Tük4; from Bio-Rad) are PE-labelled mouse antibodies directed against human CD14. Both mAbs showed a similar staining pattern for human and camel PBMC. In both species, only the monocytes population was stained positively with both CD14 antibodies. The expression pattern of CD14 (data shown only for the clone M5E2) on human and camel PBMC is shown in Fig.5. The mouse mAb 347403 (clone L243; from BD) is an APC-labelled antibody directed against human HLA-DR antigen.

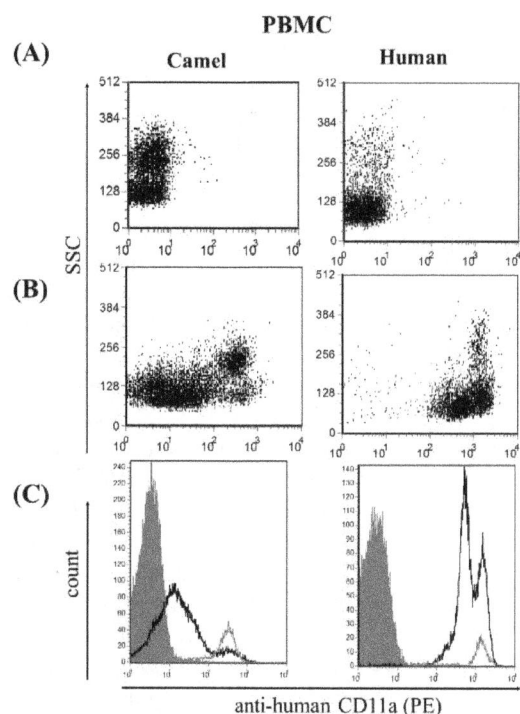

Fig. 3. Analysis of the expression pattern of CD11a on camel and human PBMC. Ficoll-separated camel or human PBMC were incubated with PE-labelled with mouse isotype control antibody (A) or the PE-labelled monoclonal antibody 555380 (clone G43-25B) specific for human CD11a (B) and analysed on the flow cytometer. The expression pattern of CD11a on camel or human PBMC was analysed by plotting SSC against CD11a expression. After gating lymphocytes and monocytes according to their forward and side scatter characteristics, the expression density of CD11a was shown in an overlapping histogram (C).

Fig. 4. Analysis of the expression pattern of CD11b on camel and human PBMC. Ficoll-separated camel or human PBMC were incubated with PE-Cy7-labelled mouse isotype control antibody (A) or the PE-Cy7-labelled monoclonal antibody 557743 (clone ICRF44) specific for human CD11b (B) and analysed on the flow cytometer. The expression pattern of CD11b on camel or human PBMC was analysed by plotting SSC against CD11b expression. After gating lymphocytes and monocytes according to their forward and side scatter characteristics, the expression density of CD11b was shown in an overlapping histogram (C).

For human PBMC the mAb 347403 stained only the monocytes population and a subpopulation of lymphocytes, which is expected to be B cells. For camel cells however, monocytes showed only week reactivity with this mAb. Only a minor subset of camel lymphocytes stained weekly positive with this mAb.

Reactivity of mAbs to human leukocyte antigens with camel granulocytes

Camel and human leukocytes were separated by hypotonic lysis of erythrocytes and were labelled with mAb to human CD antigens. Camel granulocytes showed reactivity only to three mAbs to human CD18, CD11a and CD11b (data not shown). The mAbs 555923 (FITC-labelled mouse anti-human CD18) and 555380 (PE-labelled mouse anti human CD11a) stained both human and camel granulocytes widely positive. However, a minor subpopulation of human granulocytes remained negative for the mAb 555923. Although the anti-human CD11b mAb 557743 stained both human and camel granulocytes positively, the reactivity of camel granulocytes was more weekly than that of human cells.

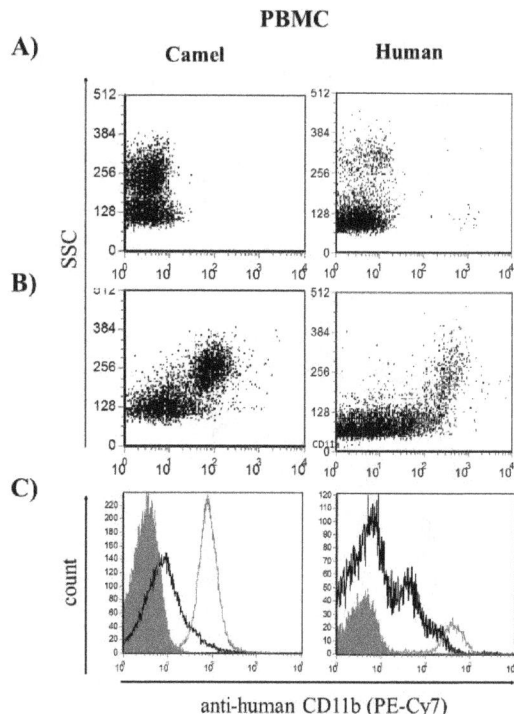

Only for human cells, a minor subpopulation of granulocytes remained negative for the mAb 557743.

Discussion

In comparison to the progress that has been made in the characterization of camel immunoglobulins (Hamers-Casterman et al., 1993; Muyldermans, 2013), few data are available on cellular immunity of camels in health or disease.

MAbs to leukocyte antigens have been considered as highly important tools for the analysis of cellular immunology in human (Maecker et al., 2012) as well as in different animal species (Hopkins et al., 1993; Lunn et al., 1998; Schafer and Burger, 2012; Duvel et al., 2014; Gerner et al., 2015). The lack of mAbs that define camel immune cells represents one of the major difficulties in studying the camel cellular immune response.

As the production of mAbs is very costly, the objective of the present study was to screen existing mAbs to human leukocyte antigens, immunoglobulin (Ig) chains and major MHC for their reactivity with camel leukocytes.

PBMC

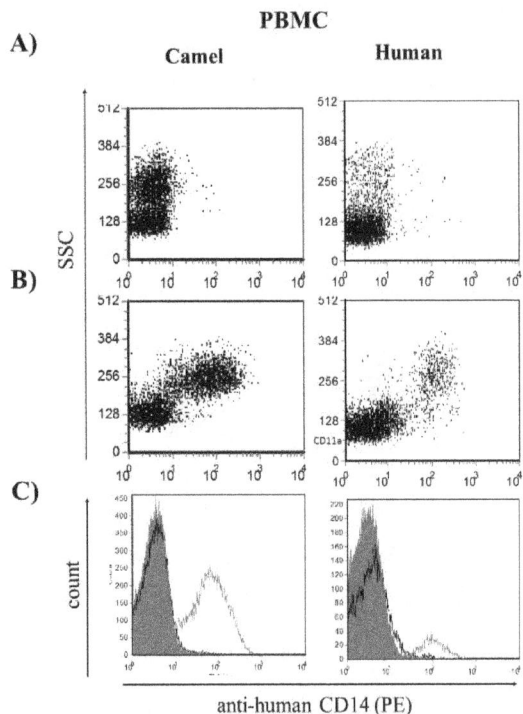

Fig. 5. Analysis of the expression pattern of CD14 on camel and human PBMC. Ficoll-separated camel or human PBMC were incubated with PE-labelled mouse isotype control antibody (A) or with the PE-labelled monoclonal antibody 555398 (clone M5E2) specific for human CD14 (B) and analysed on the flow cytometer. The expression pattern of CD14 on camel or human PBMC was analysed by plotting SSC against CD14 expression. After gating on lymphocytes or monocytes according to their forward and side scatter characteristics, the expression density of CD14 was shown in an overlapping histogram (C).

Two-parameter flow cytometry has been proven as a useful tool to study the cross-reactivity of mAbs developed against leukocyte differentiation antigens of one species with leukocyte antigens of other species (MacHugh et al., 1991; Naessens et al., 1993; Maecker et al., 2012). The specificity of a mAbs to a given antigen can be predicted according to the flow-cytometric pattern of expression of that molecule on labeled leukocytes (MacHugh et al., 1991; Naessens et al., 1993; Davis et al., 2007; Davis and Hamilton, 2008).

CD18 is the common β_2-chain (β_2-integrin) for all three forms of CD11 (a, b, c) (Harris et al., 2000). It has been shown that CD18 is expressed on all human leukocytes (Drbal et al., 2000) which is in accordance with our results of staining human PBMC and granulocytes with the mouse mAb 555923 (clone 6.7). Similar to their human counterparts, camel PBMC and granulocytes showed expressed CD18. As the patterns of reactivity for camel and human PBMC and granulocytes were identical so the homology of the proteins stained may be assumed.

Human CD11a is expressed together with CD18 as a hetero-dimer termed as leukocyte function antigen 1 (LFA-1). LFA-1 is the most important integrin expressed by all human leukocytes that regulate cell migration through binding to ICAM-1,-2 or-3 (van Kooyk and Figdor, 2000). As camel PBMC and granulocytes stained weekly than their human counterparts with the mAb 555380 (clone G43-25B) specific for human CD11a, it is likely that this mAb has a lower affinity for camel CD11a. However, the staining pattern of cell populations in both species with a higher staining density for human and camel granulocytes, monocytes and a subset of lymphocytes indicates that this antibody detects CD11a in camels.

CD11b is expressed as a hetero-dimer with CD18 (also termed Mac-1 or CR3) mainly on myeloid cells (granulocytes and monocytic cells) (Imhof and Aurrand-Lions, 2004; Nicholson et al., 2007) with a lower expression on lymphocytes like NK cells, $\gamma\delta$ T cells and a small subset of CD8+ T cells (Fiorentini et al., 2001; Graff and Jutila, 2007). The higher staining intensity of human and camel granulocytes and monocytes with the mAb 557743 (clone ICRF44) specific for human CD11b and the weaker staining of lymphocytes indicates that this mAb recognizes CD11b in both species.

CD14 is a co-receptor for bacterial lipopolysaccharides and is mainly expressed on blood monocytes (Hussen et al., 2013). Three clones of antibodies specific to human CD14 have been tested for cross-reactivity with camel leukocytes. Only the two mAbs 555398 (clone M5E2) and MCA1568PE (clone Tük4) stained camel monocytes but not granulocytes or lymphocytes, which indicates that these mAbs recognize camel CD14.

Human MHC class II antigen (HLA-DR) is constitutively expressed on professional antigen-presenting cells like dendritic cells, B cells, and monocytes (Abeles et al., 2012). The mAb 347403 (clone L243), which stained human monocytes and a population of lymphocytes, induced only a weak staining response in camel monocytes and lymphocytes. It is likely that this mAb has a low affinity to camel MHC-II molecules.

In summary, the present study aimed at providing the field of immunology with new antibodies to camel leukocyte antigens. Although some useful mAbs (about 10 % of studied 52 mAb) have been identified in the present study, which may contribute to fill the gap of available reagents for studying the immune response of camels to infectious pathogens and their response to vaccination, there is a clear need for developing mAbs to more camel leukocyte antigens. Also further cross-reactivity studies using mAbs against leukocyte antigens of animals with close sequence homology to camels like cattle or pigs could be helpful in identifying more cross-reactive antibodies.

Acknowledgements

The cooperation and assistance of the Al Omran slaughter house personal is greatly acknowledged

Conflict of interest

The authors declare that there is no conflict of interest.

References

Abeles, R.D., McPhail, M.J., Sowter, D., Antoniades, C.G., Vergis, N., Vijay, G.K., Xystrakis, E., Khamri, W., Shawcross, D.L., Ma, Y., Wendon, J.A. and Vergani, D. 2012. CD14, CD16 and HLA-DR reliably identifies human monocytes and their subsets in the context of pathologically reduced HLA-DR expression by CD14(hi) /CD16(neg) monocytes: Expansion of CD14(hi) /CD16(pos) and contraction of CD14(lo) /CD16(pos) monocytes in acute liver failure. Cytometry A 81(10), 823-834.

Al-Mohammed Salem, K., Badi, F.A., Al Haroon, A.I. and Alluwaimi, A.M. 2012. The Cellular Populations of Normal Camel (Camelus dromedaries) Milk. Open J. Vet. Med. 2, 262-265.

Davis, W.C., Davis, J.E. and Hamilton, M.J. 1995. Use of monoclonal antibodies and flow cytometry to cluster and analyze leukocyte differentiation molecules. Methods Mol. Biol. 45, 149-167.

Davis, W.C., Drbal, K., Mosaad, A.E., Elbagory, A.R., Tibary, A., Barrington, G.M., Park, Y.H. and Hamilton, M.J. 2007. Use of flow cytometry to identify monoclonal antibodies that recognize conserved epitopes on orthologous leukocyte differentiation antigens in goats, llamas, and rabbits. Vet. Immunol. Immunopathol. 119(1-2), 123-130.

Davis, W.C. and Hamilton, M.J. 2008. Use of flow cytometry to develop and characterize a set of monoclonal antibodies specific for rabbit leukocyte differentiation molecules. J. Vet. Sci. 9(1), 51-66.

Drbal, K., Angelisova, P., Cerny, J., Pavlistova, D., Cebecauer, M., Novak, P. and Horejsi, V. 2000. Human leukocytes contain a large pool of free forms of CD18. Biochem. Biophys. Res. Commun. 275(2), 295-299.

Duvel, A., Maass, J., Heppelmann, M., Hussen, J., Koy, M., Piechotta, M., Sandra, O., Smith, D.G., Sheldon, I.M., Dieuzy-Labaye, I., Zieger, P. and Schuberth, H.J. 2014. Peripheral blood leukocytes of cows with subclinical endometritis show an altered cellular composition and gene expression. Theriogenology 81(7), 906-917.

Fiorentini, S., Licenziati, S., Alessandri, G., Castelli, F., Caligaris, S., Bonafede, M., Grassi, M., Garrafa, E., Balsari, A., Turano, A. and Caruso, A. 2001. CD11b expression identifies CD8+CD28+ T lymphocytes with phenotype and function of both naive/memory and effector cells. J. Immunol. 166(2), 900-907.

Gerner, W., Talker, S.C., Koinig, H.C., Sedlak, C., Mair, K.H. and Saalmuller, A. 2015. Phenotypic and functional differentiation of porcine alphabeta T cells: current knowledge and available tools. Mol. Immunol. 66(1), 3-13.

Graff, J.C. and Jutila, M.A. 2007. Differential regulation of CD11b on gammadelta T cells and monocytes in response to unripe apple polyphenols. J. Leukoc. Biol. 82(3), 603-607.

Hamers-Casterman, C., Atarhouch, T., Muyldermans, S., Robinson, G., Hamers, C., Songa, E.B., Bendahman, N. and Hamers, R. 1993. Naturally occurring antibodies devoid of light chains. Nature 363(6428), 446-448.

Harris, E.S., McIntyre, T.M., Prescott, S.M. and Zimmerman, G.A. 2000. The leukocyte integrins. J. Biol. Chem. 275(31), 23409-23412.

Hopkins, J., Ross, A. and Dutia, B.M. 1993. Summary of workshop findings of leukocyte antigens in sheep. Vet. Immunol. Immunopathol. 39, 49-59.

Hussen, J., Duvel, A., Sandra, O., Smith, D., Sheldon, I.M., Zieger, P. and Schuberth, H.J. 2013. Phenotypic and functional heterogeneity of bovine blood monocytes. PLoS One 8(8), e71502.

Hussen, J., Koy, M., Petzl, W. and Schuberth, H.J. 2016. Neutrophil degranulation differentially modulates phenotype and function of bovine monocyte subsets. Innate Immun. 22(2), 124-137.

Imhof, B.A. and Aurrand-Lions, M. 2004. Adhesion mechanisms regulating the migration of monocytes. Nat. Rev. Immunol. 4(6), 432-444.

Lunn, D.P., Holmes, M.A., Antczak, D.F., Agerwal, N., Baker, J., Bendali-Ahcene, S., Blanchard-Channell, M., Byrne, K.M., Cannizzo, K., Davis, W., Hamilton, M.J., Hannant, D., Kondo, T., Kydd, J.H., Monier, M.C., Moore, P.F., O'Neil, T., Schram, B.R., Sheoran, A., Stott, J.L., Sugiura, T. and Vagnoni, K.E. 1998. Report of the Second Equine Leucocyte Antigen Workshop, Squaw valley, California, July 1995. Vet. Immunol. Immunopathol. 62(2), 101-143.

MacHugh, N.D., Bensaid, A., Howard, C.J., Davis, W.C. and Morrison, W.I. 1991. Analysis of the reactivity of anti-bovine CD8 monoclonal antibodies with cloned T cell lines and mouse L-cells transfected with bovine CD8. Vet. Immunol. Immunopathol. 27(1-3), 169-172.

Maecker, H.T., McCoy, J.P. and Nussenblatt, R. 2012. Standardizing immunophenotyping for the Human Immunology Project. Nat. Rev. Immunol. 12(3), 191-200.

Muyldermans, S. 2013. Nanobodies: natural single-domain antibodies. Annu. Rev. Biochem. 82, 775-797.

Naessens, J., Olubayo, R.O., Davis, W.C. and Hopkins, J. 1993. Cross-reactivity of workshop antibodies with cells from domestic and wild ruminants. Vet. Immunol. Immunopathol. 39(1-3), 283-290.

Nicholson, G.C., Tennant, R.C., Carpenter, D.C., Sarau, H.M., Kon, O.M., Barnes, P.J., Salmon, M., Vessey, R.S., Tal-Singer, R. and Hansel, T.T. 2007. A novel flow cytometric assay of human whole blood neutrophil and monocyte CD11b levels: upregulation by chemokines is related to receptor expression, comparison with neutrophil shape change, and effects of a chemokine receptor (CXCR2) antagonist. Pulm. Pharmacol. Ther. 20(1), 52-59.

Schafer, H. and Burger, R. 2012. Tools for cellular immunology and vaccine research the in the guinea pig: monoclonal antibodies to cell surface antigens and cell lines. Vaccine 30(40), 5804-5811.

van Kooyk, Y. and Figdor, C.G. 2000. Avidity regulation of integrins: the driving force in leukocyte adhesion. Curr. Opin. Cell Biol. 12(5), 542-547.

Zidan, M., Kassem, A. and Pabst, R. 2000a. Megakaryocytes and platelets in the spleen of the dromedary camel (Camelus dromedarius). Anat. Histol. Embryol. 29(4), 221-224.

Zidan, M., Schuberth, H.J. and Pabst, R. 2000b. Immunohistology of the splenic compartments of the one humped camel (Camelus dromedarius). Vet. Immunol. Immunopathol. 74(1-2), 17-29.

22

Prevalence and antimicrobial resistance of *Bacillus cereus* isolated from beef products in Egypt

Reyad Shawish[1] and Reda Tarabees[2,*]

[1]Department of Food Hygiene and Control, Faculty of Veterinary Medicine, University of Sadat City, Sadat City, Egypt

[2]Department of Bacteriology, Mycology and Immunology, Faculty of Veterinary Medicine, University of Sadat City, Sadat City, Egypt

Abstract

Foodborne pathogens have the main concern in public health and food safety. *Bacillus cereus* food poisoning is one of the most important foodborne pathogens worldwide. In the present study, a total of 200 random beef product samples were collected from different supermarkets located at Menofia and Cairo governorates were examined for the presence of *B. cereus*. In addition, the presence of some virulence encoding genes was evaluated using Multiplex PCR. Finally, the antibiogram testing was conveyed to illustrate the resistance pattern of the confirmed *B. cereus*. The data showed that *B. cereus* was recovered from 22.5%, 30%, 25%, 37.5% and 15% of the minced meat, burger, sausage, kofta, and luncheon respectively. Among the 20 examined isolates 18/20 (90%) were harbor *hblC* enterotoxin encoding gene compared with 20/20 (100) were have *cytK* enterotoxin encoding gene. The isolated strains of *B. cereus* were resistant to penicillin G and sensitive to oxacillin, clindamycin, vancomycin, erythromycin, gentamicin, ciprofloxacin, and ceftriaxone. In all, the obtained data showed the importance of emerging *B. cereus* in disease control and prevention programs, and in regular clinical and food quality control laboratories in Egypt.

Keywords: Antimicrobial susceptibility, *Bacillus cereus*, Beef products, Multiplex PCR, Virulence genes.

Introduction

Processed beef products such as minced meat, kofta, sausage, burger, and luncheon are gaining common popularity as easily quick prepared meat meals that can solve the problem of the high price fresh meat shortage which is not within the reach of large numbers of low-income families. The contamination of these beef products with the foodborne pathogens is still the main worry for public health, amongst contamination with *B. cereus* is one of the most important foodborne pathogens causing food poisoning among the food consumers all-inclusive.

B. cereus is an aerobic spore-forming Gram-positive bacterium normally disseminated in the environment. It is usually isolated from the soil, plant materials, raw meat and processed meat products (Carlin F *et al.*, 2010; Ceuppens *et al.*, 2013). Schedule identification of *B. cereus* is generally comprised isolation on selective media, revealing of motility, hemolysis prototype on blood agar, and acidification of glucose (Stenfors Arnesen *et al.*, 2008).

Although *B. cereus* is implicated in many foodborne illness outbreaks in many countries worldwide, however only a few cases are reported because the symptoms are mostly similar to *Staphylococcus aureus* and *Clostridium perfringens* food poisoning (Stenfors Arnesen *et al.*, 2008; Bottone, 2010; Bennett *et al.*,

2013). *B. cereus* has been incriminated as a cause of two types of food poisoning, emetic and diarrheal syndromes (Drobniewski, 1993).

The pathogenesis of *B. cereus*-induced food poisoning is mostly still indistinct. The microorganism conveys an expansive number of potentially toxic components, including hemolysins, phospholipases, and proteases (Drobniewski, 1993; Beecher, 2001) nevertheless, the precise role of some is still ambiguous. The emetic and the diarrheal syndromes are still the foremost worries for the public health apprehension and the full appreciative of their pathogenesis is imperative. These syndromes are mainly manifested via the release of two core toxins, a heat-labile diarrheal enterotoxin, and heat- stable emetic enterotoxin (Stenfors Arnesen *et al.*, 2008).

The diarrheal syndrome manifested via the release of one or three diarrheal enterotoxins: the tripartite toxins hemolysin BL (HBL) and non-hemolytic enterotoxin (Nhe), the two forms of cytotoxin K (cytK-1 and cytK-2) and possibly enterotoxin T and enterotoxin FM (Moravek *et al.*, 2006). HBL, a three-components toxin, that is encoded by *hblD* and *hblC* genes respectively, and a binding component B encoded by *hblA* gene. The presence of all three components is necessary for the toxin activity (Lindback and Granum, 2006).

***Corresponding Author:** Reda Tarabees. Department of Food Hygiene and Control, Faculty of Veterinary Medicine, University of Sadat City, Sadat City, Egypt. Email: *reda.tarabees@vet.usc.edu.eg*

The deceptive of *B. cereus* induced food poisoning symptoms and the lack of the clear-cut surveillance statistics in Egypt. This makes the indulgent of the pathogenesis of *B. cereus* food poisoning confusing. Therefore, the current study was undertaken to estimate the incidence of toxigenic *B. cereus* in some beef products collected at the retail level in Egypt using PCR. Additionally, the antibiotic resistance pattern of 20 *B. cereus* isolates was assessed using disc infusion method.

Material and Methods

Sampling

A total of 200 beef product samples (40 each of minced meat, burger, sausage, kofta, and luncheon) were collected from different supermarkets located at Menofia and Cairo governorates and examined bacteriologically. The presence of toxigenic *B. cereus* was confirmed using PCR based on the presence of virulence encoding genes.

Preparation of samples

The collected samples were transferred instantly under full aseptic conditions for bacteriological isolation and identification of *B. cereus*. Briefly, 25 grams of each product were transferred to 225 ml of 0.1% sterile buffered peptone water (Oxoid, UK), then stomached for 2 minutes to provide a homogenate. The homogenate was heat-treated at 80°C for 10 minutes to kill all the vegetative bacteria and recover of the *Bacillus* spores (Rahimi *et al.*, 2013). One ml of the original dilution transferred to a sterile tube containing 9 ml of sterile buffered peptone and incubated at 34°C for 24 hrs as a primary enrichment.

Isolation and characterization of Bacillus cereus

The bottles showed turbidity as an indication of *B. cereus* growth were streaked over a dry surface of *Bacillus cereus* selective agar medium (Oxoid, UK) by a bent glass rod and the plates were incubated at 30°C for 24-48 hrs. Suspected typical colonies were later picked up onto sheep blood agar (Oxoid, UK) and incubated at 34°C for 24 hrs to observe hemolysis (Tallent *et al.*, 2012).

Typical colonies of *B. cereus* that showed β hemolysis were further identified based on the biochemical activities (Holbook and Anderson, 1980; Bottone, 2010; Tallent *et al.*, 2012).

Genotypic characterization of B. cereus enterotoxins genes hblC and cytK

The multiplex PCR was carried out according to Ngamwongsatit *et al.* (2008). The PCR reactions containing 12.5 μl PCR Master Mix, 1 μl of each primer (0.4 μM *hlb*C and 0.2 μM *cyt*K as final concentration), of 5 μl of DNA templates and RNase-free water was added to a final volume of 25 μl. The PCR conditions were, 94 °C/ 5 min; 30 cycles of (94°C for 45 sec, annealing at 54-56°C for 1 min in case of *hbl*C and at 58°C in case of *cyt*K, elongation at 72°C for 2 min)

followed by 72°C for 5 min. 94°C for 45 sec, annealing at 54 and 56°C for 1 min in case of *hbl*C and at 58°C in case of *cyt*K, elongation at 72°C for 2 min and final extension at 72°C for 5 min. The products of PCR were separated by electrophoresis on 1.5% agarose gel (AppliChem, Germany) to determine the fragment sizes. The nucleotides sequences of the primers are shown in the Table 1.

Antimicrobial susceptibility test

The antibiotic susceptibility testing was performed using the disc diffusion method (Chon *et al.*, 2012). All the isolates were grown in brain heart infusion broth (Oxoid) for 18 hrs at 34°C and then spread on Mueller-Hinton agar (Oxoid, UK) and left for 15 minutes. Then, eight commercial antibiotic discs (Oxoid, UK) were used: penicillin (10 units), oxacillin (1.0 mg/ml) vancomycin (30 mg/m), clindamycin (2.0 mg/ml), erythromycin (15 mg/ml), gentamicin (10 mg/ml), Ciprofloxacin (5μg) and Ceftriaxone (30 μg), and the plates were then incubated at 37 °C for 18–24 hrs (Chon *et al.*, 2012).

Results

Prevalence of B. cereus in the examined beef products

The data presented in Table 2 showed the prevalence rate of *B. cereus* in the examined beef products. Among the examined beef products, only 52 out of 200 (26%) were positive for *B. cereus*. The highest prevalence rate was recorded in case of beef kofta 15/40 (37.5%), while the lowest rate was in case of beef luncheon 6/40 (15%).

Genotypic characterization of enterotoxigenic genes using Multiplex PCR

The data obtained in Table 3 demonstrated the incidence rate of the *hbl*C and *cyt*K enterotoxigenic genes in the examined *B. cereus* isolates. Among the examined isolates, 18/20 (90%) were harbor *hbl*C enterotoxin encoding gene compared with 20/20 (100%) were found to have *cyt*K enterotoxin encoding gene and exhibited a specific band size (Fig. 1).

Antibiotic sensitivity testing

The data presented in Table 4 showed the antibiotic resistance pattern of the examined *B. cereus* isolates. A total of 51 isolates were tested for their antibiotic sensitivity prototype against 8 commercial antibiotic discs. The data demonstrated that all the isolates (51/51) were resistant to penicillin G (100%) and sensitive to other antibiotics 51/51 (100%).

Discussion

Contamination of meat products with toxigenic *B cereus* is one of the underestimated foodborne illness worldwide (Ceuppens *et al.* 2013). In Egypt, there is no accurate surveillance data about the numbers of *B. cereus* induced food poisoning cases. The lack of accurate data may be because of the resemblance of the symptoms with the other foodborne pathogens (Normanno *et al.*, 2007).

Table 1. Primers nucleotides sequences used for multiplex PCR amplification of *B. cereus* entrotoxins genes.

Target gene	Primer	Size in bp	Primer sequence (5'—3')	T°C	Product size in bp	conc(µM)
*hbl*C	FHblC	19	CCTATCAATACTCTCGCAA	54	695	0.4
	RHblC	20	TTTCCTTTGTTATACGCTGC	56		
*cyt*K	FCytK	20	CGACGTCACAAGTTGTAACA	58	565	0.2
	R2CytK	20	CGTGTGTAAATACCCCAGTT	58		

Table 2. Prevalence rate of *B. cereus* in the examined beef products (40 of each).

Beef products	Positive sample		Negative sample	
	No	%	No	%
Minced meat	9	22.5	31	77.5
Beef burger	12	30	28	70
Beef sausage	10	25	30	75
Beef kofta	15	37.5	25	62.5
Beef luncheon	6	15	34	85
Total	52	26	148	74
Minced meat	No	%	No	%

Table 3. Molecular detection of enterotoxigenic genes of *B. cereus* isolated from examined samples.

Target gene	No of examined isolate	Positive isolate	%
*hbl*C	20	18	90
*cyt*K	20	20	100

Table 4. Antibiotics resistant of *B. cereus* isolated beef products (*n*=51).

Antibiotic tested	Resistant	Intermediate	Sensitive
Penicillin G	51(100.0)	0 (0.0)	0 (0.0)
Oxacillin	0 (0.0)	0 (0.0)	51(100.0)
Vancomycin	0 (0.0)	0 (0.0)	51(100.0)
Clindamycin	0 (0.0)	0 (0.0)	51(100.0)
Erythromycin	0 (0.0)	0 (0.0)	51(100.0)
Gentamicin	0 (0.0)	0 (0.0)	51(100.0)
Ciprofloxacin	0 (0.0)	0 (0.0)	51(100.0)
Ceftriaxone	0 (0.0)	0 (0.0)	51(100.0)

The contamination of beef products probably occurred during handling and preparation or post-processing contamination. In addition, keeping the products unrefrigerated for several hours enhances the multiplication of *B. cereus* and hence the liberation of enterotoxin. The study herein was aimed to estimate the accurate incidence rate of toxigenic *B. cereus* and its antibiotic susceptibility pattern in some beef products collected from different localities in Egypt. The data obtained will probably highlight the emergence of *B. cereus* as a serious underestimated cause of foodborne illness and will help in understanding its pathogenesis.

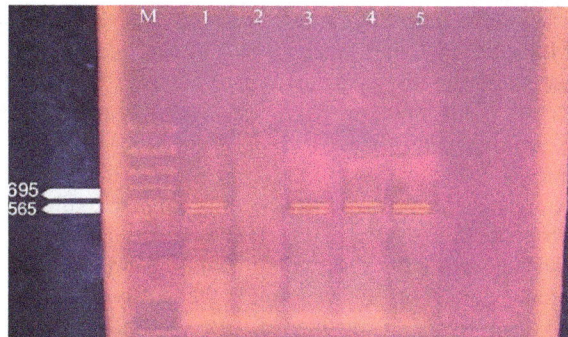

Fig. 1. Genotypic characterization of enterotoxins encoding genes *hhl*C and *cyt*K using specific primers sets. Lane (M): DNA Ladder (10bp); Lane (1): positive control; Lane (2): negative control; Lanes (3-5) *Bacillus cereus* exhibited a specific band size of 595 bp and 565 bp representing *hbl*C and *cyt*K enterotoxin-encoding genes respectively.

The data obtained in the Table 2 demonstrated that the highest incidence rate was recorded in beef kofta and the lowest was in the case of minced meat. This outcome is similar to that obtained by Mohamed and Ghanyem (2015), and higher compared with that obtained by Heikal *et al*. (2006). Conversely, this result is lower than the result obtained by Eid *et al*. (2008).

Processed ready to eat beef products are considered the main source of infection with *B. cereus* and more caution need to be taken in order to minimize the contamination of such products. The selection of fresh and clean flesh, decontamination of the mincing machine, grinders, equipment and knives used in the processing of such products will auspiciously decrease the incidence of *B cereus* foodborne illness cases among the consumers (FDA, 2012; Torky, 1995, 2004). The higher incidence rate of the *B. cereus* in kofta and minced meat in comparison with luncheon can be explained as luncheon during the processing steps the product was subjected to a high temperature that significantly decreases the number of *Bacillus* spores (Torky, 1995).

Additionally, during the processing of minced meat and kofta, additives, seasoning, and spices were added, these additives are considered a potential risk factor can increase the number of *Bacillus* spores and hence magnitude the incidence of food poisoning. Therefore more consideration should be taken during processing of raw meat and kofta, and only use additives from a trustful source. Moreover, these additives should be regularly tested for the presence of *Bacillus* spores.

Schedule examination of beef products for the presence of *Bacillus* spores is requisite. Isolation and identification of *Bacillus* using traditional methods (culturing on selective media and biochemical testing of the confirmed isolates) is still the key element for the confirmation of the infection. The severity of infection with *Bacillus* is conveyed via the liberation of an array of virulence encoding genes.

Multiplex PCR has emerged as the fast and reliable technique for the confirmation of enterotoxigenic *B. cereus* (Guinebretiere *et al.*, 2006; Ombui *et al.*, 2008). Recently, Ngamwongsatit *et al.* (2008) have developed and evaluated a group of newly efficient primers used for detection of the genes encoding enterotoxin production in 100% of the tested *B. cereus* and *B. thuringensis* strains assuming that, the presence of either gene is an indication for the presence of the whole operon (Ngamwongsatit *et al.*, 2008).

In the current work, the existence of the enterotoxin-encoding genes *hbl*C and *cyt*K was assessed in 20 *B. cereus* isolates using specific primers sets that previously approved by Ngamwongsatit *et al.* (2008). The data presented in Table 3 and Figure 1 demonstrated that 18 isolates (90%) and 20 isolates (100%) were positive for *hbl*C and *cyt*K gene, respectively. This outcome is in accordance with that obtained previously obtained by Awny *et al.* (2010). Collectively, emerging of the multiplex PCR as a rapid technique for the affirmation of toxigenic *B. cereus* in food will probably command the pathogenesis of *B. cereus* induced-food poisoning in Egypt.

A total of 51 *B. cereus* isolates were further tested for their antimicrobial susceptibility (Table 4). All the tested isolates were resistant to penicillin G, whereas sensitive to oxacillin, clindamycin, vancomycin, erythromycin, gentamicin, ciprofloxacin, and ceftriaxone. The data obtained herein with the others (Fenselau *et al.*, 2008; Organji *et al.*, 2015; Jawad *et al.*, 2016) showed that *B. cereus* has a broad range of antibiotic susceptibility and validate the resistance to penicillin G by comparing to susceptibility to clindamycin, vancomycin, and erythromycin.

Conclusion

From the obtained data, many conclusions could be drawn, contamination of beef products with *B. cereus* increase the potential of foodborne infections among the consumers. The cleanliness of the equipment, processing machines, knives, and only use additives from trustful sources are measures significantly will minimize the infection with *Bacillus* spores. Schedule antibiotic susceptibility testing of *B. cereus* isolates recovered from beef products will guide choosing the appropriate antibiotic. Also, the data authenticate the significance of counting *B. cereus* in disease control and prevention programs, and in regular clinical and food quality control laboratories in Egypt.

Conflict of interest
The authors declare that there is no conflict of interest.

References

Awny, N.M., Abou Zeid, A.A.M. and Abdo, A.M. 2010. Prevalence of toxigenic bacteria in some Egyptian food. The Fifth Scientific Environmental Conference, Zagazig University.

Beecher, D.J. 2001. The *Bacillus cereus* group. In P. C. B. Turnbull ed., Gastro-intestinal infections: toxin-associated diseases. Academic Press, London, pp: 1161-1190.

Bennett, S.D., Walsh, K.A. and Gould, L.H. 2013. Foodborne disease outbreaks caused by *Bacillus cereus*, *Clostridium perfringens*, and *Staphylococcus aureus*-then United States, 1998-2008. Clin. Infect. Dis. 57(3), 425-433.

Bottone, E.J. 2010. *Bacillus cereus*, a volatile human pathogen. Clin. Microbiol. Rev 23(2), 382-398.

Carlin, F., Brillard, J., Broussole, V., Clavel, T., Duport, C., Jobin, M., Guinebretière, M.H., Auger, S., Sorokine, A. and Nguyen-The, C. 2010. Adaptation of *Bacillus cereus*, a ubiquitous worldwide-distributed foodborne pathogen, to a changing environment. Food Res. Int. 43(7), 1885-1894.

Ceuppens, S., Boon, N. and Uyttendaele, M. 2013. Diversity of *Bacillus cereus* group strains is reflected in their broad range of pathogenicity and diverse ecological lifestyles. FEMS Microbiol. Ecol. 84(3), 433-450.

Chon, J. W., Kim, J. H., Lee, S. J., Hyeon, J. Y., Song, K.Y. and Park, C. and Seo, K.H. 2012. Prevalence , phenotypic traits and molecular characterization of emetic toxin-producing *Bacillus cereus* strains isolated from human stools in Korea. J. Appl. Microbiol. 112, 1042-1049.

Drobniewski, F.A. 1993. *Bacillus cereus* and related species. Clin. Microbiol. Rev. 6(4), 324-338.

Eid, A.M., Eleiwa, N.Z.H. and Zaky, E.M.S. 2008. Prevalence of *Bacillus cereus* in some ready-to-eat meat products. 9th Vet. Med. Zag. Conference. 20-22 August, Port-Said.

Fenselau, C., Havey, C., Teerakulkittipong, N., Swatkoski, S., Laine, O. and Edwards, N. 2008. Identification of B-lactamase in antibiotic-resistant *Bacillus cereus* spores. Appl. Environ. Microbiol. 74, 904-906.

Food and Drug Administration (FDA). 2012. *Bacillus cereus*. Downloaded from http://www.fda.gov/ Food/Science Research/Laboratory Methods/ Bacteriological Analytical Manual BAM/ ucm 070875.

Guinebretiere, M., Fagerlund, A., Granum, P.E. and Nguyen, C. 2006. Rapid discrimination of cytK-1 and cytK-2 genes in Bacillus cereus strains by a novel PCR system. FEMS Microbiol. Lett. 59(1), 74-80.

Heikal, G.I., Khafagi, N.I.M. and Mostafa, N.Y.2006. *Bacillus cereus* in some ready to cook meat products. Benha Vet. Med. J. 17(2), 343-350.

Holbook, R. and Anderson, J.M. 1980. An improved selective and diagnostic medium for isolation and enumeration of *Bacillus cereus* in foods. Can. J. Microbiol. 26(7), 254-261.

Jawad, N., Abd Mutalib, S. and Abdullah, A. 2016. Antimicrobial resistance pattern of *Bacillus cereus* strains Isolated from fried rice samples. Int. J. Chem.Tech. Res. 8(1), 160-167.

Lindback, T. and Granum, P.E. 2006. Detection and Purification of *Bacillus cereus* Enterotoxins. In: Adley, C.C. Food-Borne Pathogens: Methods and Protocols. Totawa, Humana Press, pp: 15-24.

Mohamed, W.S. and Ghanyem, H.R. 2015. Effect of some preservative on *Bacillus cereus* isolated from some meat products. Assiut Vet. Med. J. 61(146), 1-7.

Moravek, M., Dietrich, R., Buerk, C., Broussolle, V., Guinebretiere, M.H., Granum, P.E., Nguyen-The, C. and Martlbauer, E. 2006. Determination of the toxic potential of *Bacillus cereus* isolates by quantitative enterotoxin analyses. FEMS Microbiol. Lett. 257(2), 293-298.

Ngamwongsatit, P., Buasri, W., Pianariyanon, P., Pulsrikarn, C., Ohba, M., Assavanig, A. and Panbangred, W. 2008. Broad distribution of enterotoxins genes (hblCDA, nheABC, cytK and entFm) among *Bacillus thuringiensis* and *Bacillus cereus* as shown by novel primers. Int. J. Food Microbiol. 121(3), 352-356.

Normanno, G., La Salandra, G., Dambrosio, A., Quaglia, N.C., Corrente, M., Parisi, A., Santagada,

G., Firinu, A., Crisetti, E. and Celano, G.V. 2007. Occurrence, characterization and antimicrobial resistance of enterotoxigenic *Staphylococcus aureus* isolated from meat and dairy products. Int. J. Food Microbiol. 115(3), 290-296.

Ombui, J.N., Gitahi, N. and Gicheru, M. 2008. Direct detection of *Bacillus cereus* enterotoxin genes in food by multiplex polymerase chain reaction. Int. J. Integ. Biol. 2(3), 172-181

Organji, S.R., Abulreesh, H.H., Elbanna, K., Osman, O.E.H. and Khider, M. 2015. Occurrence and characterization of toxigenic *Bacillus cereus* in food and infant feces. Asian Pac. J. Trop. Biomed. 5(7), 515-520.

Rahimi, E., Abdos, F., Momtaz, H., Baghbadorani, Z.T. and Jalali, M. 2013. *Bacillus cereus* in infant foods: prevalence study and distribution of enterotoxigenic virulence factors in Isfahan Province, Iran. Sci. World J. doi:10.1155/2013/292571.

Stenfors Arnesen, L.P., Fagerlund, A. and Granum, P.E. 2008. From soil to gut: *Bacillus cereus* and its food poisoning toxins. FEMS Microbiol. Rev. 32(4), 579-606.

Tallent, S.M., Rhodehamel, E.J., Harmon, S.M. and Bennett, R.W. 2012. *Bacillus cereus*. In: Bacteriological analytical manual. USA: US Food and Drug Administration; 2012. Available at: https://www.fda.gov/Food/FoodScienceResearch/LaboratoryMethods/ucm070875.htm

Torky, A.A.S. 1995. Bactero- toxological studies of *Bacillus cereus* in meat products. Master Thesis, Meat and Milk Hygiene, Cairo, Cairo University.

Torky, A.A.S. 2004. Trials for inhibition of some food poisoning microorganism in meat products. PhD thesis, Meat and Milk Hygiene. Cairo, Cairo University.

23

Biosecurity and geospatial analysis of mycoplasma infections in poultry farms at Al-Jabal Al-Gharbi region of Libya

Abdulwahab Kammon[1,*], Paolo Mulatti[2], Monica Lorenzetto[2], Nicola Ferre[2], Monier Sharif[3], Ibrahim Eldaghayes[1] and Abdunaser Dayhum[1]

[1]*Faculty of Veterinary Medicine, University of Tripoli, P.O. Box 13662, Tripoli, Libya*
[2]*Istituto Zooprofilattico Sperimentale delle Venezie, Viale dell'Universita, 10, Legnaro, Padova 35020, Italy*
[3]*Faculty of Veterinary Medicine, University of Omar Al-Mukhtar, Albeida, Libya*

Abstract
Geospatial database of farm locations and biosecurity measures are essential to control disease outbreaks. A study was conducted to establish geospatial database on poultry farms in Al-Jabal Al-Gharbi region of Libya, to evaluate the biosecurity level of each farm and to determine the seroprevalence of mycoplasma and its relation to biosecurity level. A field team of 7 Veterinarians belongs to the National Center of Animal Health was assigned for data recording and collection of blood samples. Personal information of the producers, geographical locations, biosecurity measures and description of the poultry farms were recorded. The total number of poultry farms in Al-Jabal Al-Gharbi Region is 461 farms distributed in 13 cities. Out of these, 102 broiler farms and one broiler breeder farm (10 houses) which were in operation during team visit were included in this study. Following collection of blood, sera were separated and tested by Enzyme-linked immunosorbent assay (ELISA) for the presence of antibodies against Mycoplasma (General antigen for M. gallisepticum and M. synoviae). The seroprevalence of Mycoplasma in the region was 28% (29 poultry farms out of 103 were infected). About 50% (23 out of 47) of poultry farms located in Garian city were infected with Mycoplasma and one significant cluster of Mycoplasma infection in the city was identified. Low level of biosecurity was found in poultry farms of the region. Out of the 103 farms included, 63% of poultry houses has a ground of soil and 44% of them has uncoated walls which may influence the proper cleaning and disinfection. Almost 100% of the farms are at risk of exposure to diseases transmitted by wild birds such as avian influenza and Newcastle disease due to absence of wild birds control program. Although, 81% of the farms have entry restrictions, only 20% have disinfectants at entry which increase the risk of exposure to pathogens. The results of this study highlight the weakness points of biosecurity measures in poultry farms of Al-Jabal Al-Gharbi region and high seroprevalence of mycoplasma. Data collected in this study will assist the Veterinary authorities to apply effective disease control strategies.
Keywords: Biosecurity, Geospatial analysis, Mycoplasma, Poultry.

Introduction

The severe economic, social and public health consequences of infectious diseases in poultry require effective plans for rapid detection and response. Geospatial database of farm locations and biosecurity measures are essential to control disease outbreaks. Attributed farm locations are needed because many infectious disease mitigation strategies, such as culling or ring vaccination, explicitly rely on spatial relationships between susceptible animal population and pathogen reservoirs (Bruhn *et al.*, 2012).

Biosecurity is the prevention or control of pathogenic microorganisms from contacting animal or human populations. In the context of modern poultry production, it is essentially keeping the birds separate from the agents causing the disease. Used properly, biosecurity will also minimize the effect of disease and contain the spread of disease, if found (Dorea *et al.*, 2010).

Avian mycoplasmosis is caused by several pathogenic mycoplasmas of which Mycoplasma gallisepticum (MG) and M. synoviae (MS) are the most important; they are the only ones listed by the OIE. MG causes chronic respiratory disease of domestic poultry, especially in the presence of management stresses and/or other respiratory pathogens. Ms causes synovitis and/or airsacculitis. Infections of mycoplasma can yield significant losses in performance and associated economics to all sectors of the poultry industry worldwide (Evans *et al.*, 2005).

In the 1999 outbreak of MG in North Carolina, Vaillancourt *et al.* (2000) found a direct connection between an MG-positive farm and a previous case when the MG-positive grower helped another grower who had MG and returned to his farm without changing clothing and boots which reflects a failure in biosecurity. Silva *et al.* (2015) found high seroprevalence rates of mycoplasma (MG & MS) in

---
*Corresponding Author: Dr. Abdulwahab Kammon. Department of Poultry and Fish Diseases, Faculty of Veterinary Medicine, University of Tripoli, P.O. Box 13662, Tripoli, Libya. Email: *abd_kammon@vetmed.edu.ly*

backyard and commercial chickens which emphasize the need of keeping chicken flocks free from disease using effective biosafety systems.

There is lack of information on poultry industry in Libya in term of geospatial data. Moreover, to our knowledge, no detailed study has been carried out to determine the level of biosecurity that is practiced by poultry producers in Al-JabalAl-Gharbi region of Libya, and much less the relationship of such practices with mycoplasma infections. The present study was conducted for this reason.

Materials and Methods

Data collection

Prior to this study, there was no database on poultry production in this region. A field team of 7 Veterinarians belongs to the National Center of Animal Health was trained and assigned for collection of data using a questionnaire containing personal information of the producers, geographical information, information of the farm, biosecurity measures and some other questions on previous diseases and control measures adopted. Blood samples were collected for the detection of antibodies against MG and MS. One hundred and two broiler farms and one broiler breeder farm (10 houses) which are located in 10 cities were included in this study (Table 1).

Table 1. Number of the poultry farms evaluated for the level of biosecurity and mycoplasma seroprevalence.

City	Frequency
Garian	47
Alasabaa	3
Kelaa	1
Yafrin	11
Rayaina	12
Zentan	6
Rujban	2
Alharaba	1
Nalut	16
Gadamis	4
Total	103

All of these farms were in operation during visit and evaluated according to the level of biosecurity practice and the presence of antibodies against Mycoplasma taking into account the relationship between biosecurity level and Mycoplasma infection. Eleven biosecurity variables were included which are related to either proper cleaning and disinfection or protection of the flock from external pathogens. The biosecurity variables evaluated were shown in Table 2. Every variable was coded as good biosecurity practice (code= 1) and bad biosecurity practice (code= 0).

Table 2. Names and description of biosecurity variables investigated.

NO	Biosecurity variable (name)	Description (Code)
1	GROUND	Ground of the poultry house (Soil=0, Concrete=1)
2	WALL	Walls of the poultry house (uncoated brick=0, coated brick=1)
3	DIS BETWEEN FARMS	Distance between farms (≤1000 meter=0, >1000 meter=1)
4	OTHER BIRD SPECIES	Other birds species in the farm (yes=0, no=1)
5	ENTRY RESTRICTION	The presence of a gate (no=0, yes=1)
6	ENTRY DISINFECTANTS	Disinfectants at the gate for cars (no=0, yes=1)
7	HOUSE DISINFECTANTS	Foot bath with disinfectants in front of the house(s) (no=0, yes=1)
8	COVERALL CLOTHS	Presence of clothes for visitors and workers (no=0, yes=1)
9	BIRD DISPOSAL	How dead birds are disposed (thrown away=0, burned and buried=1)
10	WILD BIRD CONTROL	Control of wild bird (no=0, yes=1)
11	RODENTS CONTROL	Control of rodents (no=0, yes=1)

Serological analysis

Twenty blood samples were collected from each poultry farm (each house) at the end of the production cycle. After collection, the blood samples were sent to the Veterinary Laboratory of the region. Sera were separated and tested by Enzyme-linked immunosorbent assay (ELISA) using Mycoplasma (MG-MS) commercial kit (Biochek®, Netherlands).

Spatial analysis

In this study a map showing all seven branches (regions) of the National Center of Animal Health was designed using QGIS 2.8.1 software (http://www.qgis.org) (Fig. 1).

The poultry farms of Al-Jabal Al-Gharbi region were also shown on the map based on their coordinates.

The spatial aggregation of positive farms was investigated through a purely spatial scan statistic, using a Bernoulli probability model (Kulldorff, 1997), which is particularly suitable for presence/absence or positive/negative data.

Farms were considered positive based on at least one positive ELISA result. A cluster of positive farms was considered significant when the simulated P-value was ≤0.05 (Dwass, 1957). The identified cluster was ranked on the basis of a likelihood function (Kulldorff and Nagarwalla, 1995; Kulldorff, 1997).

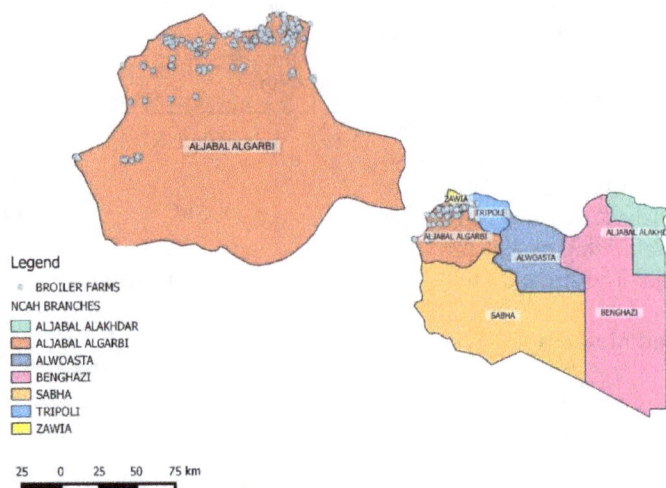

Fig. 1. A map showing the 7 branches of the National Center of Animal Health and poultry farms of Al-Jabal Al-Gharbi region.

Table 3. Number of poultry farms in different cities in Al-Jabal Al-Gharbi region.

City	No. of farms/housesat operation during study				No. of empty farms (out of operation during team visit)	Total
	Broilers	Layers	Breeders	Quails		
Nalut	16	1	0	0	144	161
Garian	60	3	1	1	59	124
Yafrin	13	1	0	0	51	65
Rayaina	17	1	0	0	27	45
Ruhaibat	0	0	0	0	15	15
Gadamis	11	0	0	0	1	12
Zentan	9	0	0	0	2	11
Jadu	0	0	0	0	7	7
Alasabaa	5	0	0	0	2	7
Mezda	0	0	0	0	6	6
Rujban	3	0	0	0	1	4
Alharaba	1	0	0	0	2	3
Kelaa	1	0	0	0	0	1
Total	136	6	1	1	317	461

Table 4. Number and percentage of poultry farms showed good biosecurity practice at every biosecurity variable.

Biosecurity variable	Garian *n=47	Alasabaa n=3	Kelaa n=1	Yafrin n=11	Rayaina n=12	Zentan n=6	Rujban n=2	Alharaba n=1	Nalut n=16	Gadamis n=4	Total n=103
Ground	20	0	0	2	6	3	0	1	4	2	38 (37%)
Wall	37	1	0	5	8	1	0	0	6	0	58 (56%)
Dis. Between farms	13	3	1	3	1	6	1	1	8	2	39 (38%)
Other bird species	44	3	1	11	10	6	2	1	12	4	94 (91%)
Entry restriction	45	3	1	2	12	6	2	1	11	0	83 (81%)
Entry disinfectants	9	0	0	5	1	1	0	0	5	0	21 (20%)
House disinfectants	45	3	1	10	12	6	2	1	16	4	100 (97%)
Coverall cloths	6	0	0	6	0	6	0	1	1	0	17 (17%)
Bird disposal	14	0	1	4	2	5	1	0	13	4	44 (43%)
Wild bird control	1	0	0	0	0	0	0	0	0	0	1 (0.97%)
Rodents control	3	0	0	9	6	1	1	0	2	0	22 (21%)

*n= number of poultry farms that participated.

The data were handled bySaTScanTM version 9.1.1 (http://www.satscan.org), while the output was visualised in ESRI™ ArcMap®version 10.1 (http://www.esri.com/).

Results and Discussion

The total number of poultry farms in Al-Jabal Al-Gharbi Region is 461 farms distributed in 13 cities (Table 3). Poultry farms showed low level of biosecurity especially the ground of the houses, distance between farms, the presence of disinfectants at the farm entry, the use of coverall cloths, disposal of dead birds and control of wild birds and rodents (Table 4). 63% of poultry houses has a ground of soil and 44% of them has uncoated walls which may influence the proper cleaning and disinfection. Almost 100% of the farms are at risk of exposure to diseases transmitted by wild birds such as avian influenza and Newcastle disease due to absence of wild birds control program (Keawcharoen et al., 2011). Although, 81% of the farms have entry restrictions, only 20% have disinfectants at entry which increase the risk of exposure to pathogens that may be transmitted by vehicles carrying feed, day old chicks, etc,. Biosecurity and biosurveillance measures have been largely successful at minimizing MG outbreaks among the breeding stock of the turkey and chicken industries (Evans et al., 2005).

Table 5 presenting the number of poultry farms infected with Mycoplasma. The prevalence of Mycoplasma (MG-MS) in the region was 28% (29 poultry farms out of 103 were infected).

Table 5. Number of poultry farms infected with Mycoplasma.

City	MG-MS**
Garian (*n=47)	23
Alasabaa (n=3)	0
Kelaa (n=1)	1
Yafrin (n=11)	1
Rayaina (n=12)	0
Zentan (n=6)	1
Rujban (n=2)	0
Alharaba (n=1)	1
Nalut (n=16)	1
Gadamis (n=4)	1
Total (n=103)	29 (28%)

*n= number of poultry farms that participated.
**MG-MS= Mycoplasma Gallisepticum and Mycoplasma Synovie (Mycoplasma general antigen).

About 50% (23 out of 47) of poultry farms located in Garian city were infected with Mycoplasma (MG-MS). This may due to the extensive production in the city. This study showed presence of other bird species mainly backyard chickens in 94% of the poultry farms (Table 4).

Backyard chickens could play important role in mycoplasma spread. Buchala et al. (2006) tested 15 free range chicken farms and found seroprevalence of 73% for MG and 100% for MS.

Pereira (2005), in a study on the prevalence of antibodies against MG and MS in 160 backyard chickens in Uberlândia, found that 102 (63.8%) were positive for MG. In the 1999 outbreak of MG in North Carolina, Vaillancourt et al. (2000) found a direct connection between an MG-positive farm and a previous case when the MG-positive grower helped another grower who had MG and returned to his farm without changing clothing and boots which reflects a failure in biosecurity. This may indicate that birds reared in farms where biosecurity programs are implemented are less contaminated than those reared in environments with no biosecurity measures (Silva et al., 2015).

Spatial analysis scanning for clusters with high rates using the Bernoulli model was conducted using SatScan Software. Geographical localization of Mycoplasma infection clusters in Al-Jabal Al-Gharbi region are shown in Figure 2.

Spatial analysis identified one significant cluster of Mycoplasma infection (P <0.01) (Fig. 2; Table 6). This cluster is mostly located within Garian's administration borders.

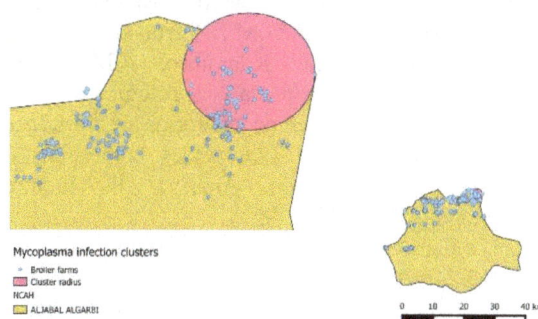

Mycoplasma infection clusters
· Broiler farms
▨ Cluster radius
NCAH
▨ ALJABAL ALGARBI

0 10 20 30 40 km

Fig. 2. Geographical localization of Mycoplasma infection clusters in Al-Jabal Al-Gharbi region.

Table 6. Characteristics of Mycoplasma cluster.

Cluster ID	Radius (km)	No. of farms included	No. of cases observed	No. of cases expected	P-value
1	21.52	29	18	2.14	0.0013

Geographic information system (GIS) and spatial analyses constitute a useful approach that supports the generation of hypotheses on drivers for disease diffusion based (Pfeiffer et al., 2008). This study showed that all poultry farms of Al-Jabal Al-Gharbi region had bad biosecurity practice which may be a good reason for wide spread of mycoplasma infections. However, there is still a possibility of vertical transmission of mycoplasma from infected parents to their progeny.

The results of this study highlight the weakness points of biosecurity measures in poultry farms of Al-Jabal Al-Gharbi region. The seroprevalence rates of mycoplasma found in the present study emphasize the need of keeping chicken flocks free from disease using effective biosecurity system. Veterinary authorities has to inforce the application of biosecurity measures to improve birds' health and welfare.

Training of producers on the importance of biosecurity and its applications is of great value. This may be achieved by conducting seminars, using media and leaflets.

Conflict of interest
The authors declare that there is no conflict of interest.

Acknowledgments

The authors acknowledge the assistance of the Veterinarians and Veterinary Laboratory Staff of Al-Jabal Al-Gharbi region for collection of data and testing of blood samples.

References

Bruhn, M.C., Munoz, B., Cajka, J., Smith, G., Curry, R.J., Wagener, D.K., and Wheaton, W.D. 2012. Synthesized Population Databases: A Geospatial Database of US Poultry Farms. Methods Rep. RTI Press. 2012 Jan 1; MR-0023-1201, 1-24.

Buchala, F.G., Ishizuka, M.M., Mathias, L.A., Berchieri Júnior, A.G.M., Cardoso, A.L.S.P., Tessari, E.N.C. and Kanashiro, A.M.I. 2006. Detecção de resposta sorológica contra Mycoplasma em aves de criatórios de "fundo de quintal" próximos a explorações comerciais do estado de São Paulo. Arquivos do Instituto Biológico 73(2), 143-148.

Dorea, F.C., Berghaus, R., Hofacre, C. and Cole, D.J. 2010. Survey of Biosecurity Protocols and Practices Adopted by Growers on Commercial Poultry Farms in Georgia, U. S. A. Avian Dis. 54, 1007-1015.

Dwass, M. 1957. Modified randomization tests for nonparametric hypotheses. Ann. Math. Stat. 28, 181-187.

Evans, J.D., Leigh, S.A., Branton, S.L., Collier, S.D., Pharr, G.T. and Bearson, S.M.D. 2005. Mycoplasma gallisepticum: Currentand Developing Means to Controlthe Avian Pathogen. J. Appl. Poult. Res. 14, 757-763.

Keawcharoen, J., van den Broek, J., Bouma, A., Tiensin, T., Osterhaus, A.D. and Heesterbeek, H. 2011. Wild Birds and Increased Transmission of Highly Pathogenic Avian Influenza (H5N1) among Poultry, Thailand. Emerg. Infect. Dis. 17(6), 1016-1022.

Kulldorff, M. 1997. A spatial scan statistic. Commun. Stat. Theory Meth. 26, 1481-1496.

Kulldorff, M. and Nagarwalla, N. 1995. Spatial disease clusters: detection and inference. Stat. Med. 14, 799-810.

Pereira, M.S. 2005. Prevalência de anticorpos contra Mycoplasma gallisepticum, Mycoplasma synoviae e Salmonella pullorum e identificação bacteriológica de Salmonella spp. em galinhas "caipiras" no município de Uberlândia [Monografia]. Uberlândia (MG): Universidade Federal de Uberlândia.

Pfeiffer, D.U., Robinson, T.P., Stevenson, M., Stevens, K.B., Rogers, D.J. and Clements, A.C.A. 2008. Spatial analysis in epidemiology. Oxford University Press, pp: 142.

Silva, C.B.C., Chagas, W.F., Santos, R.F., Gomes, L.R., Ganda, M.R. and Lima, A.M.C. 2015. Seroprevalence of Salmonella and Mycoplasma in Commercial Broilers, Backyard Chickens, and Spent Hens in the Region of Triângulo Mineiro, State of Minas Gerais, Brazil. Brazilian J. Poult. Sci. 17(1), 57-62.

Vaillancourt, J.-P., Martinez, A., Smith, C. and Ley, D. 2000. The epidemiology of Mycoplasma gallisepticumin North Carolina. In: Proc. 35th National Meeting on Poultry Health and Processing, Ocean City, MD, pp: 34-36.

24

Expression of various sarcomeric tropomyosin isoforms in equine striated muscles

Syamalima Dube[1], Henry Chionuma[1], Amr Matoq[2], Ruham Alshiekh-Nasany[1], Lynn Abbott[1], Bernard J. Poiesz[1] and Dipak K. Dube[1,*]

[1]*Department of Medicine, SUNY Upstate Medical University, 750 East Adams Street, Syracuse, New York 13210, USA*
[2]*University of Florida, College of Medicine-Jacksonville, Suite 1130, 841 Prudential Drive, Jacksonville, FL 32207, USA*

Abstract

In order to better understand the training and athletic activity of horses, we must have complete understanding of the isoform diversity of various myofibrillar protein genes like tropomyosin. Tropomyosin (TPM), a coiled-coil dimeric protein, is a component of thin filament in striated muscles. In mammals, four TPM genes (TPM1, TPM2, TPM3, and TPM4) generate a multitude of TPM isoforms via alternate splicing and/or using different promoters. Unfortunately, our knowledge of TPM isoform diversity in the horse is very limited. Hence, we undertook a comprehensive exploratory study of various TPM isoforms from horse heart and skeletal muscle. We have cloned and sequenced two sarcomeric isoforms of the *TPM1* gene called TPM1α and TPM1κ, one sarcomeric isoform of the *TPM2* and one of the *TPM3* gene, TPM2α and TPM3α respectively. By qRT-PCR using both relative expression and copy number, we have shown that TPM1α expression compared to TPM1κ is very high in heart. On the other hand, the expression of TPM1α is higher in skeletal muscle compared to heart. Further, the expression of TPM2α and TPM3α are higher in skeletal muscle compared to heart. Using western blot analyses with CH1 monoclonal antibody we have shown the high expression levels of sarcomeric TPM proteins in cardiac and skeletal muscle. Due to the paucity of isoform specific antibodies we cannot specifically detect the expression of TPM1κ in horse striated muscle. To the best of our knowledge this is the very first report on the characterization of sarcmeric TPMs in horse striated muscle.

Keywords: Absolute copy number, Horse, qRT-PCR, Relative expression, TPM.

Introduction

Tropomyosins, a family of actin-biding proteins, are present in all eukaryotes from yeast to humans. They play a critical role(s) in regulating the function of actin filaments in both muscle and nonmuscle cells (Lees-Miller and Helfman, 1991; Pittenger *et al.*, 1994; Pieples and Wieczorek, 2000; Perry, 2001; Denz *et al.*, 2004; Gunning *et al.*, 2008).

Sarcomeric tropomyosin is a component of the thin filament whereas muscle myosin isoforms comprise the thick filament in myofibrils. The dynamic interaction between the thick and thin filaments results in muscle contraction, which is triggered by nerve impulses that in turn stimulate the release of Ca^{2+} in the cytosol. Tropomyosin attached troponin(s) then binds to Ca^{+2} and undergoes a massive conformational change that aids the myosin associated ATPase activity to hydrolyze ATP and release energy. The energy thus released initiates muscle contraction. Muscle contraction is a function that various animals, including humans, exploit to move, stretch, and even keep themselves warm. Hence, various myofibrillar proteins including tropomyosin play critical role(s) in muscle contraction that is essential for walking, running, and exercising.

The horse is a unique and incredible athlete with remarkable capabilities. In fact, athletic performance is a vital criteria used for the selection of superior horses. It is well established that athletic performance of animals including humans can be improved by proper and rigorous physical exercise/training, which again depends on the expression of various genes related to energy metabolism as well as muscle contraction (McGivney *et al.*, 2009; Eivers *et al.*, 2010, 2012). However, very little is known about exercise-related gene expression patterns in equine muscles for example heart, and skeletal muscles.

Some myofibrillar protein genes like, TNNC2 (Tn-C type 2) ACTN1 (alpha actin, skeletal muscle) and TPM1 (tropmyosin 1) were found to be up regulated in equine skeletal muscle after exercise (Eivers *et al.*, 2012). TPM1 and TPM2 along with the transcripts of some other myofibrillar protein genes are among the most highly abundant transcripts in equine skeletal muscle (McGivney *et al.*, 2010). Yet, to the best our knowledge, none of the sarcomeric TPM isoforms from equine heart and skeletal muscles have been cloned or sequenced. Nor have extensive studies been done to evaluate the full repertoire of TPM sarcomeric isoforms expressed in equine cardiac and skeletal muscles.

In vertebrates, tropomyosin is encoded by four tropomyosin genes *TPM1, TPM2, TPM3*, and *TPM4* (Lees-Miller and Helfman, 1991; Pittenger *et al.*, 1994; Pieples and Wieczorek, 2000; Perry, 2001; Denz *et al.*, 2004; Gunning *et al.*, 2008) except for zebrafish where six tropomyosin genes are present (Booth *et al.*, 1998; McGivney *et al.*, 2010). In mammalian systems the TPM sarcomeric isoforms deemed to be important in heart and skeletal muscle includeTPM1α , TPM1κ , TPM2α , and TPM3α (Lees-Miller and Helfman, 1991; Perry, 2001; Gunning *et al.*, 2008; Dube *et al.*, 2016). Hence, in this study, we have cloned and sequenced the above sarcomeric tropomyosin cDNAs from equine striated muscles. Recently, we have described sarcomeric TPM4α expression in human hearts and, to a much more limited degree, human skeletal muscle (Dube *et al.*, 2016).

However, in several mammals, for example rodents, the *TPM4* gene is truncated. As a result, the *TPM4* gene does not code a sarcomeric isoform in rodents. Also, the predicted isoforms of the horse *TPM4* gene (GenBank mRNA accession # XM_014734753.1) did not include the sarcomeric isoform because of a stop codon in exon 2. Further, no definitive role on muscle contraction in mammals has yet been assigned for TPM4α , the sarcomeric isoform of the *TPM4* gene. Hence, in this study, we have not included TPM4α.

Materials and Methods

Conventional and nested RT-PCR for amplification of TPM1α, TPM1κ, TPM2α and TPM3α

Total RNAs from whole horse (*Equus ferus caballus*) heart and skeletal muscle were procured from Zyagen (San Diego, CA) and BioChain (Newark, CA). 1st strand cDNA was made using oligo (dT)12-15 using SuperScript II (Life Technologies, Grand Island, NY) following manufacturer's specifications as described earlier (Thurston *et al.*, 2009; Nan *et al.*, 2015). First, PCR amplification for TPM1α and TPM1κ were carried out with the P1 and P2 primer-pair (Table 1 and Fig. 1).

For nested PCR, the first amplified DNAs from heart and skeletal muscle were diluted 200 fold with distilled water and 2 μl from each sample was amplified with the P5 and P2 primer-pair for TPM1κ amplification and P3 and P2 primer-pair for TPM1α amplification. P8 was used as probe for both isoforms. The primer combinations P5 and P6; P1 and P7 were used in the direct sequencing of TPM1κ. Nucleotide sequences of

various primer-pairs used for amplification of different isoforms are provided in Table 1.

Following amplification the DNA product was run on a 1.5% agarose gel. DNA bands of appropriate size(s) were extracted using the MinElute Gel Extraction kit provided by QIAGEN. One portion of isolated DNA was used for determination of nucleotide sequences and a portion of the isolated DNA was ligated into a T/A cloning vector (Invitrogen) using the manufacturer's specifications as previously described (Thurston *et al.*, 2009; Nan *et al.*, 2015).

This resulting ligation mixture was then used for the transformation of competent One Shot *E. coli* cells (provided by Invitrogen) as per the manufacturer's protocol. For identification of the particular isoform we performed colony hybridization with [^{32}P]-labeled Exon 2b specific probe for TPM1α or exon 2a specific probe for TPM1κ, as listed in Table 1. The hybridization positive colonies were picked up; grown overnight and plasmid DNA were isolated using the QIAprep Spin Miniprep kit (QIAGEN). The isolated plasmid DNA as well as the gel extracted DNA (as stated above) were sequenced at the Cornell University Core DNA sequencing facility. For amplification of TPM2α and TPM3α we employed TPM2α and TPM3α specific primer-pairs designed using the predicted sequences available in GenBank. The amplified DNAs were cloned into T/A cloning vector (Invitrogen) and subsequently sequenced as stated above.

Real-time quantitative RT-PCR.

qRT-PCR analyses of cDNA templates were performed using the LightCycler 480 Real-Time PCR System as described before (Dube *et al.*, 2014; Nan *et al.*, 2015). Reactions were carried out in a 384-well plate using the LightCycler 480 SYBR Green I Master kit (Roche). Briefly, each well contained a total volume of 10 μl reaction solution, of which 2 μl was cDNA template and 8 μl was SYBR green mix (5 μl 1 x SYBR green Master mix, 2.8 μl of PCR-grade water, and 0.2 μl of 10 μM primer pair). Primers for real-time PCR for various TPM isoforms are listed in Table 1. In case of TPM1α and TPM1κ, cDNA was made with an oligonucleotide specific for exon 9a/b that allowed us to make an isoform specific cDNA corresponding to the mRNA containing exon 9a/b as in various sarcomeric isoforms. Amplification in the absence of a cDNA template was also evaluated to insure a lack of signal due to primer dimerization and extension or carryover. Data were analyzed using both relative and absolute quantification methods. Relative quantification of qRT-PCR data was performed using the delta CT (sample CT minus 18S rRNA CT) and delta delta CT (sample delta CT minus comparator delta CT) methods (Pfaffl, 2001; Livak and Schmittget, 2001).

Table 1. Primer-pairs and probes used for amplification and detection of TPM1α, TPM1κ,TPM2α, and TPM3α.

Isoform: TPM1α & TPM1κ	As indicated in Fig. 1	Type of amplification		Nucleotide sequence
		Con RT-PCR	qRT-PCR	
MTPM1-1A(+)	P1	X	-	5′-ATGGACGCCATCAAGAAGAA-3′
MTPM1-2A(+)	P5	X		5′-CGGAGGACGAGCGGGACGGG-3′
MTPM1-2A probe	P4		X	5′-GAGCTGCACAAGGCGGAGGACAG-3′
MTPM1-2B (+)	P3		X	5′-ATGAACTGGACAAATACTCTGAG-3′
MTPM1-2A(-)	P7			5′-TGTCCTCCGCCTTGTGCAG-3′
MTPM1-3-4(-)	P6		X	5′-TCAATGACTTTCATGCCTCT-3′
MTPM1-9A(-)	P2	X		5′-CGCTCTCAACGATATGACTT-3′
TPM2α				
MTPM2-1A(+)		X		5′-ATGGACGCCATCAAGAAGAAG-3′
MTPM2-9A(-)		X		5′-TCAGAGGGAGGTGATGTCATTGA-3′
TPM2 (+)			X	5′-CTCAAGGAGGCAGAGACCCG-3′
TPM2 (-)			X	5′-GGCCACACTGGTGGGGGCTC-3′
MTPM2 Exon 3 probe				5′-ATTCAGCTGGTTGAGGAGGAGCTGG-3′
TPM3α				
MTPM3-1A(+)		X		5′-CGCCTGGCCACTGCCCTGCAA-3′
MTPM3-9A(-)		X		5′-GAGTCTGGTCCAGCATCCTT-3′
TPM3 (+)			X	5′-CTTGGAGCGCACAGAGGAAC-3′
TPM3 (-)			X	5′-GATCCAGAACAGAGCAGAAAC-3′
MTPM3 Exon 2 probe				5′-GAGAAGAAGGCTGCTGAT-3′

A comparative value was calculated using the formula $X^{-\text{delta delta CT}}$, where "$E$" equals the efficiency of specific primer pairs. This is similar to the $2^{-\text{delta delta CT}}$ method but corrects for the assumption that the reaction is occurring with 100% efficiency. Efficiencies (E) were determined using dilution series of isoform-specific plasmid clones with respective isoform-specific primers pairs.

The LightCycler 480 software plotted the CT at each concentration against the logarithm of the dilutions of the clone, generating a linear regression curve that calculated efficiency based on the formula $E = 10^{[-1/\text{slope}]}$. Efficiency of 18S rRNA was determined by serial dilution of horse cDNAs generated with specific primers (Dube *et al.*, 2014; Nan *et al.*, 2015).

For determination of absolute copy number, optical density was taken of various horse isoform specific clones (for example, TPM1α, TPM1κ, TPM2α, and TPM3α separately using a spectrophotometer. The copy number per volume of clone in solution was determined using the equation number of copies = (ng of plasmid DNA x 6.02×10^{23})/(bp length of plasmid x 1×10^{9} x 650), which was simplified by Andrew Staroscik at the URI Genomics and Sequencing Center. A dilution series of each clone was done for 1×10^{1}–1×10^{4} copies of template, which was used to create a standard curve after amplification (Booth *et al.*, 1998; Livak and Schmittgen, 2001; Nan *et al.*, 2015). For better accuracy, each sample in the dilution series was run in triplicate.

Western blot

Horse heart and horse skeletal thigh muscle protein extracts were obtained from ZYAGEN. Protein concentration was verified using the BioRad protein reagent kit. For each sample in a total reaction mixture of 30 µl was made, 5 µl protein sample, 7.5 µl NuPage LDS sample buffer (4x), 15.5 µl distilled water and 2 µl NuPage sample reducing agent (10x). The samples were run on NuPage 4-12% Bis Tris gel and then transferred to nitrocellulose membrane according to the manufacturer's instruction as described earlier (Thomas *et al.*, 2010).

The membrane was stained with Ponceau S solution in order to verify the transfer of the protein onto the membrane itself. The Ponceau stained membrane paper was then blocked in 5% milk protein solution for ~1 hour at room temperature to prevent non-specific binding. Primary antibody (for example CH1 or anti GAPDH) with appropriate dilution in 5% milk was incubated at 4°C overnight with constant shaking. The membrane paper was washed three times in TBST solution. Secondary antibody was then applied to the membrane. Secondary antibody used for GAPDH, CH1 was anti-Mouse IgG. After the application of secondary antibody the nitrocellulose membrane was again washed three times with TBST. Electrochemiluminescence (ECL) was applied by using equal amounts of BioRad ClarityTM Western ECL substrates. Imaging was done using BioRad chemi MP Imaging system. In the case that the signal from the

ECL process was too weak the blot was exposed to x-ray film.

Statistical Analysis

The means, standard deviations, and comparative analyses of each data set for statistical significance were done using paired Student's *t*-test. Western Blot analyses for protein expression with extracts of various mammalian systems (Yuan, *et al.*, 2006).

Results

Evaluation of expression of TPM1α and TPM1κ in horse cardiac and skeletal muscles using conventional as well as nested RT-PCR.

Figure 1 shows the exon composition of TPM1α and TPM1κ. The only difference between these two TPM1 isoforms is in exon 2. For identification, we first used conventional RT-PCR with a primer-pair that amplifies both TPM1α and TPM1κ.

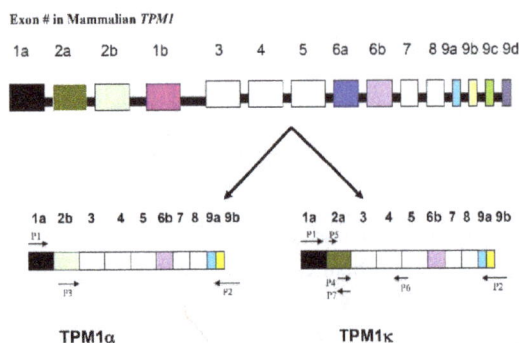

Fig. 1. Alternatively spliced two sarcomeric *TPM1* isoforms.

The results presented in Figure 2A (panel a-b) show the amplified DNA in heart (lane 1) and skeletal muscle (lane 2). In the next step, we amplified the previous amplicons with isoform specific primer-pairs as described under methods section. The results in Figure 2B (panel a-b) show that TPM1α is expressed in both heart (lane 1) and skeletal muscle (lane 2). Similarly, the results in panel Figure 2B (panel c-d) show that TPM1κ is also expressed in both cardiac and skeletal muscle. The expression patterns of the two isoforms were further confirmed by determining the nucleotide sequences of the gel extracted DNA.

Further, we cloned the DNA amplified by the generic primer-pair into T/A cloning vector and identified the particular isoform by PCR amplification of the DNA of each colony directly with an isoform specific primer-pair. We identified colonies (3 from each isoform), isolated DNA from each colony, and determined nucleotide sequences. The cloned DNAs for each isoform were subsequently used as the template for determining the absolute copy number of the particular transcript expressed in cardiac and skeletal muscle cells by qRT-PCR.

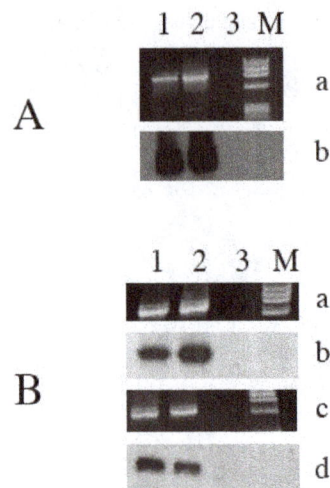

Fig. 2. Agarose gel electrophoresis of amplified TPM1α and TPM1κ DNAs by nested RT-PCR. **(A):** The PCR products generated by the generic primer-pair MTPM1-1A(+)/MTPM1-9A(-) contains both TPM1α and TPM1κ. (Panel a): Ethidium bromide staining of the amplified DNA ran onto agarose gel. Panel b. Hybridization with [^{32}P] labeled TPM1exon 3 probe. **(B):** The final amplified DNA (Fig. 2A) was diluted 200 fold and 2 μl of diluted DNA was used for amplification with TPM1α and TPM1κ specific primer-pairs. (Panel a): The PCR amplified DNA with TPM1α – specific primer –pair MTPM1-2B (+)/MTPM1-9A(-) were separated by agarose gel electrophoresis and finally stained with ethidium bromide. (Panel b): Southern hybridization with [^{32}P] labeled TPM1exon 3 probe. (Panel c): Amplified DNA with TPM1κ specific primer pair [MTPM1-2A(+)/MTPM1-9A(-)] were separated by agarose gel electrophoresis and stained subsequently with ethidium bromide. (Panel d): Southern hybridization with [^{32}P] labeled TPM1exon 3 probe. For (A) and (B): (Lane 1): RNA from 3 horse heart; (Lane 2): RNA from horse skeletal muscle; (Lane 3): Primer control.

The nucleotide as well as deduced amino acid sequences of TPM1α and TPM1κ is shown in Figure 3 and Figure 4, respectively. It is to be noted that the deduced amino acid sequences of horse TPM1α is ~100% similar with human, mouse, and bovine TPM1α sequences (Table 2), whereas there are four amino acid changes in horse exon 2a (Fig. 5), which is the integral part of TPM1κ isoform. In order to determine the expression of TPM1κ protein in horse heart and skeletal muscle, we used a TPM1κ specific antibody that was raised in rabbits against a 15-mer peptide from the exon 2a of human TPM1κ (Rajan *et al.*, 2010) (Fig. 6). Unfortunately, we failed to detect TPM1κ expression both in hearts and skeletal muscle of horse. It is to be noted that in horse TPM1κ, there are three changes in the 15-mer peptide from human TPM1κ exon 2A used for raising antibody in rabbits (Fig. 6). Hence, antibody against human TPM1κ protein may not recognize the horse TPM1κ protein. Alternatively, the expression level of TPM1κ protein is extremely low in equine striated muscle used in this study.

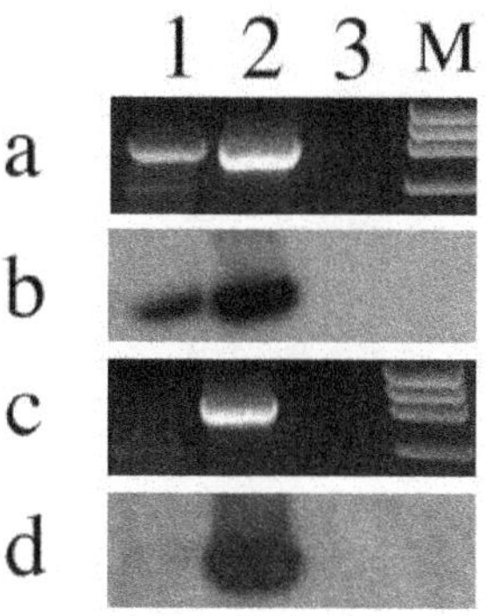

Fig. 3. Agarose gel electrophoresis of amplified TPM2α and TPM3α DNAs by conventional RT-PCR. (Panel a): The PCR amplified DNA with TPM2a specific primer-pair MTPM2-1A(+)/MTPM9A(-) were separated by agarose gel electrophoresis and subsequently stained with ethidium bromide. (Panel b): Southern hybridization with [^{32}P] labeled TPM2 exon 3 probe Table 1). (Panel c): The PCR amplified DNA with TPM3a specific primer-pair MTPM3-1A(+)/MTPM3-9A(-) were separated by agarose gel electrophoresis and subsequently stained with ethidium bromide. (Panel d): Southern hybridization with [^{32}P] labeled TPM 3 exon 2 probe (Table 1). (Lane 1): RNA from 3 horse heart; (Lane 2): RNA from horse skeletal muscle; (Lane 3): Primer control.

```
  1- ATGGACGCCATCAAGAAGAAGATGCAAATGCTGAAGCTCGACAAGGAGAACGCCTTGGAT-60
     M  D  A  I  K  K  K  M  Q  M  L  K  L  D  K  E  N  A  L  D
 61- CGAGCGGAGCAGGCAGAGGCCGATAAGAAGGCGGCTGAGCACAGGAGCAAACAGCTGGAA-120
     R  A  E  Q  A  E  A  D  K  K  A  A  E  D  R  S  K  Q  L  E
121- GATGAGCTAGTGTCGCTGCAAAAGAAACTCAAGGGCACCGAAGATGAACTGGACAAATAC-180
     D  E  L  V  S  L  Q  K  K  L  K  G  T  E  D  E  L  D  K  Y
181- TCCGAGGCTCTCAAAGATGCCCAGGAGAAGCTGGAGCTGGCGGAGAAAAAGGCCACCGAC-240
     S  E  A  L  K  D  A  Q  E  K  L  E  L  A  E  K  K  A  T  D
241- GCTGAAGCCGATGTGGCCTCTCTGAACAGACGCATCCAGCTGGTTGAGGAAGAGCTGGAT-300
     A  E  A  D  V  A  S  L  N  R  R  I  Q  L  V  E  E  E  L  D
301- CGTGCCCAGGAGCGTCTGGCCACAGCCCTGCAGAAGCTGGAGGAAGCCGAGAAGGCAGCA-360
     R  A  Q  E  R  L  A  T  A  L  Q  K  L  E  E  A  E  K  A  A
361- GATGAGAGCGAGAGAGGCATGAAAGTTATTGAGAGCCGAGCCCAAAAGGATGAAGAGAAA-400
     D  E  S  E  R  G  M  K  V  I  E  S  R  A  Q  K  D  E  E  K
401- ATGGAAATTCAGGAGATCCAACTCAAAGAGGCCAACCACATTGCTGAAGATCCCGACCGC-460
     M  E  I  Q  E  I  Q  L  K  E  A  K  H  I  A  E  D  A  D  R
461- AAGTATGAAGAGGTGGCCCGTAAGCTGGTCATCATTGAGAGTGACTTGGAACGTGCAGAG-500
     K  Y  E  E  V  A  R  K  L  V  I  I  E  S  D  L  E  R  A  E
501- GAACGGGCTGAGCTCTCAGAAGGCAAATGTGCCGAGCTTGAAGAAGAATTGAAAACTGTG-560
     E  R  A  E  L  S  E  G  K  C  A  E  L  E  E  E  L  K  T  V
561- ACGAACAACTTGAAGTCACTGGAGGCTCAGGCTGAGAAGTACTCACAGAAGGAAGACAAA-600
     T  N  N  L  K  S  L  E  A  Q  A  E  K  Y  S  Q  K  E  D  K
601- TATGAGGAAGAGATCAAGGTCCTTTCTGACAAGCTGAAGGAGGCTGAGACTCGGGCTGAA-660
     Y  E  E  E  I  K  V  L  S  D  K  L  K  E  A  E  T  R  A  E
661- TTTGCAGAGAGGTCAGTAACTAAATTGGAGAAAAGCATTGATGACTTAGAAGACGAGCTG-700
     F  A  E  R  S  V  T  K  L  E  K  S  I  D  D  L  E  D  E  L
701- TACGCTCAGAAACTGAAGTACAAAGCCATCAGCGAGGAGCTGGACCACGCTCTCAACGAT-760
     Y  A  Q  K  L  K  Y  K  A  I  S  E  E  L  D  H  A  L  N  D
761- ATGACT
     M  T
```

Fig. 4. Nucleotide and deduced amino acid sequences of Horse TPM1α. Nucleotide sequence of the PCR amplified DNA with the primer-pair MTPM1-1A (+)/TPM1-9A (-) as well as the cloned cDNA displayed the same nucleotide sequence as shown above. The deduced protein/amino acid sequences appear below the nucleotide sequence.

Cloning and sequencing of TPM2α and TPM3α using conventional RT-PCR

Primer-pairs used for amplification of TPM2α and TPM3α by RT-PCR with RNA from heart and skeletal muscle, designed by aligning various published mammalian and non-mammalian TPM2 and TPM3 sequences, are listed in Table 1.

```
    ATGGACGCCATCAAGAAGAAGATGCAAATGCTGAAGCTCGACAAGGAGAACGCCTTGGAT
  1 ---------+---------+---------+---------+---------+---------+ 60
    M  D  A  I  K  K  K  M  Q  M  L  K  L  D  K  E  N  A  L  D  -
    CGAGCGGAGCAGGCAGAGGCCGATAAGAAGGCGGCTGAGGACAGGAGCAAACAGCTGGAA
 61 ---------+---------+---------+---------+---------+---------+ 120
    R  A  E  Q  A  E  A  D  K  K  A  A  E  D  R  S  K  Q  L  E  -
    GAGGAGGACATCGCAGCGATGGAGAAGCTAATGCGGGCGTCGGAGGACGAGCGGGACCGG
121 ---------+---------+---------+---------+---------+---------+ 180
    E  E  D  I  A  A  M  E  K  L  M  R  A  S  E  D  E  R  D  R  -
    GTGCTGGAGGAGCTGCACAAGGCGGAGGACAGCCTCCTGGCCGCCGACGAGGCCGCCGCC
181 ---------+---------+---------+---------+---------+---------+ 240
    V  L  E  E  L  H  K  A  E  D  S  L  L  A  A  D  E  A  A  A  -
    AAGGCTGAAGCCGATGTGGCCTCTCTGAACAGACGCATCCAGCTGGTTGAGGAAGAGCTG
241 ---------+---------+---------+---------+---------+---------+ 300
    K  A  E  A  D  V  A  S  L  N  R  R  I  Q  L  V  E  E  E  L  -
    GATCGTGCCCAGGAGCGTCTGGCCACAGCCCTGCAGAAGCTGGAGGAAGCCGAGAAGGCA
301 ---------+---------+---------+---------+---------+---------+ 360
    D  R  A  Q  E  R  L  A  T  A  L  Q  K  L  E  E  A  E  K  A  -
    GCAGATGAGAGCGAGAGAGGCATGAAAGTTATTGAGAGCCGAGCCCAAAAGGATGAAGAG
361 ---------+---------+---------+---------+---------+---------+ 420
    A  D  E  S  E  R  G  M  K  V  I  E  S  R  A  Q  K  D  E  E  -
    AAAATGGAAATTCAGGAGATCCAACTGAAAGAGGCCAAGCACATTGCTGAAGATGCCGAC
421 ---------+---------+---------+---------+---------+---------+ 480
    K  M  E  I  Q  E  I  Q  L  K  E  A  K  H  I  A  E  D  A  D  -
    CGCAAGTATGAAGAGGTGGCCCGTAAGCTGGTCATCATTGAGAGTGACTTGGAACGTGCA
481 ---------+---------+---------+---------+---------+---------+ 540
    R  K  Y  E  E  V  A  R  K  L  V  I  I  E  S  D  L  E  R  A  -
    GAGGAACGGGCTGAGCTCTCAGAAGGCAAATGTGCCGAGCTTGAAGAAGAATTGAAAACT
541 ---------+---------+---------+---------+---------+---------+ 600
    E  E  R  A  E  L  S  E  G  K  C  A  E  L  E  E  E  L  K  T  -
    GTGACGAACAACTTGAAGTCACTGGAGGCTCAGGCTGAGAAGTACTCACAGAAGGAAGAC
601 ---------+---------+---------+---------+---------+---------+ 660
    V  T  N  N  L  K  S  L  E  A  Q  A  E  K  Y  S  Q  K  E  D  -
    AAATATGAGGAAGAGATCAAGGTCCTTTCTGACAAGCTGAAGGAGGCTGAGACTCGGGCT
661 ---------+---------+---------+---------+---------+---------+ 720
    K  Y  E  E  E  I  K  V  L  S  D  K  L  K  E  A  E  T  R  A  -
    GAATTTGCAGAGAGGTCAGTAACTAAATTGGAGAAAAGCATTGATGACTTAGAAGACGAG
721 ---------+---------+---------+---------+---------+---------+ 780
    E  F  A  E  R  S  V  T  K  L  E  K  S  I  D  D  L  E  D  E  -
    CTGTACGCTCAGAAACTGAAGTACAAAGCCATCAGCGAGGAGCTGGACCACGCTCTCAAC
781 ---------+---------+---------+---------+---------+---------+ 840
    L  Y  A  Q  K  L  K  Y  K  A  I  S  E  E  L  D  H  A  L  N  -

    GATATGACTTCCATATAA
841 ---------+-------- 858
    D  M  T  S  I  *  -
```

Fig. 5. Nucleotide and deduced amino acid sequences of Horse TPM1κ. The deduced protein/amino acid sequences appear below the nucleotide sequences. It is to be noted that the copy number of TPM1κ compared to the copy number of TPM1α is significantly lower. Hence, using the T/A cloning system, it was extremely difficult to get the full length TPM1κ cDNA clone from the amplified products using generic primer-pair. Instead, we cloned the partial TPM1κ DNA (amplified by P1/P2 primer-pair as shown in Fig. 1) into T/A cloning vector and sequenced it. The rest of the N-terminus sequencing was done as follows: cDNAs were made with RNA from horse heart and skeletal muscle made using P2 primer, which is located in exon 9a/b (Fig. 1) and the amplification was done with the two sets of primer-pairs – P1/P7 and P4/P6. The amplified DNAs were separated by agarose gel electrophoresis and stained with ethidium bromide. DNA was extracted from the desired band using gel extraction kit as described under the Methods section. Isolated DNAs were sequenced from both sides with appropriate oligonucleotides.

```
                41                                     80

*Coiled-coil    fgabcdefgabcdefgabcdefgabcdefgabcdefgabc
  Hum.TPM1 κ    EDIAAKEKLLRVSEDERDRVLEELHKAEDSLLAAEEAAAK
  Mus.TPM1 κ    ............A.......................D.T...
  Equ.TPM1 κ    .....M...M.A.......................D.....
  Hum.TPM1 α    DELVSLQKKLKGTEDELDKYSEALKDAQEKLELAEKKATD
```

Fig. 6. Alignment of the peptide sequences encoded by exon 2a of the TPM1 gene from human, horse, and mouse. Double underlined 15 mer peptide of human TPM1κ is the peptide used for raising antibody (Rajan *et al.*, 2010). Please note the differences in the amino acid residues between different species. For comparison, we have included the TPM1.exon 2b sequences (part of TPM1α) also at the end. (*) Position refers to the location in leucinezipper coiled-coil motif; *a* and *d* are the interface residues; *e* and *g* are outer residues that may interact across the coiled-coil; *b*, *c* and *f* are on the far side from the coiled-coil interface (Rajan *et al.*, 2010).

Table 2. Percent similarity in nucleic acid as well as amino acid sequences of different sarcomeric isoforms from horse, human, bovine, and monkey

Gene/ Isoform	Comparison	% Similarity	
		N.A.	A.A.
TPM1α	Horse v Human	95.98	99.647
	Horse v Mouse	93.86	100
	Horse v Bovine	95.63	99.647
	Horse v Monkey	96.15	100
TPM1κ	Horse v Human	95.32	98.59
	Horse v Mouse	93.22	98.94
TPM2α	Horse v Human	95.07	99.647
	Horse v Mouse	94.836	100
	Horse v Bovine	95.775	100
	Horse v Monkey	95.657	99.647
TPM3α	Horse v Human	97.427	100
	Horse v Mouse	92.723	98.947
	Horse v Bovine	97.066	100
	Horse v Monkey	96.959	100

(N.A.): Nucleic acid; (A.A.): Amino acids.

The amplified DNAs were run in agarose gel as stated under TPM1α. The bands of appropriate size(s) (not shown) were gel eluted and sequenced. The nucleotide sequence data confirmed the corresponding sarcomeric tropomyosin expressed in heart and skeletal muscle. Expression analyses were carried out by qRT-PCR using relative expression and copy number determination as given in the following section. Amplified DNA was also cloned in a T/A cloning vector and a particular isoform was detected by PCR using an isoform specific primer-pair as described under TPM1α and TPM1κ. DNA for TPM2α and TPM3α were isolated from the colony carrying the plasmid with the particular amplified DNA.

Isolated DNAs were subsequently used for determining the nucleotide sequences. The nucleotide as well as deduced amino acid sequences for TPM2α and TPM3α are given in Figure 7 and Figure 8, respectively. Comparison of nucleotide as well as deduced amino acid sequences with other mammalian TPM2α and TPM3α sequence is presented in Table 2. Similarity in amino acid sequences of horse TPM2α with human and other mammals is near 100 percent and the percent similarity at the nucleotide level is ~95%. Similarly, the nucleotide as well as deduced amino acid sequences of horse TPM3α when compared to other mammalian system, are also very conserved. At the amino acid level they are about 100% similar.

Relative expression of TPM1α, TPM1κ, TPM2α, and TPM3α in horse heart and skeletal muscle

qRT-PCR analyses were carried out using the 2-(ddCt) method to determine the relative expression of TPM1α or TPM1κ and 18S rRNA was used as the reference gene in making this determination.

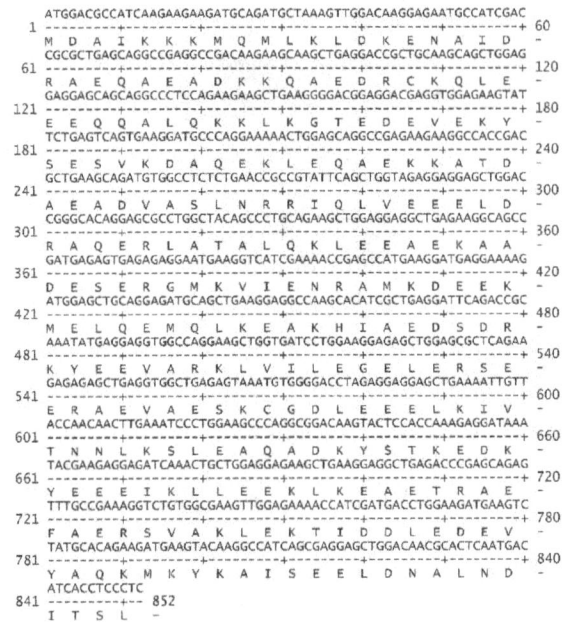

Fig. 7. Nucleotide and deduced amino acid sequences of the Horse TPM2α.

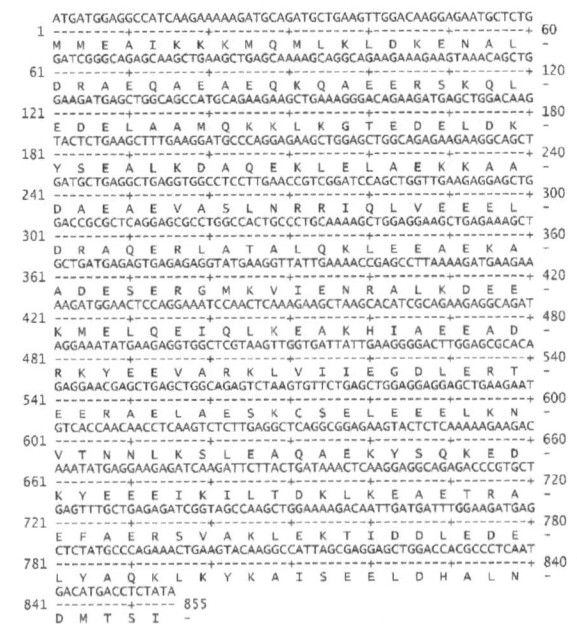

Fig. 8. Nucleotide and deduced amino acid sequences of the Horse TPM3α.

In order to eliminate the effect of other TPM isoforms, the cDNA was made with a gene and isoform specific primers.

The results show the unique melting temperatures for TPM1α (top, Fig. 9A) relative to TPM1κ (bottom). Agarose gel electrophoresis was also performed with the qRT-PCR amplified DNA of both these isoforms (Fig. 9B). Ethidium bromide staining shows a single band for each amplified DNA.

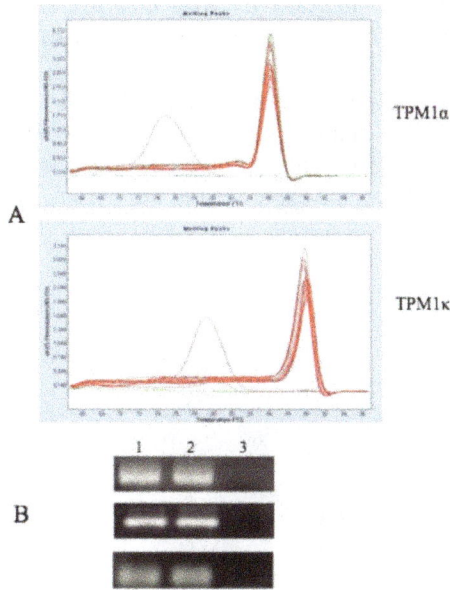

Fig. 9. Melt curves of qRT-PCR and the agarose gel electrophoresis of PCR amplified DNA stained with ethidium bromide. **(A):** Melt curves for amplified horse TPM1α and TPM1κ DNA. The melting points of TPM1α and TPM1κ are different. The multiple curves represent the products from multiple replicates of the RT-PCR assay. **(B):** PCR products separated by agarose gel electrophoresis and subsequently stained with ethidium bromide. The results demonstrate amplification of a single product for TPM1α (top panel) or TPM1κ (middle panel) or 18S rRNA amplification (bottom panel). (Lane 1): Heart; (Lane 2): Skeletal muscle; (Lane 3): Primer control.

The results indicate that the primer-pairs used for amplification for TPM1α or TPM1κ are specific. Panel A in Figure 10 depicts that TPM1α expression in horse skeletal muscle is ~1.65 fold higher compared to cardiac muscle (p=0.02578). On the contrary, the expression of TPM1κ is a little higher in heart when compared to skeletal muscle (Fig. 10, Panel B). However, the small difference is statistically significant as determined by Student's T-Test (p = 0.01859).

We also performed qRT-PCR for determining the relative expression level of TPM2α and TPM3 α transcripts using the 2^{DDCT} method. First we determined the efficiency of each of the primer pairs used for the amplification of TPM2α and TPM3α respectively. We then determined the melt curve for each isoform, and also analyzed the size of each amplified DNA by agarose gel electrophoresis followed by ethidium staining (Fig. 11).

Finally, we performed the qRT-PCR amplification for determining relative expression. The results as depicted in Figure 12 show that expression of TPM2 α is ~3.6 fold higher in horse skeletal muscle compared to cardiac muscle.

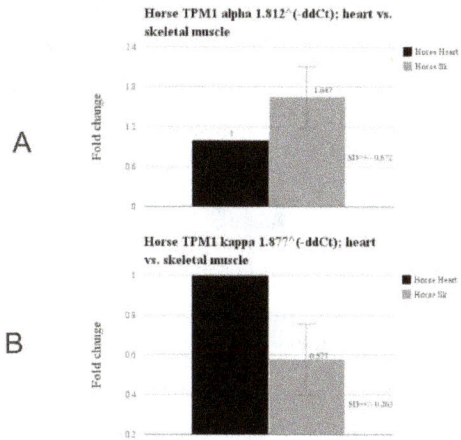

Fig. 10. Relative Expression of TPM1α and TPM1κ transcripts in heart and skeletal muscle by qRT-PCR. **(A):** Fold change of TPM1α in skeletal muscle vs heart Calculated p value as determined by Student's T-test = 0.025. **(B):** Fold change of TPM1κ in skeletal muscle vs heart Calculated p value as determined by Student's T-test = 0.0189.

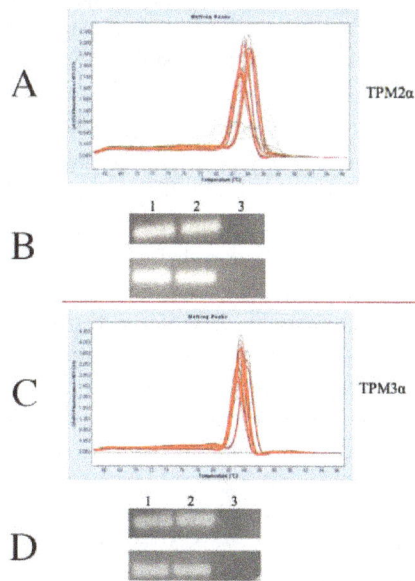

Fig. 11. Melt curves of qRT-PCR and the agarose gel electrophoresis of PCR amplified DNA stained with ethidium bromide. **(A):** Melt curves for amplified horse TPM2α DNA. The multiple curves represent the products from multiple replicates of the RT-PCR assay. **(B):** PCR products separated by agarose gel electrophoresis and subsequently stained with ethidium bromide. The results demonstrate amplification of a single product for TPM2α (top panel) or 18S rRNA amplification (bottom panel). **(C):** Melt curves for amplified horse TPM3α DNA. The multiple curves represent the products from multiple replicates of the RT-PCR assay. **(D):** PCR products separated by agarose gel electrophoresis and subsequently stained with ethidium bromide. The results demonstrate amplification of a single product for TPM2α (top panel) or 18S rRNA amplification (bottom panel). For (B) and (D): (Lane 1): Heart; (Lane 2): Skeletal muscle; (Lane 3): Primer control.

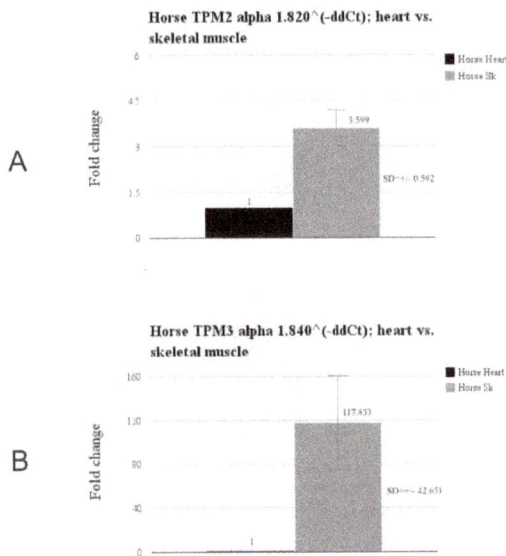

Fig. 12. Fold changes (primer efficiency (eff.)^-ddCt) of horse TPM2α and TPM3α in heart (H) vs. skeletal muscle (Sk). **(A):** Horse TPM2α eff. = 1.820 (mean value for 2 separate experiments each being in triplicate). **(B):** Horse TPM3α eff. = 1.812 (mean value for 2 separate experiments each being in triplicate).

However, the relative expression of TPM3 α is about 117 fold higher in skeletal muscle compared to heart. The relative expression experiment using 2^{DDCT} shows that the expression level of most of the sarcomeric TPM isoforms is higher in equine skeletal muscle compared to heart except for the expression of TPMκ, which is higher in cardiac muscle. In order to verify the results we determined the absolute copy number of various TPM isoforms in heart and skeletal muscles. To determine the absolute copy number of a particular isoform we had to use an isoform specific cloned cDNA as the template for calculating the standard curve. We also determined the standard curve for TPM2α and TPM3α using respective cDNA template and isoform specific primer-pair (Fig. 11).

Determination of the absolute copy number of transcripts of TPM1α, TPM1κ, TPM2α, and TPM3α in equine heart and skeletal muscle

The results presented in Table 3 show the absolute copy number of TPM1α, TPM1κ, TPM2α, and TPM3α expressed in heart and skeletal muscle. The results are in good agreement with our results on relative expression as presented in the preceding section. In brief, the copy numbers of each of three isoforms, TPM1α, TPM2α, and TPM3α are higher in skeletal muscle. On the contrary, the copy number of TPM1κ is higher in heart. It is to be noted that the expression level of TPM1κ in equine heart is very low (1.34 X 10²/μg of total RNA) and it is even lower in skeletal muscle.

Western blot analyses for detection of sarcomeric tropomyosin expression in equine heart and skeletal muscle.

Our Western blot results with extracts from horse hearts and skeletal muscle using the CH-1 monoclonal antibody that recognizes all sarcomeric tropomyosin proteins, shows the expression in hearts (lane 1, panel b, Fig. 13).

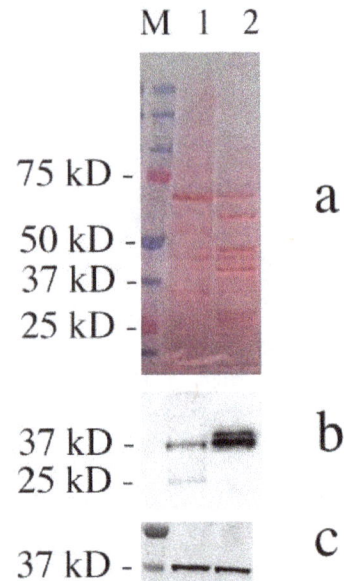

Fig. 13. Western blot analyses of sarcomeric tropomyosin in horse heart and skeletal muscle extracts. (Panel a): Ponceu staining of the blot. (Panel b): Staining with CH1 monoclonall antibody. (Panel c): staining with anti-GAPDH antibody. (Lane M): Molecular weight marker; (Lane 1): Heart ; (Lane 2): Skeletal muscle.

Because CH1 recognizes all sarcomeric isoforms for example, TPM1α, TPM1κ, TPM2α, and TPM4α, the results do not help determine expression of a particular TPM isoform. As mammalian hearts are known to generate overwhelming amount of TPM1a (~95% of the total sarcomeric TPMs) (Rajan *et al.*, 2010), one can assume that the ~37 kD band represents TPM1α. At this point it is extremely difficult to assign an identity to the `25 kD band.

To the best of our knowledge, sarcomeric tropomyosin is not low molecular weight TPM. However, there are reports in the literature and also our unpublished results that strongly support that the low molecular weight TPM with exon 9a are expressed in mammalian striated muscles. As a matter fact, the predicted sequence of tropomyosin alpha-1 chain isoform X1 with exon 9a of horse is available in the data base (NCBI Reference Sequence: XP_005603060.1). It is possible that the low molecular band may represent such an isoform.

Table 3. Quantitative RT-PCR of horse TPM1α, TPM1κ, TPM2α, and TPM3α by determining absolute copy number.

Tissue / organ	TPM1α	TPM1κ	TPM2α	TPM3κ	Ratio TPM1α : TPM2α	Ratio TPM1α : TPM3α
Heart	$4.25 \times 10^4 +$ 9.1×10^2	1.34×10^2	$2.43 \times 10^5 +$ 2.2×10^3	1.93×10^3 $+1.1 \times 10^2$	0.17	22
Sk muscle	$1.86 \times 10^4 +$ 8.4×10^2	0.46×10^2	$2.47 \times 10^6 +$ 1.9×10^4	1.54×10^6 2.1×10^4	0.007	0.012
Ratio H : Sk	2.28	2.9	0.098	0.001		

Sarcomeric tropomyosin expression in equine skeletal muscle (lane 2, panel b, Fig. 13) is relatively higher compared to heart. Multiple bands are also visible in the skeletal muscle – the higher band is ~39 kD and the lower band ~37 kD. The broadness of the lower band (~37 kD) suggests the presence of more than one protein/iosform. It is to be noted that the higher band in the skeletal muscle may represent TPM2α or TPM1κ, each of which run slower compared to TPM1α or TPM3α. The lower band may represent TPM1α and TPM3α because the electrophoretic mobility of the two are similar (Pieples and Wieczorek, 2000; Rajan *et al.*, 2010). The results with CH1 monoclonal antibody show that the overall sarcomeric TPM protein expression in equine skeletal muscle is higher compared to heart. while GAPDH expression is similar in heart and skeletal muscle. (compare lane 1 and 2, panel c, Fig. 13).

Discussion

Tropomyosin (TPM) belongs to a multigene family of actin binding proteins. In vertebrates, tropomyosins are encoded by four genes designated as *TPM1, TPM2, TPM3,* and *TPM4*, which generate more than 50 isoforms via alternate splicing and/or using different promoters. To the best of our knowledge no sarcomeric tropomyosin has been cloned and sequenced from an equine species. Nor has the full isoform expression repertoires been defined. Hence, we undertook a comprehensive study on the characterization of all sarcomeric tropomyosins from horse hearts and skeletal muscle.

Sarcomeric tropomyosin includes TPM1α and TPM1κ, which are the alternatively spliced products of the *TPM1* gene. The difference between these two isoforms is in exon 2. TPM1α contains exons 1a, 2b, 3, 4, 5, 6b, 7, 8, 9a/b whereas TPM1κ includes all the exons as in TPM1α except for exon 2b; instead it has exon 2a. The sarcomeric isoform of TPM2 and TPM3 are designated as TPM2α and TPM3α, respectively.

In this study, we have not included *TPM4* because the role(s) of TPM4α in muscle contraction is not well defined in mammals as in the case of avian (Fleenor *et al.*, 1992), amphibians (Hardy *et al.*, 1995; Spinner *et al.*, 2002), and aquatic animals like fish (Schevzov *et al.*, 2011). In some mammals for example in rodents, TPM4α is not expressed. In humans, however, we have recently reported the expression of TPM4α transcripts in hearts and skeletal muscle. In fact, we have also reported the potential of TPM4α protein expression in human hearts (Spinner *et al.*, 2002). However, we do not know yet the function it may perform in cardiac contractility of human striated muscles.

For the first time, we have cloned and sequenced TPM1α and TPM1κ from horse heart and skeletal muscle. Interestingly, the amino acid sequences of horse TPM1α is ~100% similar with human TPM1α isoform (Fig. 6). As there are some differences in exon 2a sequences of horse and human TPM1 gene, there are some differences in TPM1κ from human and horse. Unfortunately, the nucleotide as well as amino acid sequences of TPM1α from *Equus caballus* (the horse species that includes all domestic horses) has not been reported in GenBank. Recently predicted sequences of two TPM1 isoforms from E caballus have been posted in the GenBank; neither of them can encode a high molecular wt tropomyosin like TPM1α.

However, the amino acid sequences of the Predicted TPM1isoform X 1 (XP_008520892.1; submitted in July 2014) from *Equus przewalskii* (another horse species that still lives in the wild of Central Asia) shows 100% similarity with our TPM1α sequence from *Equus caballus*. Seven predicted TPM1 isoform sequences from *Equus przewalskii* (known as Przewalski horse) are available in GenBank. Unfortunately none of the seven isoforms have exon 2a like sequences. So, we cannot compare our TPM1κ sequence from *Equus caballus* with predicted TPM1κ from Przewalski horse. Tropomyosin is an alpha helical coiled-coil dimeric protein. The coiled-coil structure is characterized by a heptapeptide repeat motif (a-b-c-d-e-f-g). The amino acid residues in the hydrophobic core positions a and *d* are the primary determinants of folding and stability as explained by Rajan *et al.* (2010).

The difference between TPM1α and TPM1κ is only in exon2. TPM1α contains exon 2b where as TPM1κ contains exon 2a. Hence, 26 out of 40 amino acid residues are different between human TPM1α and TPM1κ. As pointed out earlier, 284 amino acid residues are identical in human and horse TPM1α. Although the TPM1α from horse and human are identical and exon 2a in horse contain four additional substitutions, the stability of the coiled-coil structure for TPM1α-TPM1κ hetero dimer as well as TPM1κ-TPM1κ homodimer may be altered. For example, L43I substitution in human TPM1κ in position *a* of the heptad may slightly destabilize of the κ/κ coiled coil relative to the α/α coiled coil. Also, this substitution causes the loss of hydrophobicity.

In horse, the same substitution will have the similar effect forming α–κ coiled coil heterodimer. L46M in position *d* unlike in humans, there will be lesser loss of the hydrophobicity and the destabilization will also be less. No SB (salt bridge) will be added like in the case of human. In the case of L50M in position "*a*" may cause some loss of hydrophobicity. V52A in a position of *c* may not affect significantly the coiled coil structure in horse TPM1κ. E75D in position *e* may not change the coiled coil structure. K77T in position *g* may stabilize the structure may still lose the hydrophobicity. At this point it's worth mentioning that the different 26 out of 40 amino acids in exon 2 changes the biding affinity of TPM1κ with F-actin.

In the absence of troponins, the binding is significantly lower compared to the binding of F-actin with TPM1α. In fact, no biding between TPM1κ and F-actin was observed in the absence of troponins. However, no differences were observed for the binding of TPM1α or TPM1κ with F-actin in the presence of troponins in vitro (Rajan *et al.*, 2010). We are planning to perform similar experiments with bacterially expressed TPM1α and TPM1κ with F-actin in vitro in future.

At this juncture one of our observations deserves added attention. The 41-mer peptide encoded by exon 2b, which is the integral part of TPM1α is highly conserved not only among mammals but most likely in all vertebrates from fish to humans (Fig. 6). On the contrary, the 4-mer peptide sequences encoded by exon 2a, which is a component of TPM1κ, have not been conserved throughout vertebrate evolution (Fig. 6). Twenty five years ago David Helfman had the same observation although at that time exon 2a was known to be part of TPM1β and exon 2b as part of TPM1α (Lees-Miller and Helfman, 1991). Currently, exon 2a is also known to be an integral part of the sarcomeric isoform TPM1κ. Although functional involvement of the tropomyosin isoforms containing the exon 2a peptide has been broadened, actin is still the only protein that is known to bind to this region of tropomyosin.

The fundamental implication and the reasons for the large divergence in amino acid residues 39-80 of TPM1κ and /or TPM1β remains a mystery as stated by David Helfman (Lees-Miller and Helfman, 1991). TPM2α protein sequences from *Equus caballus* are identical with the predicted TPM2 isoform X 1 published in GenBank (XP_003364171). Our TPM2α protein sequence from horse is almost identical with human and other mammalian TPM2α (Table 2). Finally, our TPM3α protein sequence is identical with Predicted tropomyosin alpha-3 chain isoform X1 [*Equus caballus*] (XP_005610140 submitted in November 2015) and also ~97-98% similar to human and other mammalian TPM3α sequences (Table 2).

We performed expression analyses of the transcripts of each of these isoforms with RNA from heart and skeletal muscle by qRT-PCR using two different approaches – relative expression and by determining absolute copy number using a standard curve of the corresponding cloned cDNA as a template. The results from both assays are comparable. Our results indicate that the relative expression of TPM1α is higher in skeletal muscle compared to heart.

On the other hand the relative expression of TPM1κ is higher in the heart. The results are consistent with our reported findings in mice (Dube *et al.*, 2014), and axolotl (Thomas *et al.*, 2010). However, when we compared the absolute copy number expression in heart and skeletal muscle, the expression of TPM1α compared to TPM1κ is much higher (~300 fold) in heart. In skeletal muscle, the expression of TPM1α compared to TPM1κ is ~4000 fold higher. In other words the copy number of TPM1κ both in heart and skeletal muscle is very low compared to TPM1α. However, the expression of TPM1κ is ~2.9 fold higher in heart whereas the expression of TPM1α in skeletal muscle compared to heart is ~4.5 fold higher. This is consistent with published results in other systems (Booth *et al.*, 1998).

Interestingly, the expression level of transcripts of TPM1α and TPM1κ is comparable in human hearts unlike in Equine system. However, at the protein level, TPM1α constitutes ~90% of the total sarcomeric trpomyosin whereas TPM1κ is ~5%. There is a sense that a control mechanism is operative at the translation level that determines the efficiency and/or priority of the various TPM transcripts (Denz *et al.*, 2004; Dube *et al.*, 2016). It's worth mentioning at this point that Rajan *et al.* (2010) generated transgenic mice overexpressing TPM1κ in a cardiac-specific manner that led to a concomitant decrease in TPM1α protein without affecting the level of total sarcomericTPM1 proteins. Incorporation of increased levels of TPM1κ protein in myofilaments leads to dilated cardiomyopathy (DCM). Physiological alterations include decreased fractional shortening, systolic and diastolic dysfunction, and decreased myofilament calcium sensitivity with no change in maximum developed tension. Also, they found that the level of expression of TPM1κ is increased in human dilated cardiomyopathy and heart failure.

In order to illustrate biological significance for expressing the TPM1k isoform these authors suggested that in terminally differentiated cells such as cardiomyocytes, there is a need for adaptation to changing environments. Increasing protein isoform diversity through processes such as alternative splicing meets this need. The TPM1κ isoform, one of the several products of the *TPM1* gene (Dube *et al.*, 2014), might provide the opportunity to modulate sarcomeric performance during changing conditions such as exercise, stress, or cardiac disease.

We now speculate that it is most likely beneficial for the athletic activity of Equines to having a lower level of TPM1κ in heart. However, we must admit that we do not know whether TPM1κ protein is expressed in equine striated muscle. Also, it is worth trying to create a transgenic mouse that will overexpress TPM1κ protein in skeletal muscle. This may also give some evidence whether TPM1κ protein is somehow associated with animal athletic activity. However, the functional role of TPM1κ is yet to be established. It is known that TPM1κ is ~5% of the total sarcomeric tropomyosin protein in human hearts, which is also true for axolotl (Thomas *et al.*, 2010).

We already reported that an anti-sense mediated down regulation of TPM1κ inhibited the cardiac contractility in axolotl in situ suggesting a critical role of TPM1κ protein in cardiac contractility. However, we do not know whether this is true for other vertebrates like humans. The expression of TPM2α and TPM3α in horse skeletal muscle is higher compared to cardiac muscle. Our findings are consistent with the published information in other mammalian systems. It is long been known that TPM3α transcripts are expressed in hearts and skeletal muscle.

It was not known that TPM3α protein is expressed in human hearts. Recently, Marston *et al.* (2013) showed that TPM3α protein is expressed in human hearts in lower quantity (< 5% of the total sarcomeric TPM protein).

Our unpublished data also support this observation. TPM3α transcripts have not been detected in mouse hearts. Although TPM3α transcripts are expressed in equine hearts and skeletal muscle, we do not know the expression patterns of the corresponding protein.

Acknowledgements

The work was supported by a grant from the Department of Medicine and Barbara Kopp Cancer Research Fund to BJP and funding from College of Health Professionals, Upstate Medical University, Syracuse, to DKD. Authors are thankful to Ms. Lori Spicer for her assistance in the preparation of the manuscript.

Conflict of interest

The authors declare that there is no conflict of interests.

References

Booth, F.W., Tseng, B.S., Fluck, M. and Carson, J.A. 1998. Molecular and cellular adaptation of muscle in response to physical training. Acta Physiol. Scand. 162(3), 343-350.

Denz, C.R., Narshi, A., Zajdel, R.W. and Dube, D.K. 2004. Expression of a novel cardiac-specific tropomyosin isoform in humans. Bioch. Biophys. Res. Commun. 320(4), 1291-1297.

Dube, D.K., Dube, S., Abbott, L., Alshiekh-Nasany, R., Mitschow, C. and Poiesz, B. 2016. Cloning, sequencing, and the expression of the elusive sarcomeric TPM4α isoform in humans. Mol. Biol. Int. doi:10.1155/2016/3105478.

Dube, S., Panebiancol, L., Matoq, A.A., Chionuma, H.N., Denz, C.R., Poiesz, B.J. and Dube, D.K. 2014. Expression of TPM1k, a novel sarcomeric isoform of the TPM1 gene in mouse heart and skeletal muscle. Mol. Biol. Int. 2014:896068.doi: 10.1155/2014 /896068.Epub.

Eivers, S.S., McGivney, B.A., Fonseca, R.G., MacHugh, D., Menson, K., Park, S.D., Rivero, J.L., Taylor, C.T., Katz, L.M. and Hill, E.W. 2010. Alterations in oxidative gene expression in equine skeletal muscle following exercise and training. Physiol. Genomics 40, 83-93.

Eivers, S.S., McGivney, B.A., Gu, J., MacHugh, D.E., Katz, L.M. and Hill, E.W. 2012. PGC-1α encoded by the PPARGC1A gene regulates oxidative energy metabolism in equine skeletal muscle during exercise. Anim. Genet. 43, 153-162.

Fleenor, D.E., Hickman, K.H., Lindquester, G.J. and Devlin, R.B. 1992. Avian cardiac tropomyosin gene produces tissue-specific isoforms through alternative RNA splicing. J. Muscle Res. Cell Motil. 13, 55-63.

Gunning, P., O'Neill, G. and Hardmen, E. 2008. Tropomyosin-based regulation of actin cytoskeleton in time and space. Physiol. Rev. 88, 1-35.

Hardy, S., Theze, N., Lepetit, D., Allo, M.R. and Thiebaud, P. 1995. The Xenopus laevis TM-4 gene encodes non-muscle and cardiac tropomyosin isoforms through alternative splicing. Gene 156, 265-270.

Lees-Miller, J. and Helfman, D. 1991. The molecular basis for tropomyosin isoform diversity. Bioessays 13, 429-437.

Livak, K.J. and Schmittgen, T.D. 2001. Analysis of relative gene expression data using real-time quantitative PCR and 2-DDCT method. Methods 25, 402-408.

Marston, S.B., Copeland, O., Messer, A.E., MacNamara, E., Nowk, K., Zampronio, C.G. and Ward, D.G. 2013. Tropomyosin isoform expression and phosphorylation in the human heart in health and disease. J. Muscle Res. Cell Motil. 34(3-4), 189-197.

McGivney, B.A., Eivers, S.S., MacHugh, D.E., MacLeod, J.N., O'Gorman, G.M., Park, S.D., Katz, L.M. and Hill, E.W. 2009. Transcriptional adaptations following exercise in thoroughbred horse skeletal muscle highlights molecular mechanisms that lead to muscle hypertrophy. BMC Genomics 10, 638. DOI: 10.1186/1471-2164-10-638.

McGivney, B.A., McGettigan, P.A., Browne, J.A., Evans, A.C., Fonseca, R.G., Loftus, B.J., Lohan, A., MacHugh, D.E., Murphy, B.A., Katz, L.M. and Hill, E.W. 2010. Characterization of the equine skeletal muscle transcriptome identifies novel functional responses to exercise training. BMC Genomics 11, 398. DOI: 10.1186/1471-2164-11-398.

Nan, C., Dube, S., Matoq, A., Mikesell, L., Abbott, L., Alshiekh-Nasany, R., Chionuma, H., Huang, X., Poiesz, B.J. and Dube, D.K. 2015. Expression of sarcomeric tropomyosin in striated muscles in axolotl treated with shz-1, a small cardiogenic molecule. Cardiovasc. Toxicol. 15(1), 29-40.

Perry, S.V. 2001. Vertebrate tropomyosin, properties and function. J. Muscle Res. Cell Motil. 22, 5-49.

Pfaffl, M.W. 2001. A new mathematical model for relative quantification in realtime RT-PCR. Nucl. Acids Res. 29, 2002-2007.

Pieples, K. and Wieczorek, D.F. 2000. Tropomyosin 3 increases striated muscle isoform diversity. Biochemistry 39, 8291-8297.

Pittenger, M.F., Kazzaz, J.A. and Helfman, D.M. 1994. Functional properties of nonmuscle tropomyosin isoforms. Curr. Opin. Cell Biol. 6, 96-104.

Rajan, S., Jagatheesan, G., Karam, C.N., Alves, M.L., Bodi, I., Schwartz, A., Buclago, C.F., D'Souza, K.M., Akhter, S.A., Boivin, G.P., Dube, D.K., Petrasheveskaya, N., Herr, A.B., Hullin, R., Liggett, S.B., Wolska, B.M., Solaro, R.J. and Wieczorek, D.F. 2010. Molecular and Functional Characterization of a Novel Cardiac-Specific Human Tropomyosin Isoform. Circulation 121, 410-418.

Schevzov, G., Whittaker, S., Fath, T., Lin, J.J. and Gunning, P.W. 2011. Tropomysin isoforms and reagents. Bioarchitecture 1, 135-164.

Spinner, B.J., Zajdel, R.W., McLean, M.D., Denz, C.R., Dube, S., Mehta, S., Choudhury, A., Nakatsugawa, M., Dobbins, N., Lemanski, L.F. and Dube, D.K. 2002. Characterization of a TM-4 type tropomyosin that is essential for myofibrillogenesis and contractile activity in embryonic hearts of the Mexican axolotl. J. Cell Biochem. 85, 747-761.

Thomas, A., Rajan, S., Thurston, H.L., Masineni, S.N., Dube, P., Bose, A., Muthu, V., Dube, S., Wieczorek, D.F., Poiesz, B.J. and Dube, D.K. 2010. Expression of a novel tropomyosin isoform in axolotl heart and skeletal muscle. J. Cell Biochem. 110, 875-881.

Thurston, H.L., Prayaga, S., Thomas, A., Guharoy, V., Dube, S., Poiesz, B.J. and Dube, D.K. 2009. Expression of Nkx2.5 in wild type, cardiac mutant, and thyroxine-induced metamorphosed hearts of the Mexican axolotl. Cardiovas.Toxicol. 9, 13-20.

Yuan, J.S., Reed, A., Chen, F. and Stewart, C.N. 2006. Statistical analysis of real-time PCR data. BMC Bioinformatics 7, 85-101.

25

Seroprevalence of Schmallenberg virus and other Simbu group viruses among the Lebanese sheep

Alain Abi-Rizk[1,*], Tony Kanaan[1] and Jeanne El Hage[1,2,3]

[1]*Faculty of Agricultural and Food Sciences, Holy Spirit University of Kaslik (USEK), P.O.Box 446, Jounieh, Lebanon*
[2]*Lebanese Agricultural Research Institute, Fanar, Bekaa P.O. Box 287, Lebanon*
[3]*Ecole Pratique des Hautes Etudes, 75014 Paris, France*

Abstract

In order to evaluate for the first time, the serological prevalence of Schmallenberg virus (SBV) and other Simbu group viruses in Lebanon, sheep originating from 15 Lebanese regions were sampled in September 2016. A total number of 750 serum samples from Awassi sheep were tested by ELISA for viral nucleoprotein antibodies. From the sampled animals, 122 animals were seropositive to SBV/Simbu group viruses. The seropositive sheep were mainly located in South Lebanon. At herd-level, a seroprevalence of 53.33% was recorded in the Seven Lebanese governorates. The animal-level seroprevalence was 16.26% and both animal and herd-level seroprevalences were negative in Mount-Lebanon. Despite that there was some serological evidence showed the presence of some Simbu group viruses in the Middle East, no study was done in Lebanon. In this study, we report for the first time the prevalence of SBV and other Simbu group viruses in Lebanon.

Keywords: Lebanon, SBV, Schmallenberg virus, Sheep, Simbu group viruses.

Introduction

Schmallenberg virus (SBV) was identified in November 2011 by Friedrich Loeffler Institute (FLI, Island of Riems, Germany) following a metagenomic analysis of a pool of blood samples coming from a farm of the town of Schmallenberg (the Rhineland of North-Westphalia, Germany) (Gibbens, 2012; Hoffmann *et al.*, 2012). The percentages of nucleotide homology presented in the new genetic sequences made it possible to classify this new virus in the family of *Bunyaviridae*, genus *Orthobunyavirus*, serogroup Simbu (Tarlinton *et al.*, 2012).

The viruses group normally noncontagious, are transmitted by hematophagous arthropods, in particular of the mosquitos and culicoides (Hoffman *et al.*, 2012; Tarlinton *et al.*, 2012).

Between the month of November 2011 and mid-March 2012, the virus was highlighted in sheep, goats and cattle in Germany, the Netherlands, Belgium, the United Kingdom, France, Italy, Luxembourg and Spain (Lievaart-Peterson *et al.*, 2012, 2015). Thus constituting the first occurrence of indigenous circulation of *Orthobunyavirus* of the serogroup Simbu in Western Europe.

However, other *Orthobunyavirus* were identified in Europe (case of the Batai virus in Germany), Africa, Asia, the Middle East, and Australia (cases of Akabane virus), either sporadically by the analysis of pools of mosquitos (Jöst *et al.*, 2011; Horne and Vanlandingham, 2014), or due to an endemic presence (case of the Tahyna virus) (Bennett *et al.*, 2011).

In fact, back in 1980 an outbreak of Akabane virus was confirmed in cattle in the Turkish Province of Aydin. Thereafter, many Middle East countries were screened for the presence of neutralizing antibodies to Akabane virus. The results showed that the virus was present in the south Turkish coast, Cyprus, the Orontes river valley in Syria and the lower Jordan River valley.

Interestingly, the fact that this virus failed to persist in southern Turkey for more than two years indicates that the Middle East may be open to epidemic rather than endemic infection.

The presence of neutralizing antibodies in the eastern Turkish Provinces of Gaziantep and Diyarbakir suggests that this might be the route whereby Akabane virus and probably other Simbu group viruses could invade the Middle East region (Taylor and Mellor, 1994).

Regarding the infection by SBV, its associated disease appears in the adult cattle by a fall of the dairy production, fever, diarrhea being able to be severe and sometimes abortions. A congenital attack is also described in lambs, calves and kids, is characterized by malformations of the arthrogryposes / hydranencéphalitis type (Lievaart-Peterson *et al.*, 2015).

Previous work conducted by the authors on brain samples collected from malformed ovine fetuses

*Corresponding Author:** Alain Abi-Rizk. Faculty of Agricultural and Food Sciences, Holy Spirit University of Kaslik (USEK), P.O.Box: 446, Jounieh, Lebanon.Email: *alainabirizk@usek.edu.lb*

(submitted for post mortem examination in December 2015), detected SBV by RT-q PCR in 2 out of the 7 tested animals (protocol generously provided by Dr. Bernd Hoffmann from the Friedrich-Loeffler-Institut). This study therefore aimed to evaluate for the first time, the seroprevalence of SBV and other Simbu group viruses in Lebanon.

Materials and Methods
Country location and background
Lebanon, located at the eastern shores of the Mediterranean, with an area of 10452 Km^2 most of it mountainous. The length is almost three times its width and it have the Mount-Lebanon and the anti-Lebanon that are parallel to each other, they are separated by the Bekaa plain. Narrows from north to south. Lebanon has 454 Km of land boundaries and a coast line of 225 Km (Ministry of Agriculture, 2009).

Blood sampling
In September 2016, a total of 750 sheep above 12 month of age belonging to 15 large herds (> 500 sheep per herd) were sampled. Farms were chosen randomly throughout the seven Lebanese governorates: Lebanon South (4 farms), Mount Lebanon (3 farms) Lebanon North (1 farm) Nabatiyeh (2 farms), Bekaa (2 farms), Baalbeck-Hermel (2 farms), Akkar (1 farm) (Table 1).

Table 1. Number of sampled sheep per governorate and region.

Governorate	Herd / Region	Number of samples
Lebanon South	Saida	50
	Tyr	50
	Koura	50
	Jezzine	50
Mount- Lebanon	Baabda	50
	Keserwan	50
	Chouf	50
Nabatiyeh	Bent jbeil	50
	Marjeoun	50
Akkar	Akkar	50
Bekaa	Bekaa	50
	Zahle	50
Lebanon North	Zgharta	50
Baalbeck-Hermel	Baalbak	50
	Hermel	50

A number of 50 blood sample was collected from each herd, representing at least 10% of individuals in each herd. Blood samples (25ml per sample) were collected from the external jugular vein and the serum was separated into 2ml crayo-vial and preserved at -20ºC until analysis.

ELISA test
In accordance with the manufacturer's instructions, all collected sera were evaluated for anti-SBV antibody using a commercially available ELISA kit (IDEXX Schmallenberg Ab Test) (IDEXX Switzerland AG Laboratories). This kit detects SBV and cross-react with other Simbu serogroups.

Briefly, all collected sera and controls were diluted 1:10 and distributed in the wells of the microtiter plate (100 µl per well). After 60 minutes of incubation in darkness at 22–24°C, all the wells were washed 3 times with 300 µl of wash solution and added 100 µl per well of the conjugate. After 60 minutes of incubation in darkness at 22–24°C, the wells were washed once again 3 times with 300 µl wash solution and added with 100 µl of TMB substrate. After 10 minutes of incubation at 22–24°C, the color reaction was stopped by adding into each well 100 µl of the Stop solution.

The plates were read with a photometer at a wavelength of 450 nm, and the optical density (OD) of the samples was analyzed in relation to the negative and the positive controls with the formula: S/P%= (sample OD-negative control OD)/(positive control OD-negative control OD). The sample is considered negative if S/P% is <30%, suspect if S/P% is between 30% and 40%, and positive if S/P% is >40%.

The true prevalence of serologically positive animals was estimated by adjusting the apparent prevalence to the sensitivity and specificity of the test as previously described (Rogan and Gladen, 1978)

Results
Schmallenberg virus or other Simbu group viruses prevalence in Lebanon
The results of the anti-SBV/Simbu group viruses antibody detection tests (Table 2) showed that 122 of the 750 tested sheep had anti-SBV/Simbu group viruses' antibodies, representing an individual prevalence of 16.26%.

Table 2: Prevalence of SBV and other Simbu viruses in Lebanon.

Item	Total	SBV + (±STDV)	Prevalence %
Sheep	750	122 (±3.53)	16.26
Herds	15	8 (±4.24)	53.33

The sheep that were tested positive were from the 8 of the 15 herds tested for SBV Simbu group viruses. The infection rate at herd level was therefore 53.33 %.

According to the results shown in Table 2, SBV/Simbu group viruses infection varied substantially between the different Lebanese governorates, with a maximum recorded in Lebanon South and Nabatiyeh, where 30% of the analyzed animal were positive, and no seropsitivity was recorded in Bekaa , Baalbeck-Hermel and Mount-Lebanon (Table 3).

Table 3: Prevalence of SBV in the different Lebanese governorates.

Governorates	Number of animals	SBV +	Prevalence %
Nabatieh	100	30 (±1.4)	30
Lebanon South	150	48 (±2.1)	32
Lebanon North	100	32 (±2.1)	32
Mount Lebanon	150	0 (±1)	0
Bekaa	100	1 (±0.5)	1
Akkar	50	11 (±0)	22
Baalbak Hermel	100	0 (±0)	0

A diverse geographical variation of the seropositivity was observed in the different Lebanese regions. In the southern part of the country, 80% of the tested herds contained SBV-seropositive sheep where in Mount-Lebanon (were the lowest population of sheep is located) the percentage of infected herds was 0% (Figure 1).

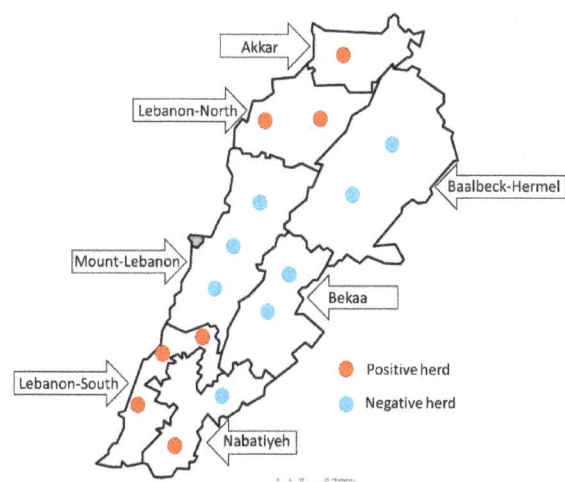

Fig. 1. Prevalence of SBV/Simbu group Viruses herds in the different Lebanese governorates.

Discussion

This is the first study that investigates the epidemiology of SBV and other Simbu group viruses' infection in Lebanon.

Herd seroprevalence in this study (53.3%) was alarming and somehow expected after the several outbreaks and sever economic losses from SBV detected from 2011 till now in many European and Mediterranean countries like Germany, France, Belgium, Italy, Spain, Greece, turkey and others.

Interestingly, our results were lower to what was previously shown in Belgium for example (above 80% of the herds) (Méroc *et al.*, 2013) and higher than Turkey (39.8%) (Azkur *et al.*, 2013).

This study present for the first time, a clear evidence that SBV and Simbu group viruses are already spread in Lebanon and that most of the Lebanese flocks had been in contact with SBV or other Simbu group viruses somehow.

The absence of severe symptoms and any vaccination program could mean that most of the Lebanese sheep have acquired a natural protective immunity against these viruses (Sailleau *et al.*, 2013). But till today, it remains unknown how long this natural immunity could last, mainly that the Lebanese , sheep and goats are kept out on pasture day and night with only a shelter against extreme weather conditions and are not protected against parasites, mosquitos, culicoides and viruses.

For that, even in highly immunized flocks, because of all newborn animals, part of the sheep population will continuously remain susceptible.

This study should be taken into consideration as part of comprehensive SBV surveillance strategy in the country, mainly because no study is done for the detection of SBV or other Simbu group viruses and thus no prevention action are made to control the spreading of these virus.

In Lebanon, around 55% of the total population of sheep is located in the Eastern part at the Bekaa Valley. In this region, the majority of herds are large, which increase the stocking density and eventually increase the likelihood of transmission knowing that no animal in this region is yet seropositive. The absence of seropositivity in the Bekaa could be related to the absence of the vectors in this region which is characterized by rainy winters and extremely dry, and hot summers. More detailed epidemiological studies are needed to elucidate other factors, such as climate variations, presence of culicoides and rearing system that could contribute to high SBV seroprevalence and a continuous surveillance must be done in order to avoid any undesirable outbreaks.

For the moment, insufficient data are present in order to establish the origin and the time of SBV and or other Simbu viruses' infection of the sheep in Lebanon. One hypothesis is that transmission could have coincided with the importation of new animals. Yet, that there is not enough evidence to implicate the animal importation as the main source of Simbu viruses. The presence SBV already confirmed by RT-q PCR and Simbu virus-specific antibodies in most of the Lebanese herds suggests that these viruses have already spread to neighboring countries such as Syria, Palestine and Cyprus.

On the other hand, SBV coming from Greece could have been already dispersed in the area before these importations.

Even if the ELISA method used in this work does not provide a definite diagnosis for the detection of SBV, it is a recommended technique when a large number of animals needs to be tested.

Further molecular detection and phylogenetic analysis of SBV and other Simbu viruses in all the Lebanese ruminants and/or culicoides midges could reveal the source of the infections in Lebanon.

Conflict of interest

The authors declare that they have no competing interests.

References

Azkur, A.K., Albayrak, H., Risvanli, A., Pestil, Z., Ozan, E., Yilmaz, O., Tonbak, S., Cavunt, A., Kadi, H., Macun, H.C., Acar, D., Ozenc, E., Alparslan, S. and Bulut, H. 2013. Antibodies to Schmallenberg virus in domestic livestock in Turkey. Trop. Anim. Health. Prod. 45(8), 1825-1828.

Bennett, R.S., Gresko, A.K., Murphy, B.R. and Whitehead, S.S. 2011. Tahyna virus genetics, infectivity, and immunogenicity in mice and monkeys. Virol. J. 8, 135. doi: 10.1186/1743-422X-8-135.

Gibbens, N. 2012. Schmallenberg virus: a novel viral disease in northern Europe. Vet. Rec. 170(2), 58.

Hoffmann, B., Scheuch, M., Höper, D., Jungblut, R., Holsteg, M., Schirrmeier, H., Eschbaumer, M., Goller, K.V., Wernike, K., Fischer, M., Breithaupt, A., Mettenleiter, T.C. and Beer, M. 2012. Novel orthobunyavirus in cattle, Europe, 2011. Emerg. Infect. Dis. 18(3), 469-472.

Horne, K.M. and Vanlandingham, D.L. 2014. Bunyavirus-Vector Interactions. Viruses, 6(11), 4373-4397.

Jöst, H., Bialonski, A., Maus, D., Sambri, V., Eiden, M., Groschup, M.H., Günther, S., Becker, N. and Schmidt-Chanasit, J. 2011. Isolation of Usutu virus in Germany. Am. J. Trop. Med. Hyg. 85(3), 551-553.

Lievaart-Peterson, K., Luttikholt, S. J. M., Van den Brom, R., & Vellema, P. 2012. Schmallenberg virus infection in small ruminants–First review of the situation and prospects in Northern Europe. Small Ruminant Res. 106(2-3), 71-76.

Lievaart-Peterson, K., Luttikholt, S., Peperkamp, K., Van den Brom, R. and Vellema, P. 2015. Schmallenberg disease in sheep or goats: Past, present and future. Vet. Microbiol. 181, 147-153.

Méroc, E., De Regge, N., Riocreux, F., Caij, A.B., van den Berg, T. and van der Stede, Y. 2013. Distribution of Schmallenberg Virus and Seroprevalence in Belgian Sheep and Goats. Transbound. Emerg. Dis. 61(5), 425-431.

Ministry of agriculture. 2009. The Agriculture in Lebanon 2008 – 2009. The National project for agriculture development – FAO. pp: 64.

Rogan, W.J., Gladen, B., 1978. Estimating prevalence from the result of a screening test. Am. J. Epidemiol. 107(1), 71-76.

Sailleau, C., Boogaerts, C., Meyrueix, A., Laloy, E., Bréard, E., Viarouge, C., Desprat, A., Vitour, D., Doceul, V., Boucher, C., Zientara, S., Nicolier, A. and Grandjean D. 2013. Schmallenberg virus infection in dogs, France, 2012. Emerg. Infect. Dis. 19(11), 1896-1898.

Tarlinton, R., Daly, J., Dunham, S., & Kydd, J. 2012. The challenge of Schmallenberg virus emergence in Europe. Vet. J. 194(1), 10-18.

Taylor, W.P. and Mellor, P.S. 1994. The distribution of Akabane virus in the Middle East. Epidemiol. Infect. 113(1), 175-185.

26

Jejuno-jejunal intussusception in a guinea pig (*Cavia porcellus*)

Tara J. Fetzer and Christoph Mans*

School of Veterinary Medicine, University of Wisconsin-Madison, 2015 Linden Drive, Madison, WI 53706, USA

Abstract

An approximately four-year-old male castrated guinea pig (*Cavia porcellus*) was presented for painful defecation with a 24-hour history of hyporexia and intermittent episodes of rolling behavior. Upon presentation the patient was quiet, alert, and responsive, and mildly hypothermic. Abdominal palpation revealed an approximately 2-cm long oblong mass within the caudal abdomen. Abdominal radiographs revealed gastric dilation without volvulus and a peritoneal mass effect. The patient was euthanized following gastric reflux of brown malodorous fluid from his nares and oral cavity. A necropsy was performed and revealed a jejuno-jejunal intussusception causing mechanical gastrointestinal ileus, and gastric dilatation without volvulus. While non-obstructive gastrointestinal stasis is common and obstructive ileus is uncommon in guinea pigs, this report shows that intestinal intussusception is a differential in guinea pigs with ileus and gastric dilatation.

Keywords: Bloat, Colic, Gastric distention, Gastrointestinal tract, Rodent.

Introduction

Gastrointestinal disease, especially ileus and gastric dilatation, are common presentations in guinea pigs. Ileus is a multifactorial condition and can be associated with hyporexia or anorexia, dental disease, pain, stress or anxiety, gastroenteritis of various etiologies, certain drugs or medications, dysbiosis, fecal impactions, chronic disease, and neoplasia (DeCubellis and Graham, 2013). Presenting signs may include anorexia, decreased fecal production, bruxism, distended and painful abdomen, decreased borborgymi, gastric tympany, dehydration, dyspnea, and shock (DeCubellis and Graham, 2013).

History and physical examination may lead to a suspicion of gastrointestinal ileus, however, abdominal imaging is required for diagnosis. Intestinal intussusception in guinea pigs has been reported in a case series of 49 unspecified spontaneous small intestinal intussusceptions in young guinea pigs from a closed breeding colony (Schoenbaum *et al.*, 1972). In addition, a case of ileocolic intussusception in a 5-month-old female guinea pig has been reported (Pellaz *et al.*, 2012).

A reducible colo-colic intussusception has been reported in a 3-day-old guinea pig, suspected to be secondary to a colonic rupture leading to adhesions and fibrinous peritonitis (Rowles *et al.*, 1993).

Case Details

An approximately 4-year-old male castrated guinea pig (*Cavia porcellus*) was presented for painful defecation with a 1-day history of hyporexia, intermittent episodes of rolling behavior, and decreased urination. The day prior to presentation the patient had been evaluated by another veterinarian for sneezing and ocular discharge. An upper respiratory infection was suspected and the animal was prescribed trimethoprim/sulphamethoxazole (17 mg/kg PO q12h) and a critical care nutritional supplemental diet. Syringe feedings were well tolerated. Urination was not witnessed within 24-hours prior to presentation. Stools were firm and dry and there was tenesmus. Intermittent rolling from side to side was noted as well. Prior to presentation the patient had no previously reported significant medical or surgical history. The diet consisted of commercial guinea pig pellets, timothy hay, dried fruits, and kale.

Upon presentation the patient was quiet, alert, and responsive. The body weight was 1.18 kg and the patient was found to have adequate muscling and body condition. The patient was hypothermic (36.6°C, physiological range: 37.2 to 39.5°C) and mildly dehydrated, heart and respiratory rate were within normal limits. Moderate pelvic limb ataxia was noted and conscious proprioception was absent in both pelvic limbs, but the remainder of his neurologic examination was normal. The abdomen was soft upon palpation with a large distended stomach and gas filled intestines appreciated. An approximately 2-cm long oblong mass effect within the caudal abdomen was palpated. The remainder of the physical examination was within normal limits.

Differentials for the abdominal mass effect included a gastrointestinal mass of unknown etiology, firm ingesta, or a firm inexpressible urinary bladder. The

*Corresponding Author: Christoph Mans. School of Veterinary Medicine, University of Wisconsin-Madison, 2015 Linden Drive, Madison, WI 53706, USA. Email: *christoph.mans@wisc.edu*

patient was sedated with midazolam (0.5 mg/kg IM) and butorphanol (0.25 mg/kg IM), in order to facilitate manual restraint for diagnostic procedures. Sedation was marked and sufficient. Abdominal radiographs revealed a severely gas distended stomach, caudally displaced intestines and cecum, and decreased abdominal serosal detail (Fig. 1 and 2).

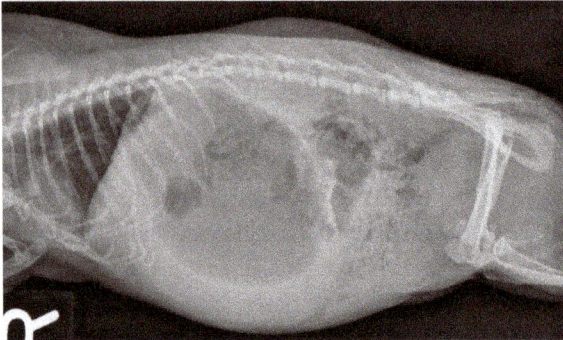

Fig. 1. Right lateral abdominal radiograph of a 4-year-old, male castrated guinea pig with gastric dilatation without volvulus and an abdominal mass effect. The stomach is severely dilated with primarily gas and a small amount of fluid. The intestines are displaced caudally.

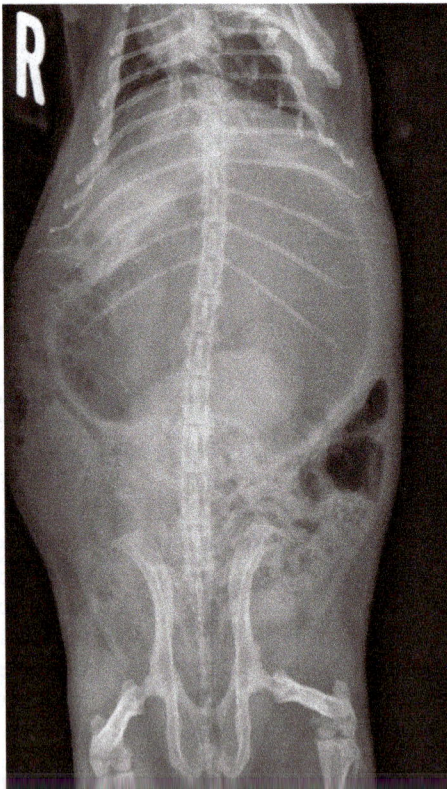

Fig. 2. Ventrodorsal abdominal radiographs of a 4-year-old, male castrated guinea pig with gastric dilatation without volvulus and an abdominal mass effect. The stomach severely dilated with primarily gas and a small amount of fluid. The intestines are displaced caudally.

Supplemental heat was provided and the patient was administered 30 ml/kg of warm lactated Ringer's solution subcutaneously.

The patient's condition did not improve over the next hour and it began refluxing copious amounts of dark brown, malodorous, fluid from both nares and the mouth. Recommendations for gastric decompression and continued intensive monitoring and supportive care, with potential surgical exploratory laparotomy were discussed.

Due to poor prognosis, humane euthanasia was elected by the owner.

A necropsy was performed and confirmed a jejuno-jejunal intussusception causing mechanical intestinal obstruction, and gastric dilatation without volvulus. Upon dissection the stomach was grossly distended measuring 11x9x3 cm, and contained approximately 160 mL of dark greenish brown malodorous fluid with approximately 50 mL of air (Fig. 3).

An 8.5-cm jejuno-jejunal firm, hyperemic, red to black discolored intussusception was noted; 35-cm distal to the pylorus (Fig. 4).

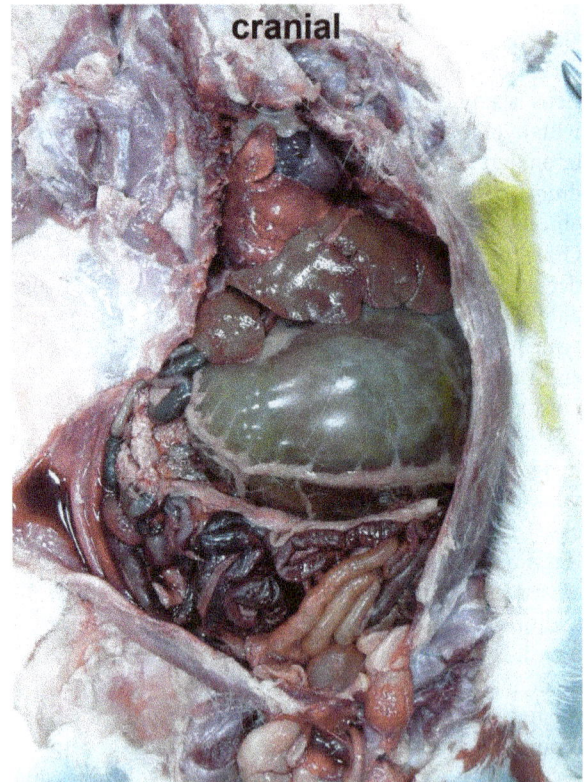

Fig. 3. Necropsy photograph of a 4-year-old, male castrated guinea pig diagnosed with gastric dilation without volvulus and a jejuno-jejunal intussusception. The stomach is severely distended causing caudal displacement of the intestines. The duodenum and jejunum (right abdomen) are dilated, hyperemic, and dark red to black in appearance consistent with necrosis.

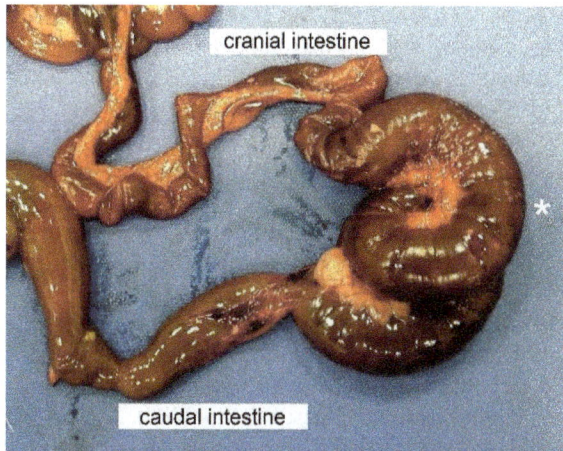

Fig. 4. Necropsy photograph of a 4-year-old, male castrated guinea pig diagnosed with an 8.5 cm jejuno-jenjunal intussusception. The intestines cranial to the intussusception (asterisk) are congested and hyperemic, with dilation and necrosis secondary to an outflow obstruction. The intestines caudal to the intussusception are normal in width and texture.

For 25-cm orad to the intussusception the jejunum and duodenum were grossly distended, congested, hyperemic, and friable. The intestines distal to the intussusception contained a scant amount of ingesta and air, but were normal in width and texture. No additional significant abnormalities were appreciated upon gross necropsy. Histopathology of the gastrointestinal tract revealed minimal multifocal enteritis. The final postmortem diagnosis was jejuno-jejunal intussuception without an identifiable primary underlying cause.

Discussion

Intussusceptions are defined as a telescoping of one portion of the intestines (intussusceptum) into other portions of the intestinal tract (intusscepiens) (Levitt and Bauer, 1992). Reported causes of intussusceptions in various species include gastrointestinal parasites, gastroenteritis of various etiologies, intestinal masses or neoplasms, abdominal surgery, and may also be idiopathic (Applewhite et al., 2001; Burkitt et al., 2009). The underlyling cause for the intussuception was not identified in the case reported in this manuscript. There are reports of intussusceptions in various species including guinea pigs (Schoenbaum et al., 1972; Rowles et al., 1993; Pellaz et al., 2012). However, dogs are the most commonly reported species to have intestinal intussusceptions in the veterinary literature (Levitt and Bauer, 1992; Applewhite et al., 2001).

Intussusceptions are more common in younger animals and the most common location is at the ileocolic junction, although they may occur anywhere in the alimentary tract and in animals of any age (Constable et al., 1997; Burkitt et al., 2009). Clinical signs are variable but usually are associated with gastrointestinal upset such as vomiting, diarrhea, decreased fecal output, anorexia, weight loss, tenesmus, colic, and abdominal distension in addition to vague signs such as depression or lethargy (Schoenbaum et al., 1972, Burkitt et al., 2009). Treatment is focused on aggressive intravenous fluid therapy, analgesics, correction of underlying cause if apparent, and ultimately surgical correction (Levitt and Bauer, 1992; Applewhite et al., 2001). Prognosis is dependent on various factors such as duration of signs prior to care, anatomic location, severity of the obstructive process, and any concurrent systemic disease (Burkitt et al., 2009). Survival rates in patients undergoing surgical correction reported in the veterinary literature for various species are 35%-80% (Levitt and Bauer, 1992; Constable et al., 1997; Burkitt et al., 2009) with recurrence rates as high as 20%-25% (Applewhite et al., 2001; Burkitt et al., 2009).

Intestinal intussusceptions are rare in guinea pigs. A case of ileocolic intussusception in a young female guinea pig has been reported (Pellaz et al., 2012). The patient presented with a 48-hour history of weakness and anorexia, and 24-hours of lack of fecal output despite syringe feeding a critical care formula. Physical examination revealed a soft mass in the abdominal cavity, which was confirmed by ultrasonography to be an intestinal intussusception. Surgical exploration revealed invagination of the ileum by 10-cm into the cecum. In addition, 5-cm proximal to the intussusception, an intraluminal mass was present in the jejunum, which was resected. The animal died four hours after surgery. Subacute necrotizing enteritis was diagnosed on histopathology of the resected intestinal mass. A complete necropsy was not performed (Pellaz et al., 2012).

A reducible colo-colic intussusception has been reported in a 3-day-old guinea pig, which was also diagnosed with congenital imperforate anus and secondary bowl rupture (Rowles et al., 1993). The authors assumed that the ruptured of the colon occurred first, leading to the development of a fibrinous peritonitis and adhesions, which may have subsequently led to the intussuception. The imperforate anus was not considered to be contributing to the rupture and intussusception of the colon, since the intestine distal to the intussusception was empty (Rowles et al., 1993).

In a case series of spontaneous small intestinal intussusception in 49 young guinea pigs from a closed breeding colony, the location of the small intestinal intussusceptions was not specified (Schoenbaum et al., 1972). While aflatoxicosis from contaminated wood shavings in the enclosure was a concurrent finding in some of the cases, the authors were unable to conclude that this was the definitive cause for the intussusceptions.

While *Eimeria caviae* oocysts and shizonts were identified from some of the initial cases of intussusception, the following successful treatment with a sulfonamide did eradicate the parasite, but further cases of intussusception occurred. Clinical signs included lethargy, abdominal pain on palpation, and acute death (Schoenbaum *et al.*, 1972).

Gastric dilatation with or without volvulus is known to occur in guinea pigs and carries a grave prognosis (Mitchell *et al.*, 2010; Dudley and Boivin, 2011; DeCubellis and Graham, 2013).

The pathogenesis of gastric dilatation and volvulus in guinea pigs is poorly understood and likely multifactorial. There is a reported higher incidence in breeding female guinea pigs (Dudley and Boivin, 2011).

Recognition of gastric dilatation with volvulus or gastric dilatation secondary to a small intestinal obstruction caused by an intussusception or other etiology, is critical. Standard therapy for gastrointestinal stasis, as discussed above, is not sufficient or even contraindicated (e.g. syringe feeding, prokinetics) for these cases and emergency surgery is warranted.

Gastric decompression via orogastric intubation or percutaneous needle puncture prior to surgical intervention has been described in the literature, but is considered controversial (DeCubellis and Graham, 2013).

Percutaneous needle decompression of the stomach is not recommended due to high risk of gastric rupture and subsequent peritonitis which may be fatal (Mitchell *et al.*, 2010; DeCubellis and Graham, 2013). Decompression was discussed with the owners of the guinea pig reported here, but was not performed due to the high risks and the owner's decision for euthanasia.

While non-obstructive gastrointestinal stasis is common and obstructive ileus is uncommon in guinea pigs, this report shows that intestinal intussusception is a differential in guinea pigs with ileus and gastric dilatation. Intussusception, in addition to foreign bodies or masses, should be a differential in any patient with a palpable mass in the abdomen.

Conflict of interest
The authors declare that they have no competing interests.

References

Applewhite, A.A., Hawthorne, J.C. and Cornell, K.K. 2001. Complications of enteroplication for the prevention of intussusception recurrence in dogs: 35 cases (1989-1999). J. Am. Vet. Med. Assoc. 219, 1415-1418.

Burkitt, J.M., Drobatz, K.J., Saunders, H.M. and Washabau, R.J. 2009. Signalment, history, and outcome of cats with gastrointestinal tract intussusception: 20 cases (1986-2000). J. Am. Vet. Med. Assoc. 234, 771-776.

Constable, P.D., St Jean. G., Hull, B.L., Rings, D.M., Morin, D.E. and Nelson, D.R. 1997. Intussusception in cattle: 336 cases (1964-1993). J. Am. Vet. Med. Assoc. 210, 531-536.

DeCubellis, J. and Graham, J. 2013. Gastrointestinal disease in guinea pigs and rabbits. Vet. Clin. Exot. Anim. 16, 421-435.

Dudley, E.S. and Boivin, G.P. 2011. Gastric volvulus in guinea pigs: Comparison with other Species. J. Am. Assoc. Lab. Anim. Sci. 50, 526-530.

Levitt, L. and Bauer, M.S. 1992. Intussusception in dogs and cats: A review of thirty-six cases. Can. Vet. J. 33, 660-664.

Mitchell, E.B., Hawkins, M.G., Gaffney, P.M. and Macleod, A.G. 2010. Gastric dilatation-Volvulus in a Guinea Pig (*Cavia porcellus*). J. Am. Anim. Hosp. Assoc. 46, 174-180.

Pellaz, V., Pellaz, U. and Müller, K. 2012. Ileozökale Invagination bei einem jungen Hausmeerschweinchen (*Cavia porcellus*). Kleintierpraxis. 57, 192-195.

Rowles, T.K., Keith, J.C. Jr., Warwick, K.E., Saunders, G.K. and Yau, E.T. 1993. Imperforate anus, colo-colic intussusception, and bowel rupture in a neonatal guinea pig. Lab. Anim. Sci. 43, 255-257.

Schoenbaum, M., Klopfer, U. and Egyed, M.N. 1972. Spontaneous intussusception of the small intestines in guinea pigs. Lab. Anim. 6, 327-330.

27

Seroprevalence and risk factors associated with bovine herpesvirus 1 and bovine viral diarrhea virus in North-Eastern Mexico

J.C. Segura-Correa[1], C.C. Zapata-Campos[2,*], J.O. Jasso-Obregón[2], J. Martinez-Burnes[2] and R. López-Zavala[2]

[1]*Campus de Ciencias Biológicas y Agropecuarias, Universidad Autónoma de Yucatán, Km. 5 Carretera Mérida-Xmatkuil, Mérida, Yucatán, C.P. 97315, México*
[2]*Facultad de Medicina Veterinaria y Zootecnia, Universidad Autónoma de Tamaulipas, Km. 5 A.P. No. 263 C.P. 87000, Mexico*

Abstract

Bovine herpesvirus 1 (BoHV-1) and bovine viral diarrhea virus (BVDV) are well known etiological agents of cattle that produce important economic losses due to reproductive failures and calf mortality, as well as enteric and respiratory disease. Tamaulipas is located northeast of Mexico, an important cattle production and the principal exporter of calf and heifer to the United States. The objectives of this study were to estimate the seroprevalence of BoHV-1 and of BVDV, and to determine the effects of risk factors on these infections. Blood samples of cattle from 57 farms from rural districts of Tamaulipas were collected. The samples were tested for antibodies against BoHV-1 and BVDV using commercial ELISA kits. Data on potential risk factors were obtained using a questionnaire administered to the farmer at the time the blood samples were taken. The seroprevalences for BoHV-1 and BVDV were 64.4% and 47.8%, respectively. In the logistic regression analysis, the significant risk factors were rural district, herd size and cattle introduced to the farm. This study confirms the high seroprevalence of BoHV-1 and BVDV in unvaccinated cattle in Tamaulipas, Mexico. The results of this study could be used for the development of BoHV-1 and BVDV prevention and control program in North-Eastern, Mexico.
Keywords: Bovine, Bovine herpesvirus 1, Bovine viral diarrhea virus, Risk factor, Seroprevalence.

Introduction

Bovine herpesvirus 1 (BoHV-1) and bovine viral diarrhea virus (BVDV) are viruses of cattle that can result in economic losses due to reproductive failures, calf mortality, enteric and respiratory disease. BoHV-1 is a virus of the family *Herpesviridae,* subfamily *Alphaherpesvirinae,* the causative agent of infectious bovine rhinotracheitis, a highly contagious, infectious disease (King *et al.*, 2012; Newcomer and Givens, 2016). Typical clinical signs associated with BoHV-1 infection include respiratory disease, but the virus can also be associated with conjunctivitis, vulvovaginitis, abortions, encephalitis and balanoposthitis. The transition from primary manifestations of infection to a latent stage of persistency is often the source of spread after virus reactivation (Viu *et al.*, 2014). BVDV is a *Pestivirus* from the family *Flaviviridae*, etiological agent of bovine viral diarrhea/mucosal disease (King *et al.*, 2012). Clinical signs include pyrexia, diarrhea and reduced production; it is a highly morbid disease but cause low mortality of infected animals (Grooms, 2004; Nardelli *et al.*, 2008). Both BVDV type 1 and 2 are present in Mexico. Infection of pregnant cows can result in transplacental fetal infection. Fetuses may be aborted, mummified, stillborn or born with severe anomalies. In many cases, immunotolerant (persistently infected) calves are born (Van Oirschot *et al.*, 1999). Also, BVDV can have immunosuppressive

effects, which predispose animals to infection by other microorganisms (Reggiardo and Kaeberle, 1981). The use of vaccines may reduce the economic losses caused by clinical disease, but does not seems to reduce the prevalence of either BVDV or BoHV-1 infections (Xue *et al.*, 2011). It is difficult to accurately estimate the real economic impact due to infected animals that often have no clinical signs of these infections. BoHV-1 and BVDV are widespread in Mexico as indicated by previous studies (Solis-Calderon *et al.*, 2003, 2005; Magaña-Urbina *et al.*, 2005; Segura-Correa *et al.*, 2010). However, state differences may exist within a country and between regions. Risk factors effects may also varied from region or farm to farm because microclimatic changes, management differences, stock densities, along with other factors (Almeida *et al.*, 2013). BVDV is spread between herds mainly by cattle movement, live vaccines use, semen and embryos, visitors, including veterinaries and artificial insemination technicians (Lindberg and Alenius, 1999). Some European studies report several risk factors associated to infection with BoHV-1 such as animal age, vaccination status, herd size, production system (dairy or beef), season and introduction of animals to the farm (Boelaert *et al.*, 2005; González-Garcia *et al.*, 2009). Several reports associated risk factor to BVDV infection such as density of cattle farms, altitude, more than six calves aged ≤ 12 months, animal purchasing and presence of veterinary assistance (Saa *et al.*, 2012; Fernandes *et al.*, 2016). Therefore, information on the epidemiology of BoHV-1 and BVDV is important to establish if tailored prevention and control programs are required for specific regions. The purpose of this study was to estimate the seroprevalence of BVDV and BoHV-1 in cattle and evaluate risk factors in northeast of Mexico.

Materials and Methods
Area of study
The state of Tamaulipas is located at northeast Mexico between 22° 13′ and 27° 40′ N and 97° 09′ and 99° 58′ W. The climate in the State varies from humid to semi-dry. Cattle production is an important activity in Tamaulipas which has a population of approximately 1,366,489 cattle and is the principal exporter of calf and heifer to the United States (SIAP, 2015). According to SAGARPA (Mexican Agricultural Department), Tamaulipas is divided into nine rural districts: Jaumave, Matamoros, Mante, Victoria, Gonzalez, Abasolo, San Fernando, Laredo and Díaz Ordaz.

Animals and sample collection
To estimate seroprevalence, the total cattle population of Tamaulipas (985, 896 heads) was taken into account (INEGI, 2007). The number of animals sampled (n=385 heads of more than 6 months) in the study was calculated considering an expected prevalence of 50%, a confidence level of 95% and a precision of 5% (Segura and Honhold, 2000). Farms and animals within farms were randomly selected. The smallest farm sampled had at least 50 animals. One to 17 heads were sampled per farm. Blood samples were collected from cattle of reproductive age (both sexes). All included animals were not vaccinated against BoHV-1 or BVDV. To identify possible risk factors associated to those diseases, a questionnaire was provided to farm owners, to collect information on putative herd and animal level risk factors. Most of the animals sampled belonged to the Zebu type crosses. There were no clinical signs in the animals recorded at sampling, conducted between May 2010 and December 2011.

Blood samples (10 mL) were collected from the coccygeal vein of each animal, using disposable needles (21 mm 1.5 mm) and vacutainer tubes. The samples were identified and transported on ice to the Diagnostic Laboratory of the Veterinary Medicine Faculty of University Autonomous from Tamaulipas. The blood samples were centrifuged at 1,500 g at 4°C for 10 min and the serum was transferred into disposable microcentrifuge tubes (Eppendorf®) and stored at –20°C until testing.

Laboratory analysis
Blood samples were tested for antibodies against BoHV-1 and BVDV using HerdCheck IBRgB Ab and HerdCheck BVDV p80 Ab ELISA kits (IDEXX laboratories Inc., Westbrook; Maine 04092 USA).

The tests were performed according to manufacturer's instructions. A blocking ELISA assay was used for the detection of IgG antibodies against BVDV in serum o plasm, and an indirect ELISA assay for the detection de antibodies anti BoHV-1 using monoclonal antibodies. The results were read in a microplate photometer, where the optical density (OD) was measured at 450 nm. The cut off OD was calculated as A = OD (corrected negative control) 2.0. All samples with an OD greater or equal than 0.25 were considered positives. The sensitivity and specificity of these tests were 100% and 99.5% respectively.

Potential risk factors
Data on potential risk factors were obtained using a questionnaire provided to the farmer at the time the blood samples were collected. The factors evaluated were rural district; herd size (50–200, 201–500, >500 animals), production system (dairy, beef), cattle introduced to the farm (no, yes), replacement origin (own farm; purchased), water origin (Tube water, reservoir, stream, well), age of cattle (6–36, 37-69 and 70-216 months) and sex (female, male).

Data analysis
Descriptive statistics were used to calculate the frequency of seropositive animals for antibodies against BoHV-1 and BVDV. A primary screening test to identify risk factors significantly related to BoHV-1 and BVDV seropositivity was performed using chi-square tests. Only those factors associated ($P < 0.10$) with the response variable were offered to the logistic binomial regression models. All statistical analyses were carried out using the SAS package (SAS, 2008).

Results
Overall seroprevalence values for BoHV-1 and BVDV were 64.4% and 47.8%, respectively. Among 385 cattle sampled, 142 animals were detected to have antibodies against both viruses and 93 were free of antibodies to both viruses. Seroprevalence and chi-square test results for BoHV-1 and BVDV are shown in Tables 1 and 2, respectively. Preliminary chi-square tests showed associations ($P < 0.10$) between the presence of antibodies to BoHV-1 and rural district, herd size, cattle introduced to the farm, replacement origin and water origin (Table 1); whereas the presence of antibodies against BVDV were associated with rural district, production system, herd size, and cattle introduced to the farm (Table 2).

In the logistic regression analyses, the significant risk factors were rural district, herd size and cattle introduced to the farm for BVDV (Table 3); and rural district and herd size for BoHV-1 (Table 4). The lowest seroprevalences for BoHV-1 and BVDV were observed in the rural district of Matamoros and the highest in Laredo and Abasolo, respectively (Tables 1 and 2). Seroprevalences of BoHV-1 and BVDV were significantly higher in large and middle herds, respectively (P<0.05). Farms that introduced animals to their herds showed higher odds of antibodies against BVDV.

Table 1. Seroprevalence by risk factor for bovine herpesvirus 1 in Tamaulipas, Mexico (n=385).

Risk factor	Number of animals	Positive		p value
		Number	%	
Rural district				<0.0001
Matamoros	10	2	20.00	
Mante	26	13	50.00	
Victoria	67	39	58.21	
Gonzalez	106	58	54.72	
Abasolo	72	46	63.89	
San Fernando	48	37	77.08	
Laredo	56	55	98.21	
Production system				0.6947
Beef	330	213	64.55	
Dairy	55	37	67.27	
Introduction of animals to the herd				<0.0001
Yes	113	90	80.53	
No	272	158	58.19	
Sex				0.9085
Female	346	225	65.03	
Male	39	25	64.10	
Age group (months)				0.3896
6-36	134	82	61.19	
37-69	139	96	69.06	
70-216	112	72	64.29	
Management				0.2910
extensive	324	214	66.05	
Intensive	61	36	59.02	
Herd size (head)				0.0170
50-200	176	101	57.39	
201-500	92	65	70.65	
>500	117	84	71.79	
Replacement origin				<0.0001
Outside	100	46	46.00	
Own herd	285	204	71.58	
Water origin				0.0064
Tube water	126	74	58.73	
Reservoir	165	101	61.21	
Stream-river	37	29	78.38	
Well	57	46	80.70	

Table 2. Seroprevalence by risk factor for bovine viral diarrhea virus in Tamaulipas, Mexico (n=385).

Risk factor	Number of animals	Positive		p value
		Number	%	
Rural district				0.0007
Matamoros	10	1	10.00	
Mante	26	11	42.31	
Victoria	67	34	50.75	
Gonzalez	106	44	41.51	
Abasolo	72	45	62.50	
San Fernando	48	15	31.25	
Laredo	56	34	60.71	
Production system				0.0503
Beef	330	151	45.76	
Dairy	55	33	60.00	
Introduction of animals to the herd				0.0685
Yes	113	63	55.75	
No	272	122	44.85	
Sex				0.6453
Female	346	164	47.40	
Male	39	20	51.28	
Age group (months)				0.7295
6-36	134	66	49.25	
37-69	139	68	48.92	
70-216	112	50	44.64	
Management				0.7473
extensive	324	156	48.15	
Intensive	61	28	45.90	
Herd size (heads)				<0.0001
50-200	176	67	38.07	
201-500	92	66	71.74	
>500	117	51	43.59	
Replacement origin				0.3776
Outside	100	44	44.00	
Own herd	285	140	49.12	
Water origin				0.1879
Tube water	126	58	46.03	
Reservoir	165	85	51.52	
Stream-river	37	12	32.43	
Well	57	29	50.88	

Table 3. Results of the logistic regression for bovine viral diarrhea virus seroconversion.

Risk factor	b	EE	OR	95% CI$_{OR}$
Rural district				
Matamoros	-1.640	1.017	0.05	0.01, 0.43
Mante	2.324	0.602	2.54	0.48, 13.4
Victoria	0.670	0.421	0.49	0.10, 2.27
Gonzalez	-1.586	0.462	0.05	0.01, 0.26
Abasolo	0.465	0.416	0.40	0.08, 1.94
San Fernando	-1.626	0.433	0.05	0.01, 0.19
Laredo	0	-	1	-
Introduce animals				
Yes	0.913	0.2700	6.21	2.15, 17.9
No	0	-	1	-
Herd size (heads)				
50-200	-1.534	0.2675	0.20	0.09, 0.46
201-500	1.474	0.2541	4.11	1.90, 8.89
>500	0	-	1	-

b: regression coefficient; EE: standard error of b; OR: odds ratios; 95%CI$_{OR}$: 95% confidence interval of OR.

Table 4. Results of the logistic regression for bovine herpesvirus 1 seroconversion data.

Risk factor	b	EE	OR	95% CI$_{OR}$
Rural district				
Matamoros	-1.1151	0.9511	0.017	0.001, 0.254
Mante	0.4730	0.5554	0.084	0.007, 0.990
Victoria	-0.4559	0.4033	0.033	0.003, 0.358
Gonzalez	-1.5031	0.4405	0.012	0.001, 0.130
Abasolo	0.2386	0.4060	0.041	0.004, 0.466
San Fernando	-0.1133	0.4136	0.047	0.005, 0.462
Laredo	0	-	1	-
Herd size (heads)				
50-200	-0.7886	0.2172	0.415	0.199, 0.869
201-500	0.6989	0.2018	1.839	0.926, 3.652
>500	0	-	1	-

Discussion

BoHV-1 and BVDV are involved in the respiratory disease complex. BVDV can induce a variety of clinical manifestations which may vary from clinically in apparent infection to acute or chronic severe disease (Baker, 1995). However, the most important economical consequence of BVDV infection is reproductive losses (De Vries, 2006). Clinical signs of BoHV-1 include symptoms of inflammatory processes in both respiratory and genital organs, and abortion (OIE, 2010).

The seroprevalence to BoHV-1 here found (64.4%) is higher than that of cattle in Yucatan, (54.4%) (Solis-Calderon et al., 2003) and Michoacán, Mexico (22%) (Magaña-Urbina et al., 2005). However, the prevalences in this study are lower than those reported by Córdova-Izquierdo et al. (2007) in humid tropics of Mexico (90%). Seroprevalences of BoHV-1 in the literature range from 7.5 up to 70.89 % (Solis-Calderon et al., 2003; Eiras et al., 2009; Gupta et al., 2010; Cedeño et al., 2011; Raizman et al., 2011; Yousef et al., 2013; Saravanajayam et al., 2015). The seroprevalence found in this study for BoHV-1, indicates that it is a widely distributed infection in the region.

The seroprevalence to BVDV determined in this study was 47.8% which is within the range 6.3 to 75% of seroprevalences reported in Mexico and other countries in Latin-America (Orjuela et al., 1991; Obando et al., 1999; Moles et al., 2002; Solis-Calderon et al., 2005; Ramirez-Vazquez et al., 2016). Differences in antibody prevalence between regions and countries could in part be explained by factors such as production system, herd size, disease-control measures, type of breeding, and age of the animal, this is important because indicates the permanence in the environment of both diseases (Orjuela et al., 1991; Mainar-Jaime et al., 2001). The BVDV infection could be controlled in the region by not allowing the introduction of persistently infected animals from infected herds. Lindberg and Alenius (1999) reported BVDV infection eradication without any other intervention than controlled introduction of new animals.

The high seroprevalences found in this study, indicates that BoHV-1 and BVDV are common in all rural districts of Tamaulipas. High seroprevalence for those infections have been reported in other parts of Mexico (Solis-Calderon et al., 2003, 2005; Magaña-Urbina et al., 2005). Animals having antibodies to BoHV-1 and BVDV may be infected by respiratory or via reproductive tract. Therefore, control measures should be installed to prevent contagion between animals of the same region and between other regions.

Risk factors

Rural district

There were significant differences between seroprevalence of a given virus in different rural districts. This heterogeneity may be related to the density of farms in each rural district; differences in prevalence between districts and by factors such as herd size, disease control measures, type of breeding and age of the animal (McDermott et al., 1997).

Herd size

Detection of significant differences in the seroprevalence among herd sizes indicates that this is an important risk factor for BoHV-1 and BVDV infections. Orjuela et al. (1991) reported in Colombia a high seroprevalence for BVDV in middle-sized farms (9.1%) when compared to small (6.2%) and large farms (3.4%); which agree with the results of this study (Tables 3 and 4), where the odds of infection was 4.11 times the level of infection in large herds. McDermott *et al.* (1997) and Van Wuyckhuise *et al.* (1998) reported; however, that large herds or herds with high stock density are associated with high odds for IBR.

Introduction of animals or cattle origin

The lack of differences in the seroprevalence of BoHV-1 between introduced or not introduced animals to the herd agrees with the results of Solis-Calderon *et al.* (2003). However, the introduction or not of animals was an important risk factor for BVDV (OR=6.21), which suggest the purchasing of persistently infected animals. Solis- Calderon *et al.* (2005) reported that purchase of cows (introduction of animals to the herd) in small herds increased the prevalence and risk of BVDV infection as compared to middle and large herd sizes. Mainar-Jaime *et al.* (2001) in dairy cattle in Spain found that the seroprevalence of purchased cows was much higher than for cows whose origin was the farm. However, seropositive animals are not the main risk of infection of BVDV, but the presence of persistently infected (seronegative) animals in the herd.

Age group of animals

Age group is a frequent reported risk factor for BoHV-1 seropositivity. De Quevedo *et al.* (1978), Orjuela *et al.* (1991), McDermott *et al.* (1997), Hage *et al.* (1998) and Solis-Calderon *et al.* (2003) reported higher seroprevalence in old animals. However, in this study, age was not a significant risk factor. The similar seroprevalence of BVDV observed among the three age-groups suggest the dissemination of persistently infected animals in the herds studied. The distribution of virus and risk factors identification are important in order to establish prevention and control programs against economically important diseases such as BVD and IBR. In conclusion, this study confirms the high seroprevalence of BoHV-1 and BVDV in non-vaccinated cattle in Tamaulipas, Mexico. The fact that animals were not vaccinated and that all age-groups had high seroprevalence indicates that the BoHV-1 and BVDV are naturally circulating in this population. So is urgently needed to establish measures for the epidemiological control and prevention of these diseases to decrease their incidence.

Conflict of interest

The authors declares that there is no conflict of interest.

Acknowledgments

The authors would like to acknowledge the FOMIX-Tamaulipas/CONACYT for financial support of this project (TAMPS-2008-C17-107297).

References

Almeida, L.L., Miranda, I.C.S., Hein, E.E., Neto, S.W., Costa, E.F., Marks, F.S., Rodenbush, C.R.,
Canal, C.W. and Corbellini, L.G. 2013. Herd-level risk factors for bovine viral diarrhea virus infection in dairy herds from southern Brazil. Res. Vet. Sci. 95, 901-902.

Baker, C.J. 1995. The clinical manifestations of bovine viral diarrhea infection. Vet. Clin. North Am. Food Anim. Pract. 11, 425-445.

Boelaert, F., Speybroeck, N., De Kruif, A., Aerts, M., Burzykowski, T., Molenberghs, G. and Berkvens, D.L. 2005. Risk factors for bovine herpesvirus-1 seropositivity. Prev. Vet. Med. 69, 285-295.

Cedeño, Q.J., Benavides, B.B., Cardenas, G. and Herrera, C. 2011. Seroprevalence and risk factors associated to BHV-1 and DVBV in dairy herds in Pasto, Colombia in 2011. Rev. Lasallista Invest. 8, 61-68.

Córdova-Izquierdo, A., Córdova-Jiménez, C., Saltijeral-Oaxaca, J., Ruiz-Lang, C., Cortes-Suarez, S. and Guerra-Liera, J. 2007. Seroprevalencia de enfermedades causantes de aborto bovino en el trópico húmedo Mexicano. Rev. Vet. 18, 139-142.

De Quevedo, J.M., Aguilar, S.A., Correa, G.P. and Berruecos, J.M. 1978. Algunos aspectos epizotiológicos de la rinotraqueitis infecciosa bovina. Tec. Pecu. Mex. 34, 61-68.

De Vries, A. 2006. Economic value of pregnancy in dairy cattle. J. Dairy Sci. 89, 3876-3885.

Eiras, C., Dieguez, F.J., Sanjuán, M.L., Yus, E. and Arnaiz, I. 2009. Prevalence of serum antibodies to bovine herpesvirus-1 in cattle in Galicia (NW Spain). Spanish J. Agric. Res. 7, 801-806.

Fernandes, L.G., Nogueira, A.H., De Stefano, E., Pituco, E.M., Ribeiro, C.P., Alves, C.J., Oliveira, T.S., Clementino, I.J. and de Azevedo, S.S. 2016. Herd-level prevalence and risk factors for bovine viral diarrea virus infection in cattle in the state of Paraiba, Northeastern. Trop. Anim. Health Prod. 48, 157-165.

González-Garcia, M.A., Arenas-Casas, A., Carbonero-Martínez, A., Borge-Rodríguez, C., García-Bocanegra, I., Maldonado, J.L., Gómez, J.M. and Perea-Remujo, J.A. 2009. Seroprevalence and risk factors associated with bovine herpesvirus type 1 (BHV-1) infection in non-vaccinated cattle herds in Andalusia (South of Spain). Spanish J. Agric. Res. 3, 550-554.

Grooms, D.L. 2004. Reproductive consequences of infection with bovine viral diarrhea virus. Vet. Clin. North Am. Food Anim. Pract. 20, 5-19.

Gupta, A.K., Chahar, A., Tanwar, R.K. and Fakhruddin K. 2010. Seroprevalence of infectious bovine rhinotracheitis in cattle. Vet. Practitioner 11, 169-170.

Hage, J.J., Schukken, Y.H., Digkstra, T.H., Barkema, H.W., VanValkengoed, P.H.R. and Wentink, G.H. 1998. Milk production and reproduction during a subclinical bovine herpesvirus infection on a dairy farm. Prev. Vet. Med. 34, 97-106.

Instituto Nacional de Estadística Geográfica e Informática (INEGI). 2007. Anuario estadístico del Estado de Tamaulipas. Síntesis geográfica de Tamaulipas. XI Censo General de Población y Vivienda. http://www.inegi.org.mx/est/contenidos/proyectos/Agro/ca2007/Resultados_Agricola/default.aspx. Accessed: 15 Feb. 2016.

King, A.M.Q., Adams, M.J., Carstens, E.B. and Lefkowitz, E.J. 2012. Virus Taxonomy: Classification and Nomenclature of Viruses: Ninth Report of the International Committee on Taxonomy of Viruses. San Diego, CA: Elsevier/Academic Press, pp: 1010.

Lindberg, A.L.E. and Alenius, S. 1999. Principles for eradication of bovine viral diarrhoea virus (BVDV) infection in cattle populations. Vet. Microbiol. 64, 197-222.

Magaña-Urbina, A., Solorio Rivera, J.L. and Segura-Correa, J.C. 2005. Rinotraqueitis infecciosa bovina en hatos lecheros de la región Cotzio-Téjaro, Michoacán, México. Tec. Pecu. Mex. 43, 27-37.

Mainar-Jaime, R.C., Berzal-Herranz, B., Arias, P. and Rojo-Vázquez, F.A. 2001. Epidemiological pattern and risk factors associated with bovine viral-diarrhoea (BVDV) infection in a non-vaccinated dairy-cattle population from the Asturias region of Spain. Prev. Vet. Med. 52, 63-73.

McDermott, J.J., Kadohira, M., O'Callaghan, C.J. and Shoukri, M.M. 1997. A comparison of different models for assessing variation in the seroprevalence of infectious bovine rhinotracheitis by farm, area and district in Kenya. Prev. Vet. Med. 32, 219-234.

Moles, L.P., Gavaldón, D., Torres, J.I., Cisneros, M.A., Aguirre, J. and Rojas, N. 2002. Seroprevalencia simultanea de Leptospirosis y tres enfermedades de importancia reproductiva en bovinos del altiplano central de la República Mexicana. Revista Salud Animal 24(2), 106-110.

Nardelli, S., Farina, G., Luchini, R., Valorz, C., Moresco, A., Dal Zotto, R. and Costanzi, C. 2008. Dynamic of infection and immunity in a dairy cattle population undergoing and eradication programme for infectious bovine rhinotracheitis (IBR). Prev. Vet. Med. 85, 68-80.

Newcomer, B.W. and Givens, D. 2016. Diagnosis and control of viral diseases of reproductive importance: Infectious Bovine Rhinotracheitis and Bovine Viral Diarrhea. Vet. Clin. North Am. Food Anim. Pract. 34, 425-441.

Obando, R.C., Hidalgo, M., Merza, M., Montoya, A., Klingeborn, B. and Moreno-López, J. 1999. Seroprevalence to bovine virus diarrhoea virus and other viruses of the bovine respiratory complex in Venezuela (Apure State). Prev. Vet. Med. 41, 271-278.

OIE Handdistatus II. 2010. Accessed 15 may 2016. http://www.oie.int/hs2/report.asp.

Orjuela, J., Navarrete, M., Betancourt, A., Roqueme, L., Cortez, E. and Morrison, R.B. 1991. Salud y productividad en bovinos de la costa norte de Colombia. World Anim. Rev. 69, 7-14.

Raizman, E.A., Pogranichniy, R., Negron, M., Schnur, M. and Tobar-Lopez, D.E. 2011. Seroprevalence of infectious bovine rinotracheitis and bovine viral diarrhea virus type 1 and type 2 in non-vaccinated cattle herds in The Pacific Region of Central Costa Rica. Trop. Anim. Health Prod. 43, 773-778.

Ramirez-Vazquez, N.F, Fernández-Silva, J.A, Villar-Argaiz, D., Landaño-Pino, J., Chaparro-Gutierrez, J. and Olivera-Angel, M.E. 2016. Seroprevalencia de la diarrea viral bovina, herpesvirus bovino y virus sincitial respiratorio en Argentina. Rev. CES. Med. Vet. Zoo. 11, 1.

Reggiardo, C. and Kaeberle, M.L. 1981. Detection of bacteremia in cattle inoculated with bovine viral diarrhea virus isolated from cases of mucosal disease. Vet. Microbiol. 13, 361-369.

Saa, L.R., Perea, A., Garcia-Bocanegra, I., Arenas, A.J., Jara, D.V., Ramos, R. and Carbonero, A. 2012. Seroprevalence and risk factors associated with bovine viral diarrhea virus (BVDV) infection in non-vaccinated dairy and dual purpose cattle herd in Ecuador. Trop. Anim. Health Prod. 44, 645-649.

Saravanajayam, M., Kumanam, K. and Balasubramaniam, A. 2015. Seroepidemiology of Infectious Bovine Rhinotracheitis in unvaccinated cattle. Vet. World 8(12), 1416-1419.

SAS, 2008. SAS/STAT User's Guide, Version 9.2. SAS Institute Inc., Cary, NC. USA.

Segura-Correa, J.C., Solorio Rivera, J.L. and Sánchez-Gil, L. 2010. Seroconversion to bovine viral diarrhoea virus and infectious bovine rhinotracheitis in dairy herds of Michoacan, Mexico. Trop. Anim. Health Prod. 42(2), 233-238.

Segura, J.C. and Honhold, N. 2000. Métodos de Muestreo para la Producción y Salud Animal. Universidad Autónoma de Yucatán. Mérida, Yucatán, México, pp: 139.

Servicio de Información Agroalimentaria y pesquera (SIAP). Ganadería. 2015. Accessed: 1 Sep. 2015 http://www.siap.gob.mx/exportacion-de-ganado-bovino/.

Solis-Calderon, J.J., Segura-Correa, V.M. and Segura-Correa, J.C. 2005. Bovine viral diarrhoea virus in beef cattle herds of Yucatan, Mexico: Seroprevalence and risk factors. Prev. Vet. Med. 72, 253-262.

Solis-Calderon, J.J., Segura-Correa, V.M., Segura-Correa, J.C. and Alvarado-Islas, A. 2003. Seroprevalence of and risk factors for infectious bovine rhinotracheitis in beef cattle herds of Yucatan, Mexico. Prev. Vet. Med. 57, 199-208.

Van Oirschot, J.T., Bruschke, C.J.M. and van Rijn, P.A. 1999. Vaccination of cattle against bovine viral diarrhoea. Vet. Microbiol. 64, 169-183.

Van Wuyckhuise, L., Bosch, I., Franken, P., Frankena, K. and Elbers, A.R.W. 1998. Epidemiological characteristics of bovine herpesvirus-1 infections determined by bulk milk testing of all Dutch daily herds. Vet. Rec. 142, 181-184.

Viu, M.A., Dias, L.R.O., Lopes, D.T., Viu, A.F.M. and Ferraz, H.T. 2014. Infectious bovine rhinotracheitis:

Review. Pub.Vet. 8(4).

Xue, W., Mattick, D. and Smith, L. 2011. Protection from persistent infection with a bovine viral diarrhea virus (BVDV) type 1b strain by a modified-live vaccine containing BVDV types 1a and 2, infectious bovine rhinotracheitis virus, parainfluenza 3 virus and bovine respiratory syncytial virus. Vaccine 29, 4657-4662.

Yousef, M.R., Mahmoud, M.A., Ali, S.M. and Al-Blowi, M.H. 2013. Seroprevalence of some bovine viral respiratory diseases among non vaccinated in Saudi Arabia. Vet. World 6(1), 1-4.

Permissions

All chapters in this book were first published in OVJ, by Tripoli University; hereby published with permission under the Creative Commons Attribution License or equivalent. Every chapter published in this book has been scrutinized by our experts. Their significance has been extensively debated. The topics covered herein carry significant findings which will fuel the growth of the discipline. They may even be implemented as practical applications or may be referred to as a beginning point for another development.

The contributors of this book come from diverse backgrounds, making this book a truly international effort. This book will bring forth new frontiers with its revolutionizing research information and detailed analysis of the nascent developments around the world.

We would like to thank all the contributing authors for lending their expertise to make the book truly unique. They have played a crucial role in the development of this book. Without their invaluable contributions this book wouldn't have been possible. They have made vital efforts to compile up to date information on the varied aspects of this subject to make this book a valuable addition to the collection of many professionals and students.

This book was conceptualized with the vision of imparting up-to-date information and advanced data in this field. To ensure the same, a matchless editorial board was set up. Every individual on the board went through rigorous rounds of assessment to prove their worth. After which they invested a large part of their time researching and compiling the most relevant data for our readers.

The editorial board has been involved in producing this book since its inception. They have spent rigorous hours researching and exploring the diverse topics which have resulted in the successful publishing of this book. They have passed on their knowledge of decades through this book. To expedite this challenging task, the publisher supported the team at every step. A small team of assistant editors was also appointed to further simplify the editing procedure and attain best results for the readers.

Apart from the editorial board, the designing team has also invested a significant amount of their time in understanding the subject and creating the most relevant covers. They scrutinized every image to scout for the most suitable representation of the subject and create an appropriate cover for the book.

The publishing team has been an ardent support to the editorial, designing and production team. Their endless efforts to recruit the best for this project, has resulted in the accomplishment of this book. They are a veteran in the field of academics and their pool of knowledge is as vast as their experience in printing. Their expertise and guidance has proved useful at every step. Their uncompromising quality standards have made this book an exceptional effort. Their encouragement from time to time has been an inspiration for everyone.

The publisher and the editorial board hope that this book will prove to be a valuable piece of knowledge for researchers, students, practitioners and scholars across the globe.

List of Contributors

J. Kouamo, W.F. Tassemo Tankou and A.P. Zoli
School of Veterinary Medicine and Sciences, University of Ngaoundere, Ngaoundere, Cameroon

G.S. Bah
Regional Center of the Institute of Agricultural Research for Development (IRAD) Wakwa., Ngaoundere, Cameroon

A.C. Ngo Ongla
DDPIA, MINEPIA (Ministry of Livestock, Fisheries and Animal Husbandry), Yaounde-Cameroon

D.B. Adams
24 Noala Street, Aranda, ACT 2614, Australia

S. Ohfuji
Department of Histopathology, Diagnostic Animal Pathology Office, Hokkaido, Japan

S.M. Azwai, E.A. Alfallani, F.T. Gammoudi, H.M. Rayes and I.M. Eldaghayes
Department of Microbiology and Parasitology, Faculty of Veterinary Medicine, University of Tripoli, Tripoli, Libya

S.K. Abolghait
Department of Food Hygiene and Control, Faculty of Veterinary Medicine, Suez Canal University, 41522 Ismailia, Egypt

A.M. Garbaj and H.T. Naas
Department of Food Hygiene and Control, Faculty of Veterinary Medicine, University of Tripoli, 13662, Tripoli, Libya

A.A. Moawad
Department of Food Hygiene and Control, Faculty of Veterinary Medicine, Cairo University, 12211 Giza, Egypt

I. Barbieri
Istituto Zooprofilattico Sperimentale della Lombardia e dell'Emilia Romagna, Via Bianchi, 9 - 25124 Brescia, Italy

B.U. Wakayo
College of Veterinary Medicine-Jigjiga University, Jigjiga Ethiopian Somali Regional State, Ethiopia

P.S. Brar and S. Prabhakar
Deptartment of Veterinary Gynaecology and Obstetrics, Guru Angad Dev Veterinary and Animal Sciences University, Ludhiana-141004, India

G.A. Fornazari, F. Montiani-Ferreira, I.R. de Barros Filho and A.T. Somma
Universidade Federal do Paraná, Programa de Pós-Graduação em Ciências Veterinárias, Rua dos Funcionários 1540, 8035-050, Curitiba, PR. Brazil

B. Moore
Veterinary Specialty Hospital of San Diego, 10435 Sorrento Valley Road, San Diego, CA 92121, USA

A.A. Morgado, M.C.A. Sucupira and G.R. Nunes
Department of Clinical Science, Faculdade de Medicina Veterinária e Zootecnia da Universidade de São Paulo, 05508 270, Sao Paulo, SP, Brazil

S.C.F. Hagen
Department of Surgery, Faculdade de Medicina Veterinária e Zootecnia da Universidade de São Paulo, 05508 270, Sao Paulo, SP, Brazil

Y. Abba, A. Tijjani and A.M.L. Mohd
Department of Veterinary Pathology and Microbiology, Faculty of Veterinary Medicine, Universiti Putra Malaysia, 43400 UPM Serdang, Selangor, Malaysia

F.F.J. Abdullah
Department of Veterinary Clinical Studies, Faculty of Veterinary Medicine, Universiti Putra Malaysia, 43400 UPM Serdang, Selangor, Malaysia
Research Centre for Ruminant Disease, Faculty of Veterinary Medicine, Universiti Putra Malaysia, 43400 UPM Serdang, Selangor, Malaysia

N.H. Bin Abu Daud and R. Bin Shaari
Faculty of Veterinary Medicine, Universiti Malaysia Kelantan, Locked Bag 36, Pengkalan Chepa, 16100 Kota Bharu, Kelantan, Malaysia

M.A. Sadiq, K. Mohammed and L. Adamu
Department of Veterinary Clinical Studies, Faculty of Veterinary Medicine, Universiti Putra Malaysia, 43400 UPM Serdang, Selangor, Malaysia

F.R. Al-Samarai and Y.K. Abdulrahman
Department of Veterinary Public Health/College of Veterinary Medicine, University of Baghdad, Iraq

F.A. Mohammed and F.H. Al-Zaidi
Department of Animal Resources, Directorate of Baghdad Agriculture, Ministry of Agriculture, Iraq

N.N. Al-Anbari
Department of Animal Resources, College of Agriculture, University of Baghdad, Iraq

A.H. Elkasapy
Department of Surgery, Faculty of Veterinary Medicine, Benha University, Egypt

I.M. Ibrahim
Department of Surgery, Anesthesiology and Radiology, Faculty of Veterinary Medicine, Cairo University, Egypt

D.I.S. Lopes and V.M. Maruo
Federal University of Tocantins (UFT), College of Veterinary Medicine and Animal Science, Araguaina, TO, Brazil

M.G. Sousa
Federal University of Paraná (UFPR), Department of Veterinary Medicine, Curitiba, Paraná, Brazil

A.T. Ramos
Federal University of Santa Catarina (UFSC), College of Veterinary Medicine, Curitibanos, Santa Catarina, Brazil

H. Beims, A. Overmann, M. Steinert and S. Bergmann
Department of Infection Biology, Institute of Microbiology, Technische Universität Braunschweig, Spielmannstr. 7, 38106 Braunschweig, Germany

M. Fulde
Center for Infection Medicine, Institute of Microbiology and Epizootics, Freie Universität Berlin, Berlin, Germany

S.K. Tmumen, M.H. Abushhiwa and M.A. Alkoly
Department of Surgery and Theriogenology, Faculty of Veterinary Medicine, University of Tripoli, Tripoli, Libya

S.A. Al-Azreg and S.R. Al-Attar
Department of Pathology and Clinical Pathology, Faculty of Veterinary Medicine, University of Tripoli, Tripoli, Libya

E.M. Bennour
Department of Internal Medicine, Faculty of Veterinary Medicine, University of Tripoli, Tripoli, Libya

Alison M. Lee, Nicola F. Fletcher, Conor Rowan and Hanne Jahns
School of Veterinary Medicine, Veterinary Science Centre, University College Dublin, Belfield, Dublin 4, Ireland

S.A. Sadaba and C.M. Corbi Botto
IGEVET – Instituto de Genética Veterinaria "Ing. Fernando Noel Dulout" (UNLP-CONICET La Plata), Facultad de Ciencias Veterinarias, Universidad Nacional de La Plata, La Plata, Argentina
Research Fellows from Consejo Nacional de Investigaciones Científicas y Técnicas (CONICET). Av. Rivadavia 1917 (C1033AAJ) CABA, Argentina

G.J. Madariaga and A. Massone
Laboratorio de Patología Especial Veterinaria, Facultad de Ciencias Veterinarias, Universidad Nacional de La Plata, La Plata, Argentina

M.H. Carino, M.E. Zappa, P. Peral García and S. Díaz
IGEVET – Instituto de Genética Veterinaria "Ing. Fernando Noel Dulout"
(UNLPCONICET La Plata), Facultad de Ciencias Veterinarias, Universidad Nacional de La Plata, La Plata, Argentina

S.A. Olguín
Cátedra de Métodos Complementarios de Diagnóstico, Facultad de Ciencias
Veterinarias, Universidad Nacional de La Plata, La Plata, Argentina

Carlos Javier Panei and Maria Gabriela Echeverria
Virology Laboratory, Faculty of Veterinary Sciences, National University of La Plata, 60 and 118, CC 296, 1900, La Plata, Argentina
National Scientific and Technical Research Council (CONICET), Argentina

Maria Laura Gos
National Scientific and Technical Research Council (CONICET), Argentina
Immunoparasitology Laboratory, Faculty of Veterinary Sciences, National University of La Plata, 60 and 118, CC 296, 1900, La Plata, Argentina

Alejandro Rafael Valera
Virology Laboratory, Faculty of Veterinary Sciences, National University of La Plata, 60 and 118, CC 296, 1900, La Plata, Argentina

Cecilia Monica Galosi
Virology Laboratory, Faculty of Veterinary Sciences, National University of La Plata, 60 and 118, CC 296, 1900, La Plata, Argentina
Scientific Research Commission of Buenos Aires Province (CIC-PBA), Argentina

Courtnay L. Baskerville, Nicholas J. Bamford and Simon R. Bailey
Faculty of Veterinary and Agricultural Sciences, The University of Melbourne, Werribee, Victoria, Australia

Patricia A. Harris
Equine Studies Group, WALTHAM Centre for Pet Nutrition, Melton Mowbray, Leicestershire, UK

G. Nagina, A. Asima and A. Shamim
PMAS Arid Agriculture University, Rawalpindi, Pakistan

U. Nemat
University of Animal and Veterinary Sciences Lahore, Pakistan

M.S. Medan
Department of Theriogenology, Faculty of Veterinary Medicine, Omar AL-Mukhtar University, AL-Bayda, Libya
Department of Theriogenology, Faculty of Veterinary Medicine, Suez Canal University, Ismailia, Egypt

T. EL-Daek
Department of Theriogenology, Faculty of Veterinary Medicine, Omar AL-Mukhtar University, AL-Bayda, Libya

Abdelmalik Ibrahim Khalafalla
Camel Research Centre, King Faisal University, Al Ahsa, Saudi Arabia
Department of Microbiology, Faculty of Veterinary Medicine, University of Khartoum, Sudan

Ramadan Omer Ramadan
Department of Clinical Studies, College of Veterinary Medicine, King Faisal University, Al Ahsa, Saudi Arabia

Annabel Rector
KU Leuven, Department of Microbiology and Immunology, Laboratory of Clinical & Epidemiological Virology, B-3000 Leuven, Belgium

Seif Barakat
Department of Pathology, College of Veterinary Medicine, King Faisal University, Saudi Arabia

Jamal Hussen and Ahmed M. Alluwaimi
Department of Microbiology and Parasitology, College of Veterinary Medicine, King Faisal University, Al Ahsaa, Saudi Arabia

Turke Shawaf
Department of Clinical Studies, College of Veterinary Medicine, King Faisal University, Al Ahsaa, Saudi Arabia

Abdulkareem Imran Al-herz and Hussain R. Alturaifi
Immunology Unit, Diagnostic Laboratory and Blood Bank, King Fahad Hospital Hufof, Al Ahsaa, Saudi Arabia

Reyad Shawish
Department of Food Hygiene and Control, Faculty of Veterinary Medicine, University of Sadat City, Sadat City, Egypt

Reda Tarabees
Department of Bacteriology, Mycology and Immunology, Faculty of Veterinary Medicine, University of Sadat City, Sadat City, Egypt

Abdulwahab Kammon, Ibrahim Eldaghayes and Abdunaser Dayhum
Faculty of Veterinary Medicine, University of Tripoli, Tripoli, Libya

Paolo Mulatti, Monica Lorenzetto and Nicola Ferre
Istituto Zooprofilattico Sperimentale delle Venezie, Viale dell'Universita, 10, Legnaro, Padova 35020, Italy

Monier Sharif
Faculty of Veterinary Medicine, University of Omar Al-Mukhtar, Albeida, Libya

Syamalima Dube, Henry Chionuma, Ruham Alshiekh-Nasany, Lynn Abbott, Bernard J. Poiesz and Dipak K. Dube
Department of Medicine, SUNY Upstate Medical University, 750 East Adams Street, Syracuse, New York 13210, USA

Amr Matoq
University of Florida, College of Medicine-Jacksonville, Suite 1130, 841 Prudential Drive, Jacksonville, FL 32207, USA

Alain Abi-Rizk and Tony Kanaan
Faculty of Agricultural and Food Sciences, Holy Spirit University of Kaslik (USEK), Jounieh, Lebanon

Jeanne El Hage
Faculty of Agricultural and Food Sciences, Holy Spirit University of Kaslik (USEK), Jounieh, Lebanon
Lebanese Agricultural Research Institute, Fanar, Bekaa, Lebanon
Ecole Pratique des Hautes Etudes, 75014 Paris, France

Tara J. Fetzer and Christoph Mans
School of Veterinary Medicine, University of Wisconsin-Madison, 2015 Linden Drive, Madison, WI 53706, USA

J.C. Segura-Correa
Campus de Ciencias Biológicas y Agropecuarias, Universidad Autónoma de Yucatán, Km. 5 Carretera Mérida-Xmatkuil, Mérida, Yucatán, C.P. 97315, México

C.C. Zapata-Campos, J.O. Jasso-Obregón, J. Martinez-Burnes and R. López-Zavala
Facultad de Medicina Veterinaria y Zootecnia, Universidad Autónoma de Tamaulipas, Km. 5 A.P. No. 263 C.P. 87000, Mexico

Index

www.ingramcontent.com/pod-product-compliance
Lightning Source LLC
Chambersburg PA
CBHW082011190326
41458CB00010B/3148